Optical Formulas

TUTORIAL

Second Edition

Optical Formulas
TUTORIAL
Second Edition

Ellen D. Stoner, MALS, ABOM

Instructor, Opticianry

Durham Technical Community College
Durham, North Carolina

With

Patricia Perkins, BSc (Hons), FBCO

Former Opticianry Program Director

Durham Technical Community College
Durham, North Carolina

Roy Ferguson, PhD

The Learning Curve
Sevierville, Tennessee

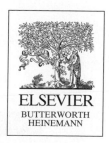

ELSEVIER
BUTTERWORTH
HEINEMANN

ELSEVIER
BUTTERWORTH
HEINEMANN

11830 Westline Industrial Drive
St. Louis, Missouri 63146

OPTICAL FORMULAS TUTORIAL, Second Edition

ISBN-13: 978-0-7506-7504-8
ISBN-10: 0-7506-7504-7

Copyright © 2005, 1997 by Elsevier Inc.

Previous edition copyrighted 1997

ISBN-13: 978-0-7506-7504-8
ISBN-10: 0-7506-7504-7

Publishing Director: Linda Duncan
Acquisitions Editor: Kathy Falk
Senior Developmental Editor: Christie Hart
Publishing Services Manager: Patricia Tannian
Designer: Paula Ruckenbrod

Printed in the United States of America

Last digit is the print number: 9 8 7 6 5 4 3 2 1

PREFACE

This text was originally designed to accompany an intensive seminar style review of formulas and basic ophthalmic optics information. The original project was conceived and written by Patricia Perkins, former Program Director of the Opticianry Program at Durham Technical Community College in North Carolina.

As the text grew, the need became apparent for a comprehensive basic description of formulas without the many pages of discussion necessary for a comprehensive textbook. Thus this text has grown to encompass most of the formulas that underlie basic ophthalmic optics theory. The book was intended to be a formula reference, not a stand-alone text, although the first edition proved useful as a textbook as well.

Because the original intention was to help licensure applicants in an examination that allows calculators but not charts, the text originally did not cover many of the non-formula techniques that are used in the field. In this second edition we are including two techniques that are in general use in the profession. These two methods, the resultant and resolving prism chart and the sine-squared method for approximating cylinder power, are occasionally helpful to the practicing optician in understanding the results provided by laboratory computers. In addition, if understood by the test taker, these two methods can aid in choosing correct answers to multiple-choice questions.

Over the course of the 7 years that the first edition of this text was available, many examination candidates wrote to say how much help the material was in preparing for examinations such as the ABO (NOCE), ABOM, and COT. As a result, in this second edition we are including practice multiple-choice questions at the end of each section (except the math review). The questions for each section are in random order rather than in the order of the subjects within the section, giving the applicant a better preparation for examinations. In the review sections all questions are potential subjects for the ABOM; the questions marked with an asterisk (*) we did *not* consider potential questions for the ABO (NOCE). We are not, however, in any way guaranteeing that the marked subjects will not appear on ABO (NOCE) or COT, nor are we attempting to provide a comprehensive selection that will cover all subjects that might appear on any of these three examinations.

This book starts with a review of basic math. If any of the first section is unfamiliar or downright foreign, the reader should consider taking a math course at a local community college! Section I is intended for those readers who need a brush-up on their basic math skills.

The reader who is familiar with optical theory may turn directly to any subject of interest in this book. Readers unfamiliar with the theory, or needing an overall review, should read the text and perform the exercises in the order given.

Because dioptric powers are commonly specified in quarter or eighth diopter steps, some opticians automatically round every dioptric value to the closest eighth. This rounding is valid for any power that the optician is going to make, order, verify, dispense, or record in the wearer's file. In many of the exercises and examples in this book, dioptric powers are rounded to hundredths, not to eighths. Rounding to hundredths occurs when the result of the calculation is an effective or actual power that will not be made, ordered, dispensed, or recorded in the wearer's file. Frequently the result will be used for another formula or calculation, such as use of the result of the oblique meridian formula in Prentice's Law to compute a prism amount. Other values, such as degrees, millimeters of thickness, and prism powers, are rounded to the significance that is consistent with the values in the problem statement. The significance to which values are rounded is indicated in each section. Readers are welcome, when using the formulas, to round to the significance they consider valid.

We enjoy receiving feedback on this text, and we would like to hear from you.

Ellen Stoner (ellen@stoner.org)
Patricia Perkins
Roy Ferguson

ACKNOWLEDGMENTS

We would like to thank the friends who spent a great deal of time finding typing and calculating errors in this second edition. Particular thanks go to Dan Brown, Terry Harris, Calvin Presnell, Richard Sheets, Amy Spiker, and Julie Sutton. Any remaining errors are strictly the responsibility of Ellen Stoner.

CONTENTS

SECTION I – MATH REVIEW

Work the exercises in this section completely. If any part of this math is new to you, or if you do not understand where the answers came from, seek help with the basic algebra and math before you attempt to understand the use of the formulas in this book.

SIGNED NUMBERS

The + and – signs can be used two ways. They signify addition and subtraction. They also signify "opposite directions." Look at these two number lines:

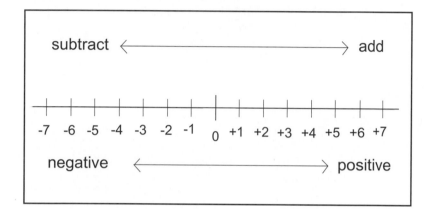

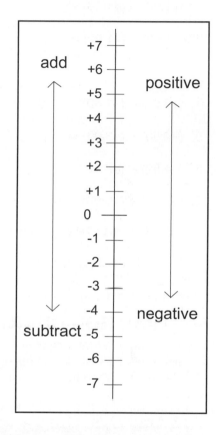

In each of these number lines a positive direction (to the right, or up) is defined and a negative direction (to the left, or down) is defined. A number line can have any orientation, and any direction can be defined as "positive." Once "positive" has been defined, "negative" means "the opposite direction."

ADDITION OF SIGNED NUMBERS

When adding numbers with the same signs, add the amounts and give the result their common sign, as below.

EXAMPLES:

1-1. $(+3.00) + (+2.00) = +5.00$. Since both numbers are positive, add 3 and 2 and use their common positive sign. Using the vertical number line above, start at the +3 and travel up two.

1-2. $(-3.00) + (-2.00) = -5.00$. Since both numbers are negative, add 3 and 2 and use their common negative sign. Using the vertical number line above, start at the –3 and travel down two.

When adding numbers with different signs, subtract the smaller amount from the larger amount and give the result the sign of the larger number, as in the following examples.

1-3. $(-2.00) + (+3.00) = +1.00$. Since the numbers have different signs, subtract 2 from 3, leaving 1, and give the result a positive sign because the larger number, 3, is positive. Using the vertical number line, start at the -2 and travel up three.

1-4. $(+2.00) + (-3.00) = -1.00$. Since the numbers have different signs, subtract 2 from 3, leaving 1, and give the result a negative sign because the larger number, 3, is negative. Using the vertical number line, start at the $+2$ and travel down three.

EXERCISES:

1. $(+1.00) + (+1.00) = $ _____

2. $(-1.00) + (-1.00) = $ _____

3. $(+3.00) + (+1.50) = $ _____

4. $(+3.00) + (-1.50) = $ _____

5. $(-4.50) + (-2.00) = $ _____

6. $(-4.50) + (+2.00) = $ _____

7. $(+7.50) + (-6.00) = $ _____

8. $(-3.25) + (+8.12) = $ _____

9. $(-10.00) + (-4.50) = $ _____

10. $(+6.75) + (+1.25) = $ _____

SUBTRACTION OF SIGNED NUMBERS

The minus sign before a number can be interpreted as meaning "opposite"; for example, -5 is the opposite of $+5$. The opposite of $+3$ is -3. The opposite of -8.75 is $+8.75$. Then what would $-(-2)$ mean? It means the opposite of -2, which is $+2$. Therefore two $-$ signs in a row make a $+$. What does $-(+3.5)$ mean? It means the opposite of $+3.5$, which is -3.5.

To subtract signed numbers, change the sign of the subtracted number and add it.

EXAMPLES:

1-5. $(+2.00) - (-4.00) = (+2.00) + (+4.00) = +6.00$ [Two minuses make a plus.]

1-6. $(-3.00) - (-2.00) = (-3.00) + (+2.00) = -1.00$

1-7. $(-3.00) - (+2.00) = (-3.00) + (-2.00) = -5.00$

EXERCISES:

11. $(+1.00) - (+1.00) = $ _____

12. $(-1.00) - (-1.00) = $ _____

13. $(+3.00) - (+1.50) = $ _____

14. $(+3.00) - (-1.50) = $ _____

15. (−4.50) − (−2.00) = _____

16. (−4.50) − (+2.00) = _____

17. (+7.50) − (−6.00) = _____

18. (−3.25) − (+8.12) = _____

19. (−10.00) − (−4.50) = _____

20. (+6.75) − (+1.25) = _____

MULTIPLICATION OF SIGNED NUMBERS

When numbers with the same signs are multiplied, the result is positive.

EXAMPLES:

1-8. (−3.00)(−2.00) = +6.00, because $3 \times 2 = 6$, and the numbers have the same signs. Or, a minus times a minus is a plus.

1-9. (+3.00)(+2.00) = +6.00

When numbers with different signs are multiplied, the result is negative.

EXAMPLES:

1-10. (+3.00)(−2.00) = −6.00, because $3 \times 2 = 6$, and the numbers have different signs.

1-11. (−3.00)(+2.00) = −6.00

EXERCISES:

21. (+1.00)(+1.00) = _____

22. (−1.00)(−1.00) = _____

23. (+3.00)(+1.50) = _____

24. (+3.00)(−1.50) = _____

25. (−4.50)(−2.00) = _____

26. (−4.50)(+2.00) = _____

27. (+7.50)(−6.00) = _____

28. (−3.25)(+8.12) = _____

29. (−10.00)(−4.50) = _____

30. (+6.75)(+1.25) = _____

DIVISION OF SIGNED NUMBERS

Division is a form of multiplication. The fraction 2/4 is the same as (2)(1/4). So, if there is a minus sign in both the numerator (top) and the denominator (bottom), the result is the same as when two minus signs are multiplied: $(−2)/(−4) = (−2)(−1/4) = +1/2 = +0.5$.

When numbers with the same signs are divided, the result is positive.

1-12. $(-3)/(-2) = +1.5$, because $3/2 = 1.5$ and the numbers have the same signs.

1-13. $(+3)/(+2) = +1.5$

When numbers with different signs are divided, the result is negative.

EXAMPLES:

1-14. $(-3.00)/(+2.00) = -1.50$, because $3/2 = 1.5$, and the numbers have different signs.

1-15. $(+3.00)/(-2.00) = -1.50$

EXERCISES: (Round to two decimal places.)

31. $(+1.00)/(+1.00) = $ _____

32. $(-1.00)/(-1.00) = $ _____

33. $(+3.00)/(+1.50) = $ _____

34. $(+3.00)/(-1.50) = $ _____

35. $(-4.50)/(-2.00) = $ _____

36. $(-4.50)/(+2.00) = $ _____

37. $(+7.50)/(-6.00) = $ _____

38. $(-3.25)/(+8.12) = $ _____

39. $(-10.00)/(-4.50) = $ _____

40. $(+6.75)/(+1.25) = $ _____

SIGNED ARITHMETIC

ADDITION
- When adding numbers with the same signs, add the amounts and give the result their common sign.
- When adding numbers with different signs, subtract the amounts and give the result the sign of the larger number

SUBTRACTION
- To subtract signed numbers, change the sign of the subtracted number and add it.

MULTIPLICATION
- When two numbers with the same signs are multiplied, the result is positive.
- When two numbers with different signs are multiplied, the result is negative.

DIVISION
- When two numbers with the same signs are divided, the result is positive.
- When two numbers with different signs are divided, the result is negative.

CALCULATORS

You will need a scientific calculator for the optics formulas in this book. Any calculator that has the sin, cos, and tan keys will do. If you are buying a calculator for this purpose, purchase the cheapest, least complicated scientific calculator you can find.

You are probably familiar with the arithmetic keys on your calculator. The subtraction key is different from the key that is used to indicate a negative number. Somewhere on your calculator is a key that looks like **+/−**, **(−)**, or **−↻+**. All scientific calculators have a key like this or something similar. Some very basic calculators (that have only +, −, ×, ÷) and some business calculators may not have a negative number key.

Calculators come in a variety of types. The sequence of keys that must be used to gain an answer to a problem depends on the type of calculator. The two basic types are called "Algebraic Notation" and "Reverse Polish Notation." In this text they are referred to as **Type A** and **Type B** calculators.

EXAMPLE:

1-16. $(-5) + (-8) = -13$. The order in which you will punch the keys is:

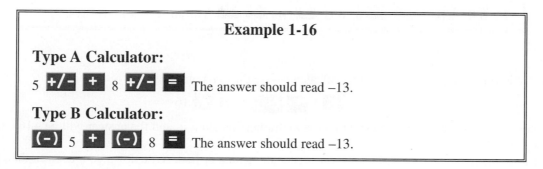

Example 1-16

Type A Calculator:

5 **+/−** **+** 8 **+/−** **=** The answer should read −13.

Type B Calculator:

(−) 5 **+** **(−)** 8 **=** The answer should read −13.

The order of punching the keys that worked shows you which type of calculator you have. You will need this information throughout the book. Also check what your negative number key is. It may not be one of the keys shown here. You may have a Type A calculator with the **(−)** key or some other key. You may have a Type B calculator with the **+/−** key or some other negative key.

EXAMPLE:

1-17. $-3 + (-14) - (-1.5)(+8) = -5$

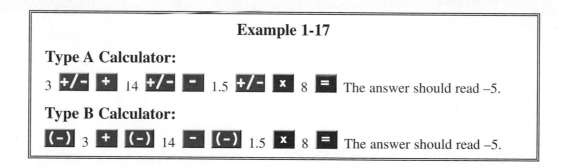

Example 1-17

Type A Calculator:

3 **+/−** **+** 14 **+/−** **−** 1.5 **+/−** **×** 8 **=** The answer should read −5.

Type B Calculator:

(−) 3 **+** **(−)** 14 **−** **(−)** 1.5 **×** 8 **=** The answer should read −5.

In the examples so far the parentheses ( ) have been included to help distinguish between a negative number and a subtraction. In the examples above you do not punch them into the calculator because the calculator does not need that distinction: the key for subtraction is different from the key for a negative number. The parentheses are also used to show multiplication. You do not punch them into the calculator for that purpose either, since the **×** key does this for you.

There are times when you will use the **(** and **)** keys on the calculator. This is when you must do some addition or subtraction *before* you do multiplication or division.

Although the problems show the + sign in some examples to show that a number is positive, you punch the $\boxed{+}$ key only when it is actually indicating addition.

EXAMPLE:

1-18. $$\frac{+16.00}{1 - (-0.005)(+16.00)}$$

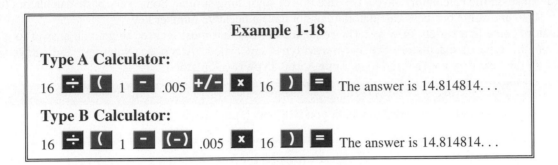

Example 1-18

Type A Calculator:

16 $\boxed{\div}$ $\boxed{(}$ 1 $\boxed{-}$ .005 $\boxed{+/-}$ $\boxed{\times}$ 16 $\boxed{)}$ $\boxed{=}$ The answer is 14.814814. . .

Type B Calculator:

16 $\boxed{\div}$ $\boxed{(}$ 1 $\boxed{-}$ $\boxed{(-)}$ .005 $\boxed{\times}$ 16 $\boxed{)}$ $\boxed{=}$ The answer is 14.814814. . .

In this fraction the denominator must be evaluated before the division occurs. If you punch in[1]:

16 $\boxed{\div}$ 1 $\boxed{-}$ $\boxed{(-)}$ 0.005 $\boxed{\times}$ 16

the calculator will divide 16 by 1, then subtract the multiplication from it, and the answer will be +16.08, which is not correct.

An alternate way to do this problem is to evaluate the denominator first, write down your answer, then punch the division into your calculator. If you punch in just the denominator[1]:

1 $\boxed{-}$ $\boxed{(-)}$ 0.005 $\boxed{\times}$ 16

you get 1.08, and if you then punch in 16 $\boxed{\div}$ 1.08, you get 14.814814. . . .

The way to punch it all into your calculator using the $\boxed{(}$ and $\boxed{)}$ keys is to punch in the numerator, punch the division key, then the $\boxed{(}$ key, then the denominator, and finally the $\boxed{)}$ key. Make sure that you punch in the $\boxed{=}$ at the end to get the final answer. If you do not punch in the equal sign, you will see only the value of the denominator of the fraction.

EXERCISES:

41. $$\frac{(+6.25)(1.53 - 1)}{(1.66 - 1)} = \underline{}$$

42. $$\frac{1.586 - 1}{0.0586} = \underline{}$$

43. $(+5)(1 + 0.067/3.32) = \underline{}$

44. $(+12.25) + (-6.25) - (0.0055/1.50)(+12.25)(-6.25) = \underline{}$

45. $$\frac{-5.00}{1 - (-0.002)(-5.00)} = \underline{}$$

---

[1] B type calculator.

Optical Formulas Tutorial

SIGNIFICANCE AND PRECISION

Some numbers are *exact numbers,* and some numbers are *approximate numbers.* Examples of exact numbers are 5 chairs or 10 houses or 3 books or 35 people. Examples of approximate numbers are 15 seconds or 3.5 meters or 186,000 miles/second or 28.4 miles/gallon.

Exact numbers are the same regardless of the exactness of counting: when you count the chairs in a room, there will not be any partial chairs. If you remove some of the pages in a book, it is still one book.

Approximate numbers depend on how carefully they are measured. A stopwatch with a second hand could be used to time an activity at 2 minutes 15 seconds. An electronic trip used to time the same activity might show 2 minutes 15.491 seconds.

The number of *significant digits* in a number means the number of "reliable" or "accurate" digits. They show how accurate the number is.

All non-zero digits are significant.

Zeros with one or more non-zero digits to both the right and left are significant (examples: 105; 30.008).

Zeros to the right of a decimal point are significant (examples: 112.300; 5.00; 1.530).

Zeros to the right of a non-decimal number are usually not significant (examples: 186,000; 1,500).

Zeros to the left of a decimal number are usually not significant (examples: 0.005; 0.128).

The *precision* of a number also indicates to what accuracy the number was measured. The number 13.25 inches has a precision of hundredths of an inch. The number 186,000 has a precision of thousands, while the number 186,282.4 is precise to the tenth.

EXAMPLES:

1-19. The measurement 85.75 mm has four significant digits and has a precision of (or is accurate to) hundredths of a millimeter.

1-20. The measurement 186,000 miles/second has three significant digits and has a precision of thousands.

1-21. The measurement 5.5 feet of ribbon has two significant digits and a precision of tenths of a foot.

1-22. The measurement 5 chairs is an exact number, so if it is used in arithmetic, its precision and significant digits are not used.

When addition and subtraction are performed with approximate numbers, the answer is rounded to the precision of the least accurate number. When multiplication and division are performed with approximate numbers, the answer is rounded to the number of significant digits of the least accurate number.

ROUNDING

Many answers will have to be rounded to a particular accuracy. Look at the *first* digit to the right of the digit you are rounding to.

If it is a 4 or less, drop it and all digits to the right of it.

If it is a 5 or more, increase the digit to the left by one, and drop all other digits to the right.

EXAMPLES:

1-23. Round to whole mm: 12.345 mm → 12 mm. (The answer will be either 12 or 13. The next digit to the right is 3, which is "4 or less," so the .345 is dropped.)

1-24. Round to one-hundredths: +12.5862 → 12.59. (The one-hundredth place is an 8. The next digit to the right is 6, which is "5 or more"; add 1 to the 8 and drop the 62.)

1-25. Round to tenths: 6.74999 → 6.7. (The 7 is in the tenths place. The next digit to the right is 4, which is "4 or less," so the 4999 is dropped.)

In Exercises 46-48: Round to two decimal places:

46. 132.5743 _____

47. 0.455555 _____

48. 1.56 _____

In Exercises 49-51: Round to whole numbers:

49. 5.500 _____

50. 4.499999 _____

51. 8.9 _____

In Exercises 52-55: Using the number 186,282.4:

52. Round to a whole number: _____

53. Round to the tens place: _____

54. Round to the one-hundreds place: _____

55. Round to the one-thousands place: _____

CONVERSIONS

METRIC-METRIC

A yard may be divided into parts. One yard contains 3 feet or 36 inches. A foot can be divided into parts. One foot contains 12 inches. A meter may be divided into parts. It is divided into decimeters, or tenths; centimeters, or hundredths; millimeters, or thousandths; and so on. Unlike English units, metrics are based on dividing each unit into tenths.

Decimeters are not used in the formulas in this book. They are included in the box below to help you remember that the decimal point moves two places between meters and centimeters.

METER ↔ DECIMETER ↔ CENTIMETER ↔ MILLIMETER

m → dm → cm → mm
1 m = 10 dm = 100 cm = 1000 mm
When converting from meters to centimeters or millimeters, move the decimal point to the right.

m ← dm ← cm ← mm
0.001 m = 0.01 dm = 0.1 cm = 1 mm
When converting from millimeters or centimeters to meters, move the decimal point to the left.

EXAMPLES:

1-26. 5.35 m = 535 cm = 5350 mm

1-27. 267 mm = 26.7 cm = 0.267 m

EXERCISES: (Do not round.)

56. Convert 5 m to mm. _____

57. Convert 2 m to cm. _____

58. Convert 50 cm to mm. _____

59. Convert 2 mm to cm. _____

60. Convert 2.45 mm to m. _____

61. Convert 4.5 cm to mm. _____

62. Convert 4.5 cm to m. _____

63. Convert 80.5 mm to m. _____

ENGLISH-METRIC

A yardstick is 3 feet or 36 inches long. A meter stick would be just slightly longer than a yardstick: it is 39.37 inches long. Therefore 1 m = 39.37 in. Under some circumstances it will be both convenient and acceptable to remember the approximation 1 m ≈ 40 in.

If you have a ruler with both inches and millimeters on it, you will notice that 1 inch is just over 2.5 cm long. In fact, 1 in = 2.54 cm = 0.0254 m.

EXAMPLES:

1-28. What would a 5 1/2 inch temple measure on a mm ruler? We have seen that 1 in = 2.54 cm = 25.4 mm. Multiply both sides of the equal sign by 5.5:
(5.5)(1 in) = (5.5)(25.4 mm) = 139.7 mm = 140 mm

1-29. How many inches are there in 1/2 meter?
1 m ≈ 40 in. Multiply both sides of the equal sign by 0.5:
(0.5)(1 m) = (0.5)(40 in) = 20 in

If an answer in feet is requested, convert to inches and divide the answer by 12. If the problem is in feet, multiply by 12 to get inches, then convert. Most of what we do in this book will involve feet, inches, meters, and millimeters.

EXERCISES: (Round answers to two decimal places.)

64. Convert 155 mm to inches. (Hint: 155 mm = how many cm? Now convert to inches.)

65. How many feet are in 155 mm? (Hint: Convert the answer in Exercise 64 to feet.)

66. Convert 6 feet to meters. (Hint: How many inches in 6 feet? Convert this number to centimeters, and then convert that answer to meters. Round to one decimal place.)

67. Convert 20 feet to meters. Round to one decimal place.

68. How many inches long is a 120-mm glasses temple? Round to two significant digits.

69. Convert the standard reading distance of 16 inches to centimeters. Round to two significant digits.

70. My computer monitor is 30 inches away from my face. How many meters is this? Round to two significant digits.

71. How many feet are in a 1-meter stick? Round to tenths of a foot.

SINE, COSINE, TANGENT

The *sine* (pronounced like "sign"), *cosine,* and *tangent* are *functions of angles*. They are abbreviated *sin*, *cos*, and *tan*. *These functions are used only when angles are involved.* If you wish to learn more about these functions than is presented here, refer to a basic trigonometry text in the library.

How you solve the equations containing angles depends on what type of calculator you have. If you do not have a calculator, or your calculator does not have the sin, cos, and tan keys, use the tables in Appendix 4 in the back of this book. If you have a calculator with a key labeled "sin," perform the test in the box below.

Try each one to determine which calculator you have

Type A Calculator:

30 `sin` The calculator should say 0.5

Type B Calculator:

`sin` 30 `=` The calculator should say 0.5.

If neither of these methods works, your calculator may be assuming that the angle is in radians or gradients. Look in the directions that came with your calculator to learn how to change the calculator to degrees from radians or gradients.

When the angle is *given* and the sine of the angle is needed, use one of these methods:

Type A. Enter the value of the angle in the calculator and then press the button labeled **sin**.

Type B. Press the button labeled **sin** on the calculator, enter the value of the angle, and then press the **equal** or **enter** button.

Appendix 4, pp. 231-232. Look for the angle in column one or five, and read to the right across the line to the next column.

EXAMPLES:

1-30. sin 45 = ?

Example 1-30

Type A Calculator:

45 `sin` The calculator should say 0.7071. . .

Type B Calculator:

`sin` 45 `=` The calculator should say 0.7071. . .

Type A. Enter **45**, press **sin**. If the calculator reads 0.707106 . . ., this is the answer.
Type B. Press **sin**, enter **45**, press =. It should show 0.707106. . . .
Appendix 4, p. 231. Find 45 at the bottom of the page in column one. Read to the right to the sine column, where it says 0.70711. This is the answer.

1-31. tan 61 = ?

Type A. Enter **61** in the calculator, press **tan**. The display should show 1.804047 . . .
Type B. Enter **tan**, **61**, =. The display should show 1.804047 . . .

Appendix 4, p. 231. Find 61 halfway down the fifth column. Read to the right to the last column, which is labeled tangent. The entry is 1.80405. This is the answer.

When the angle is *not given*, but the sine is given, you need the **sin⁻¹** key. It is usually the shifted version of the sine key.

Type A. Enter the value in your calculator, press the **second** or **inverse** or **shift** button, and then press the **sin** button.

Type B. Press the **second** or **inverse** or **shift** button on your calculator, press the **sin button**, enter the value, and then press the **equal** or **enter** button.

Appendix 4, pp. 231-232. Look for the value in column two or six, and read back to the left one column to the angle. The exact value may not be present; you may have to choose the closest one.

You will be able to find only one of the keys: **inverse**, **second**, or **shift**. Use it together with the **sin** key to get the **sin⁻¹** key.

EXAMPLES:

1-32. sin a = 0.24192. What is angle a?

Example 1-32

Type A Calculator:

0.24192 **sin⁻¹** The calculator should say 13.99. . .

Type B Calculator:

sin⁻¹ 0.24192 **=** The calculator should say 13.99. . .

Type A. Enter the value **0.24192** in your calculator. Press **second** (or **inverse** or **shift**), then **sin**. The calculator shows 13.999888 . . . . This rounds to 14 degrees.

Type B. Press **second** (or **inverse** or **shift**), then **sin**, then enter the value **.24192**, then press =. The calculator shows 13.999888 . . . . This rounds to 14 degrees.

Appendix 4, p. 231. Read down the column labeled sine on p. 231 until you come to 0.24192. Read to the left; the angle is 14 degrees.

1-33. cos β = 0.45. What is angle β?

Type A. Enter the value **.45** in your calculator. Press **second** (or **inverse** or **shift**), then **cos**. The calculator shows 63.256 . . . . This rounds to 63 degrees.

Type B. Press **second** (or **inverse** or **shift**), then **cos**, then enter the value **0.45**, then press =. The calculator shows 63.256 . . . . This rounds to 63 degrees.

Appendix 4, p. 231. Read down the cosine column on p. 231 until you come to 0.45. It does not appear in the first cosine column; it is partway down the second cosine column. You will find 0.45399 and 0.43837. Since 0.45 is closer to 0.45399 than it is to 0.43837, use the angle that corresponds to 0.45399, which is 63 degrees.

To enter negative values when you are using a calculator, use the **+/−**, **(−)**, or **⟲+** key with the number. Do not use the subtraction key **−**.

EXERCISES:

In Exercises 72-77, round answers to five decimal places. Round angles to the nearest whole angle.

72. sin 36 = ? _____

73. cos 89 = ? _____

74. tan 1 = ? _____

75. sin 180 = ? _____

76. cos 144 = ? _____

77. tan 92 = ? _____

78. sin a = 0.588; angle a = ? _____

79. cos β = 0.588; angle β = ? _____

80. tan δ = 0.36397; angle δ = ? _____

81. tan θ = –0.36397; angle θ = ? _____

82. cos α = –0.15643; angle α = ? _____

83. sin a = 0.50; angle a = ? _____
     Note: If you are using the tables in Appendix 4, there are two angles with this sine.

84. sin^2 45 = ? _____
     Note: This means find the sine of 45 degrees, and then square the amount. Sin 45 = ? Once you find this
     answer, press the x^2 key. Another notation meaning the same thing is $(sin\ 45)^2$.

SCIENTIFIC NOTATION

Occasionally we will work with numbers that are "very large" or "very small." In these cases we may use scientific
notation: a number from 1 to 9, times ten to a power. For example: one million: 1,000,000 can be written 1.00×10^6.
The $\times 10^6$ means: "Move the decimal point six places to the left."

Similarly, 10^{-6} means: "Move the decimal point six places to the right," so $1.00 \times 10^{-6} = 0.000,001$.

Every time you move the decimal point to the right, you subtract one from the exponent. Every time you move
the decimal point to the left, you add one to the exponent.

EXAMPLES:

1-34. 3.80×10^{-9} meters = 0.000,000,003,80 meters

1-35. 7.65×10^{14} waves = 765,000,000,000,000 waves

1-36. The distance from the earth to the sun is about 150 million kilometers. This is $150,000,000 = 1.5 \times 10^8$ km.

ADDITION AND SUBTRACTION

When you are adding and subtracting numbers in scientific notation without a calculator, the numbers must have the
same exponent. When using the calculator, you do not need to convert to the same exponent.

If there is a **10^X** key (this key may be above the log key and require using the shift or 2nd key with the log key),
you would enter the number 1.23×10^8 this way:

Type A: 1.23 **×** 8 **10^X**
Type B: 1.23 **10^X** 8

The easiest way is using the **EXP** key, which may be near the decimal point at the bottom of the number pad,
or the **EE** key. For both calculator types, 1.23×10^8 is entered 1.23 **EXP** 8.

Round the result to the precision of the least accurate number. That will usually (but not always) be the number
with the larger exponent.

1-37. $1.23 \times 10^8 + 3.456 \times 10^7$: convert to the same exponent.

$$
\begin{array}{ccc}
1.23 \times 10^8 & & 12.3 \times 10^7 \\
+\ 0.3456 \times 10^8 & \text{or} & +\ 3.456 \times 10^7 \\
\hline
1.5756 \times 10^8 & & 15.756 \times 10^7 = 1.5756 \times 10^8
\end{array}
$$

Example 1-37

Type A Calculator:

1.23 **EXP** 8 **+** 3.456 **EXP** 7 **=** The calculator should say 157560000.

Type B Calculator:

1.23 **EXP** 8 **+** 3.456 **EXP** 7 **=** The calculator should say 157,560,000.

Then, because the precision is two decimals on the 10^8 number, we round to 1.58×10^8. That is the precision of the least accurate number when both numbers have been converted to the same exponent.

1-38. Subtract 8.993×10^{-4} from 9.231×10^{-3}.

$$
\begin{array}{ccc}
9.231 \times 10^{-3} & & 92.31 \times 10^{-4} \\
-\ 0.8993 \times 10^{-3} & \text{or} & -\ 8.993 \times 10^{-4} \\
\hline
8.3317 \times 10^{-3} & & 83.317 \times 10^{-4} = 8.3317 \times 10^{-3}
\end{array}
$$

Then, because the precision is three decimals on the 10^{-3} number, we round to 8.332×10^{-3}. That is the precision of the least accurate number when both numbers have been converted to the same exponent.

MULTIPLICATION

When multiplying numbers in scientific notation without a calculator, multiply the numbers and add the exponents. Then round the answer to the number of significant digits of the least accurate number.

1-39.
$$
\begin{aligned}
&(1.23 \times 10^8)(3.456 \times 10^7) \\
&= (1.23)(3.456) \times 10^{7+8} \\
&= 4.25088 \times 10^{15}
\end{aligned}
$$

This answer rounds to 4.25×10^{15} because one of the original numbers has only three significant digits.

Example 1-39

Type A Calculator:

1.23 **EXP** 8 **×** 3.456 **EXP** 7 **=** The calculator should say 4.25088^{15}.

Type B Calculator:

1.23 **EXP** 8 **×** 3.456 **EXP** 7 **=** The calculator should say 4.25088^{15}.

DIVISION

When dividing numbers in scientific notation without a calculator, divide the numbers and subtract the exponent of the divisor (bottom number) from the exponent of the numerator (top number). Then round the answer to the number of significant digits of the least accurate number.

EXAMPLE:

1-40. $(8.993 \times 10^{-3})/(9.231 \times 10^{-4})$
   $= (8.993)/(9.231) \times 10^{-3-(-4)}$
   $= 0.9739008 \times 10^1$
   $= 9.739$

EXERCISES:

In Exercises 85-88 write in scientific notation, with three digits of significance:

85. 3,000,000 meters/second _____

86. 186,000 miles/second _____

87. 745,000,000,000,000 waves/second _____

88. 0.000,000,380 meters _____

In Exercises 89-91 write out normally:

89. 1×10^{-9} meters _____

90. 5.4×10^{14} Hz _____

91. 2.99792×10^8 meters _____

92. $4.00 \times 10^8 + 4.557 \times 10^9 =$ _____

93. $4.557 \times 10^9 - 4.00 \times 10^8 =$ _____

94. (20×10^{-6}) * $(3.5 \times 10^{-2}) =$ _____

95. $(3.00 \times 10^8)/(660 \times 10^{-9}) =$ _____

SECTION II – THEORY OF LIGHT

Two concepts are used to describe the propagation of light:

- Waves
- Rays

PROPERTIES OF WAVES

Four properties are used to describe a wave:

- Wavelength: the distance from a point on a wave to the corresponding point on the next wave
- Frequency: the number of waves that pass in 1 second
- Speed: the distance that the wave will travel in a second
- Amplitude: the distance from the centerline to the peak or to the valley of the wave

WAVELENGTH

One *wavelength* is the distance from a point on one wave to the corresponding point on the next wave. In this book the Greek letter lambda (λ) will be used to represent the wavelength.

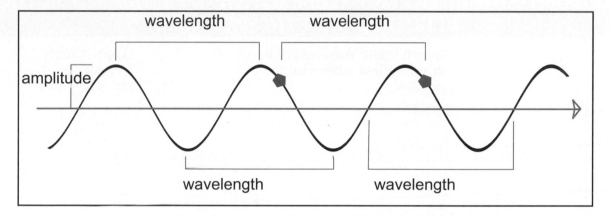

Waves of electromagnetic energy range from several hundred meters long to several billion in 1 meter. Waves of visible light are measured in *nanometers,* or **nm**. There are 1 billion nanometers in 1 meter.

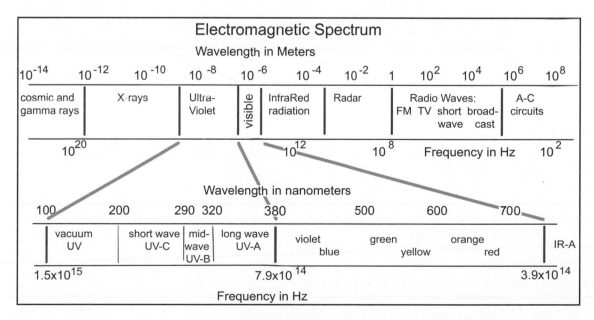

$$1 \text{ NANOMETER} = 1 \times 10^{-9} \text{ meters*}$$
$$= 0.000,000,001 \text{ meter}$$
$$= 1/1,000,000,000 \text{ meter}$$

*See the discussion of scientific notation in Section I, pp. 12 to 14.

FREQUENCY

Frequency is the number of vibrations of a given wavelength in 1 second. In the electromagnetic spectrum, longer waves vibrate fewer times in 1 second than shorter waves. The shorter the wavelength, the higher the frequency. The longer the wavelength, the lower the frequency. The unit of measurement for frequency is called the *hertz* (Hz).

1 HERTZ = 1 complete wave per second

Frequencies for visible light are large values and vary for each color of the spectrum.

RELATIONSHIP BETWEEN WAVELENGTH AND FREQUENCY IN THE ELECTROMAGNETIC SPECTRUM

	Approximate Wavelength in Air (in nm unless otherwise specified)	Approximate Frequency (in $\times 10^{14}$ Hz)
UV-C	200-290 nm	10.3-15.0
UV-B	290-320	9.4-10.3
UV-A	320-380	7.9-9.4
Violet	400	7.5
Blue	460	6.5
Green	510	5.9
Yellow	560	5.4
Orange	610	4.9
Red	660	4.5
IR-A	760-1400	2.1-3.9
IR-B	1400-3000 nm	1.0-2.1
IR-C	3×10^{-3} mm - 1 mm	0.003-1.0

See the discussion of scientific notation in Section I, pp. 12-14.
The higher the frequency of an element of the electromagnetic spectrum, the shorter the wavelength and the higher the energy. The lower the frequency of an element of the electromagnetic spectrum, the longer the wavelength and the lower the energy.

VELOCITY

Velocity is the rate or speed at which light waves travel. In a vacuum all waves in the electromagnetic spectrum travel at the same speed.

In a vacuum all elements of the EMS travel at:
- 3×10^8 meters per second
(more accurately 299,792,458 meters/second)
- 186,000 miles per second
(more accurately 186,282 miles/second)

Light travels slightly slower in air than in a vacuum, but the difference is not enough to concern us in this book. A wave in the electromagnetic spectrum will slow down as it leaves air and enters a material. The wavelengths in the electromagnetic spectrum do not all slow to the same speed in a particular material, however. White light is broken down into colors when it travels through a prism because the shorter blue waves slow more than the longer red waves. This is called *dispersion*.

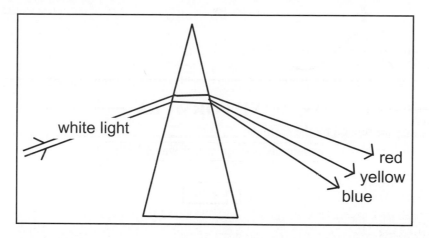

AMPLITUDE

The *amplitude* is the displacement of the peak or the valley from the centerline, or the maximum that the particle travels from its resting point if there is no wave. Amplitude is not an important concept for the theory of light.

ATTRIBUTES OF WAVES

- *Divergence*. Waves diverge from their source.
- *Infinity*. Waves that travel far enough from their source become parallel to each other. *Optical infinity* is defined as 6 meters or 20 feet.

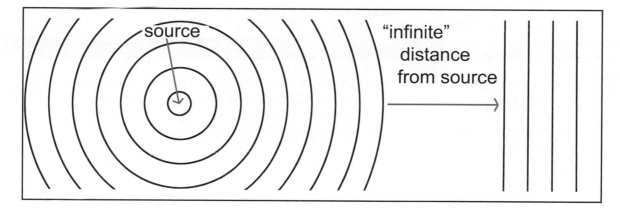

- *Constructive interference*. Two waves exactly in sync with each other will augment each other.

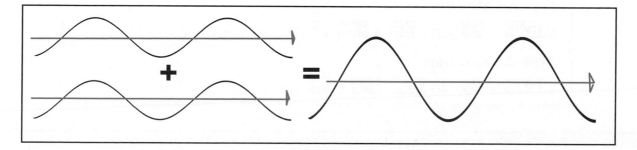

- *Destructive interference.* Two waves exactly out of sync with each other will cancel each other.

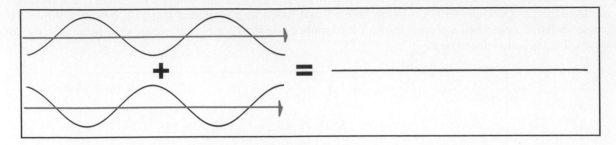

WAVE FORMULA

The properties of a wave are related by the formula

$$\boxed{\text{velocity} = \text{frequency} \times \text{wavelength}}$$

For any given color, only the frequency remains constant as the wave travels from one material to another.

$$\boxed{v = f\lambda}$$

or

$$\boxed{f = \frac{v}{\lambda}}$$

or

$$\boxed{\lambda = \frac{v}{f}}$$

where:
v = velocity of the wave: how far a peak travels in a unit of time
f = frequency of the wave: how many peaks pass in a unit of time
λ = wavelength of the wave: how far apart the peaks are

EXAMPLES:

2-1. What is the frequency of a ray of blue light that has a wavelength in air of 460 nm, or 460×10^{-9} meters/wave? (In these exercises use $v = 3.00 \times 10^8$ meters/second[1] for the velocity of light.)
$f = v/\lambda$
$\quad = (3.00 \times 10^8)/(460 \times 10^{-9})$
$\quad = (3/460) \times 10^{+8+9}$ waves/second
$\quad = 0.0065217 \times 10^{17}$ Hz
$\quad = \mathbf{6.52 \times 10^{14}\ Hz}$

Example 2-1

Type A Calculator:

3 **EXP** 8 **÷** 460 **EXP** 9 **+/−** **=** The calculator should say 6.5217^{14}.

Type B Calculator:

3 **EXP** 8 **÷** 460 **EXP** **(−)** 9 **=** The calculator should say 6.5217^{14}.

---

[1]See the discussion of scientific notation in Section I, pp. 12-14.

　　　　　　　　Optical Formulas Tutorial

2-2. If a ray of red light has a wavelength of 660 nm, what is its frequency in air?

$f = v / \lambda$

$\quad = (3.00 \times 10^8)/(660 \times 10^{-9})$

$\quad = 0.00455 \times 10^{17}$

$\quad = \mathbf{4.55 \times 10^{14}\ Hz}$

2-3. To what does the wavelength of red light (λ = 660 nm) change when the wave is traveling from air to crown glass, where the wave travels at 1.97×10^8 meters/second, if its frequency is 4.55×10^{14} Hz?

$\lambda = v / f$

$\quad = (1.97 \times 10^8)/(4.55 \times 10^{14})$

$\quad = 0.433 \times 10^{8-14}\ 0.433 \times 10^{-6}$

$\quad = 433 \times 10^{-9} = \mathbf{433\ nm}$

EXERCISES: (Round all answers to three digits.)

1. A ray of yellowish light has a wavelength of 588 nm in a vacuum. What is its frequency?

2. A ray of light has a frequency of 5.10×10^{14} Hz. What is its wavelength in polycarbonate, where the ray travels at 1.89×10^8 meters/second?

3. What is the wavelength of the ray of light having a frequency of 5.10×10^{14} Hz, while it travels through water where the wave travels at 2.26×10^8 meters/second?

4. A ray of the electromagnetic spectrum has a frequency of 8.33×10^{14} Hz. What is the wavelength of this ray in a vacuum? What part of the electromagnetic spectrum is this ray?

———————————————— DIFFRACTION ————————————————

Diffraction is the bending of waves when they pass the edge of a very small slit. Diffraction is a result of wave motion. Regardless of the distance of the source of a wave, when the wave passes through a very small opening in a barrier, the wave acts as if the opening is a new source of the wave.

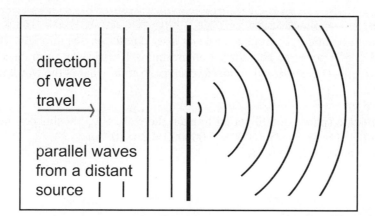

By use of a diffraction grating containing very thin slits set very close together, plus some trigonometry, the actual wavelength of a monochromatic light source can be calculated.

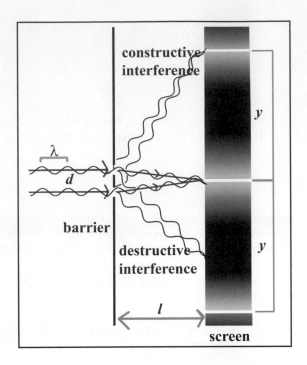

$$\lambda = \frac{dy}{l}$$

where:

λ = wavelength of the monochromatic incident light, in nanometers

d = distance between the slits on the diffraction grating, in meters

y = distance between the first two areas of constructive interference, in meters

l = distance from the diffraction grating to the screen, in meters

EXAMPLE:

2-4. A beam of monochromatic light from a speaker's laser pointer passes through a diffraction grating with slits that are spaced at 500 per mm. The diffraction grating is 10 cm away from the screen. If the distance between the first two areas of constructive interference is 35 mm, what is the wavelength of the light? What color is the laser beam?

The formula is $\lambda = dy/l$.

Step 1: Since the slits are spaced at 500 per millimeter, there are 500,000 slits per meter. Therefore the spacing between the slits, d, is $1/500{,}000 = 0.000002 = 2 \times 10^{-6}$ m

Step 2: y = 35 mm = 0.035 m = 3.5×10^{-2} m

Step 3: l = 10 cm = 0.1 m

Therefore:

$\lambda = dy/l$

$= (2 \times 10^{-6})(3.5 \times 10^{-2})/(0.1)$

$= 7 \times 10^{-8}/0.1$

$= 70 \times 10^{-8}$

$= 700 \times 10^{-9}$ m

$= 700$ nm, which is a deep red light wave

EXERCISE:

5. A monochromatic beam of light is passed through a grating having 600 slits per millimeter. The distance between the first two areas of constructive interference is 33 mm when the screen on which the interference pattern is projected is 10 cm away. What is the wavelength of the monochromatic beam of light? What color is the beam of light?

PHOTONS, RAYS, PENCILS, AND BEAMS

A *photon* is a particle of light. It is the smallest amount of light possible. A *ray* is the path of a single photon of light from a single point on a light source. A photon will travel in a straight line unless it changes speed or passes a barrier.

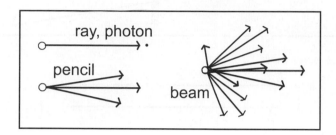

A *pencil* of light is a group of rays divergent from a single point on a light source.

A *beam* of light is composed of the group of pencils originating from all of the points on a light source.

ATTRIBUTES OF RAYS

Rays spread out from the source. Rays are *divergent* from the source. Divergent rays have *negative* vergence.

Photons travel in straight lines. This is called the *Law of Rectilinear Propagation.* There are, however, particular circumstances that cause a ray to bend.

Rays of the electromagnetic spectrum travel at a definite and constant speed in any given homogeneous medium or material.

SPEED OF VISIBLE LIGHT*

186,000 miles per second in air
122,000 miles per second in crown glass
140,000 miles per second in water
124,000 miles per second in CR-39

*The speed of light in a material is based on the speed of a particular frequency of yellow, $\lambda = 588$ nm.

—————— **VERGENCE** ——————

Divergent lines are lines that spread apart as if originating from a point. They have *negative vergence. Convergent* lines are lines that come together to meet at a point, then diverge again as they continue on their path. Convergent rays have *positive vergence.* Convergent rays of light will cross at a *real* point.

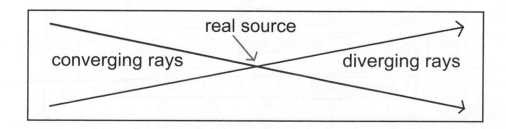

Sometimes divergent rays of light have to be projected back to a *virtual* point or source. It is *as if* the point of origin of the rays were there.

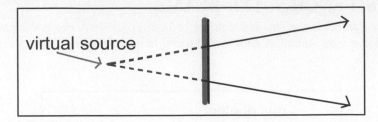

Parallel lines are lines that never meet.

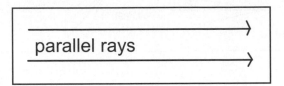

The farther light travels from its source, the less vergence it has, and the rays of light eventually become essentially parallel. Light rays originating from a distance of *20 feet* or *6 meters* or more are considered to be parallel. This is the definition of **optical infinity**.

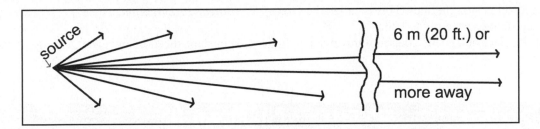

To quantify vergence, we must define both the source and the observation point. Vergence is the inverse of the distance that the observation point is from the source.

$$\text{vergence} = \frac{1}{\text{distance}_{\text{meters}}}$$

In the diagram, screen 1 is distance d from the source of the rays, so the vergence of the rays at screen 1 is D = 1/d. Screen 2 is distance t from the source, so the vergence of the same rays at screen 2 is T = 1/t. Convention in physics textbooks uses a capital letter for the vergence and a small letter for the distance from the source to the observation point. The distance is measured in meters.

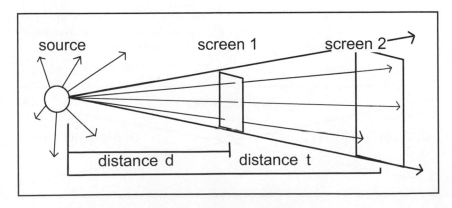

2-5. On earth we are a very large number of meters away from the sun, the source of daylight. So the vergence of the sun's rays on earth is 1/(very large number) = very close to zero.[2] Thus the essentially parallel rays that reach the earth from the sun have a vergence of 0.

2-6. When you stand 6.56 feet from a light source, you are 2 meters from the light.[3] The rays from the light source have a vergence of 1/2 = 0.5 when they enter your eye.

2-7. When you hold a piece of paper at 16 inches from your face, the rays that reflect from the page and enter your eye are coming from 0.4 meter.[3] The rays reflecting from the paper surface have a vergence of 1/0.4 = 2.5 when they enter your eye.

EXERCISES:

6. A projector is 6 meters from a screen. What is the vergence of the light rays from the projector when they fall on the screen?

7. A light source is distance y from a lens. What is the vergence of the light when it reaches the lens?

8. Light has a vergence of 5 when it falls on an object. What is the distance of the object from the light source?

ILLUMINATION

Illumination varies with the square of the distance of the object from the light source:

$$E = \frac{I}{d^2}$$

where:
E = intensity of the light on the object, in lux (lx) [or foot-candles]
I = intensity of the light at the source, in lumens (lm)
d = distance of the light source from the object in meters [or feet]

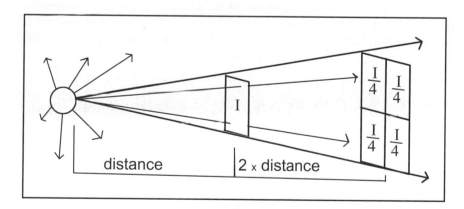

Light intensity used to be measured in foot-candles, which was the intensity of light generated by one candle on a 1-square-foot surface 1 foot away. The formula using foot-candles is the same as above, but distance is measured in feet if intensity is in foot-candles. Intensity is now more commonly measured in *lux*. One lux is one *lumen* (related to a candle) on a one square meter screen 1 meter away. One lux is approximately 10 foot-candles. (Actually, one lux = 10.76 foot-candles.)

---

[2]The distance from the earth to the sun is 150,000,000 kilometers = 150,000,000,000 meters = 1.5×10^{11} m, so the vergence is 0.000,000,000,0067 = 6.7×10^{-12}, a very small number.
[3]For conversion of feet to meters, see p. 9 in Section I.

Illumination is a measurement of how much light is incident on a surface. It *is not* a measurement of how bright the surface appears to the observer. If the surface is pure flat black, none of the incident light will reflect off the surface. Therefore the surface will *appear* dark, regardless of the intensity of the illumination or the distance of the surface from the light source.

EXAMPLES:

2-8. A book is 1 meter (about 3.25 feet) from a 100-lumen source. The intensity of light falling on the book is found with $E = I/d^2 = 100/1^2 = 100$ lux.

2-9. If the book is 2 meters (about 6.5 feet) from the 100-lumen source, the intensity of the light falling on the book is $100/2^2 = 100/4 = 25$ lux.

EXERCISES: (Round answers to whole numbers.)

9. A 1000-lumen light source is 4 meters from the center of a large screen. The edge of the screen is 5 meters from the light source.
   a. What is the intensity of light falling on the center of the screen?
   b. What is the intensity of light falling on the edge of the screen?

10. A slit lamp has a 300,000-lumen light source.
   a. What intensity of light falls on the patient's eye when it is 30 cm away from the source?
   b. What intensity of light falls on the eye when it is 40 cm from the source?

———— ABSORPTION, REFLECTION, REFRACTION ————

Three things may happen when light travels from one material to another material:

- Absorption
- Reflection
- Refraction

Absorption is what occurs when a photon of light enters a material but does not exit again. Absorption of photons in the electromagnetic spectrum may result in thermal, electrical, or chemical changes. These are different forms of energy. Dark colors absorb more than light colors. Most materials absorb infrared waves as heat. Absorption is why we wear dark colors in the winter and light colors in the summer, and it is the reason that blacktop becomes very hot in the summer sun. Photosynthesis is an example of a chemical change, and so is the change of photochromatic glasses lenses from light to dark when exposed to UV light. The solar cells in many small calculators are an example of the conversion of visible light to electrical energy.

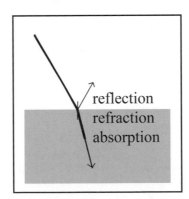

Reflection occurs when a light ray is turned back into the incident material instead of traveling on into the new material. If the surface of the new material is relatively smooth, any two rays that are reflected from the surface will continue to travel with the same relationship to each other that they originally had. Reflection from a smooth surface changes the direction of the rays but not their vergence, which is their relationship to each other. *Regular* or *specular* reflection comes from a shiny or reflective surface. If the surface is not smooth, the rays reflect in a random manner with respect to each other and the result is *diffuse* reflection.

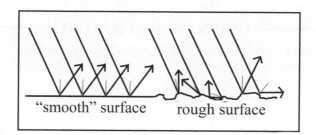

"smooth" surface   rough surface

The light that is reflected by an object results in color perception. An object appears to be black if it absorbs all of the wavelengths of the visible spectrum and reflects little or no light. An object appears to be white if it reflects diffusely all of the wavelengths of the visible spectrum. An object appears to be red if it reflects light from the red portion of the spectrum and absorbs all others.

Refraction is the bending or change in direction of light when it passes from one transparent material to another transparent material of a different optical density.

FACTORS AFFECTING REFRACTION

- *The material itself.* Each transparent material has a different optical density, which affects how much it slows a light ray down. So each material has a particular refracting ability.
- *The obliquity of the incident light ray.* Light rays incident normal (meaning perpendicular) to a surface slow down, but do not change direction. Rays incident at any other angle will change direction, or be bent. The greater the angle at which the ray meets the surface, the more it is bent or changes direction.
- *The frequency (or wavelength) of the incident light ray.* Light rays with different frequencies (directly related to wavelengths) travel at different speeds in any particular material. Only in a vacuum do all frequencies travel at the same speed.

─────────── LAW OF REFLECTION ───────────

When a ray of light is reflected from a surface, whether it is rough or smooth, the angle of reflection will equal the angle of incidence.

angle incidence = angle reflection

The normal, an imaginary line perpendicular to the surface, is used to measure the angles of incidence and reflection. Because the angles are equal, for a smooth surface the vergence of incident light is not changed. Two rays striking the surface at an angle to each other will leave the surface at the same angle to each other. See the left side of the drawing. For each of the rays in the drawing, the reflecting angle is equal to the incident angle.

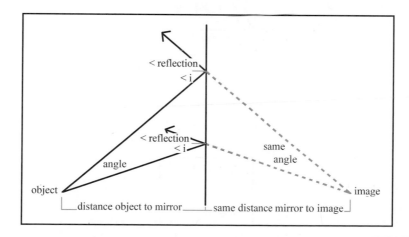

This is why an image in a flat mirror appears to be the same distance behind the mirror that the object is in front of the mirror. The formulas dealing with reflection from flat and curved surfaces are discussed in Section VII, Image Formation.

LAWS OF REFRACTION

1. A ray of light striking a transparent surface ***normal*** (perpendicular) to the surface will not be bent, but the speed of the light will be changed because of the change in optical density of the material. See the upper ray in the figure below.
2. Light passing obliquely (at an angle other than perpendicular) from a material of *lesser* optical density (faster) to a material of *greater* optical density (slower) will be bent *toward* the normal. See the left side of the lower ray in the figure below.
3. Light passing obliquely from a material of *greater* optical density (slower) to a material of *lesser* optical density (faster) will be bent *away* from the normal. See the right side of the lower ray in the figure below.

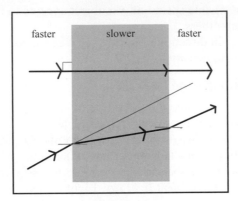

Note: The larger of the angle of incidence and the angle of refraction is on the side where the speed of light is faster. **LAFS:** **L**arge **A**ngle, **F**ast **S**ide.

The angle between the light ray and the normal to the surface between the two materials is called the ***angle of incidence,*** or $\angle i$. The angle at which the ray emerges into the second material is the ***angle of refraction,*** or $\angle r$. The angle between the path of the refracted ray and the path the ray would have taken if it had not bent is the ***angle of deviation***, or $\angle d$.

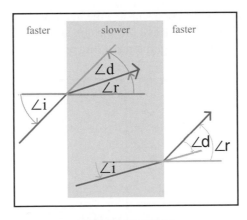

$$\angle i = \angle r + \angle d$$
$$\angle d = \angle i - \angle r$$
$$\angle r = \angle i - \angle d$$

EXAMPLES:

2-10. If the angle of incidence is 20 degrees and the angle of refraction is 15 degrees, by how much is the ray deviated?

Optical Formulas Tutorial

∠d = ∠i − ∠r
    = 20 − 15
∠d = 5 degrees
Note that ∠i is greater than ∠r, so the ray is traveling from a faster material to a slower material.

2-11. If the ray is deviated by −18 degrees from its original path, and the angle of incidence is 48 degrees, what is the angle of refraction?
∠r = ∠i − ∠d
    = 48 − (−18)
    = 48 + 18
∠r = 66 degrees
Note that ∠i is smaller than ∠r, so the ray is traveling from a slower to a faster material.

2-12. If the angle of deviation is 16 degrees and the angle of refraction is 40 degrees, what is the angle of incidence?
∠i = ∠r + ∠d
    = 40 + 16
∠i = 56 degrees

EXERCISES:

11. If a ray of light traveling through air is incident on a plane surface at 20 degrees and is deviated 5 degrees from its original path by the new material, what is the angle of refraction?

12. If a ray of light entering a plane glass block from air is deviated from its path by 10 degrees and its angle of refraction is 5 degrees, what was the angle of incidence of the ray of light?

13. If a ray of light leaving a material and traveling into air is incident on the surface at 15 degrees and it is refracted at an angle of 33 degrees, what is the angle of deviation? (Why is this angle negative?)

14. If a ray of light traveling from glass into air has an angle of incidence of 25 degrees and is deviated −4 degrees, what is its angle of refraction?

INDEX OF REFRACTION

The index of refraction of a transparent material is a ratio that compares the speed of light in a vacuum to the speed of light as it moves through the material. The speed of light in a vacuum is 186,000 miles per second, or 3×10^8 meters per second. Although a ray of light will be slowed when it enters air from a vacuum, it is not slowed enough to affect our calculations, so the speed of light is approximated at 186,000 miles/second and 3×10^8 meters/second in either air or vacuum. (We actually use the speed of a yellow wave, λ = 588 nm, for the index of refraction.)

The small letter *n* is the symbol for index of refraction in this book. Some books use the Greek letter *mu* (μ) for this.

$$n = \frac{\text{speed of light in a vacuum}}{\text{speed of light in the material}}$$

Alternatively,

$$\text{speed of light in the material} = \frac{\text{speed of light in a vacuum}}{n}$$

The amount of refraction or bending of light by a material is dependent on the speed of light through the material. The more the ray is slowed, the more it is bent or refracted.

The higher the index of refraction is, the slower the light travels through the material, and the more the ray is bent. This is why a higher index lens is thinner than a lower index lens of the same power and same minimum thickness. The material slows the light more, so the curve on the lens bends the light more than the same curve would do on a lower index lens.

INDICES FOR SOME COMMON OPHTHALMIC MATERIALS

Air = 1.00
Water = 1.33
CR-39 = 1.498 or 1.50
(Tools in most laboratories are calibrated to 1.53.)
Trivex* = 1.53
Crown glass = 1.523
Polycarbonate = 1.586
Barium glass ≈ 1.60 (depending on content)
Flint glass ≈ 1.70 (depending on content)
High-index plastics: available in many indices
High-index glass: available in many indices
Cornea of the eye = 1.37 (average)
Lens of the eye = 1.42 (average)
Aqueous, vitreous, and tear film = 1.34 (average)

*Trivex is registered to PPG Industries. Technical information is from http://corporate.ppg.com/PPG/opticalprod/en/monomers/products/Properties.htm.

EXAMPLES:

2-13. What is the speed of light in miles/second in a barium glass with an index of 1.60? Round the answer to thousands, three significant digits.
Speed = 186,000/1.60 = 116,000 miles/second

2-14. What is the speed of light in meters/second for a material of index 1.60? Round the answer to two decimal places, three significant digits.
Speed = $3 \times 10^8/1.60 = 1.88 \times 10^8$ m/second

Example 2-14, Option 1	**Example 2-14, Option 2**
Type A Calculator:	**Type A Calculator:**
3 EXP 8 ÷ 1.60 = The calculator should say 187,500,000, which is 1.88×10^8.	3 ÷ 1.60 = The calculator should say 1.875, to which you append $\times 10^8$.
Type B Calculator:	**Type B Calculator:**
3 EXP 8 ÷ 1.60 = The calculator should say 187,500,000, which is 1.88×10^8.	3 ÷ 1.60 = The calculator should say 1.875, to which you append $\times 10^8$.

2-15. What is the index of refraction of a material that slows yellow light to a speed of 76,500 miles/second? (This is in the range of a diamond and is close to an upper limit for the index of refraction.) Round to three significant digits.
Index = 186,000/76,500 = 2.43

2-16. What is the index of a material that slows yellow light to a speed of 2.26×10^8 meters/second?
Index = $3 \times 10^8/2.26 \times 10^8 = 1.33$
The $\times 10^8$ is in both the numerator and the denominator of the fraction, and therefore it cancels.

EXERCISES:

In the following exercises all numbers use three significant digits and therefore the answers should be rounded to three significant digits.

15. If yellow light has a speed of 118,000 miles/second in a transparent material, what is the index of refraction of that material? What is the speed in this material in meters/second?

16. What is the refractive index of a material if the speed of yellow light passing through it is 109,000 miles/second? What is the speed in this material in meters/second?

17. How fast will yellow light travel through a material of refractive index 1.53? Answer in both miles/second and meters/second.

18. What is the index of refraction of a material if yellow light travels at 1.81×10^8 meters/second in it? What is the speed of light in miles/second in this material?

19. How fast will yellow light travel through a material of refractive index 1.42? Answer in both meters/second and miles/second.

SNELL'S LAW

When a ray of light travels from one material, the ***incident*** material, to another material, the ***refracting*** material, the direction of the ray will be changed according to Snell's Law:

$$n_i(\sin \angle i) = n_r(\sin \angle r)$$

where:
n_i = the index of refraction of the incident material
n_r = the index of refraction of the refracting material
$\angle i$ = the angle that the incident light ray makes with the normal (perpendicular) to the surface
$\angle r$ = the angle that the refracted light ray makes with the normal (perpendicular) to the surface
Which side is the incident side and which side is the refracting side depends on whether the ray is entering the slower material or the faster material. Notice again that the larger angle is on the fast side—LAFS: Large Angle, Fast Side.

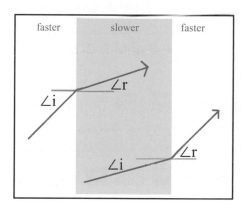

EXAMPLES:

2-17. If a ray of light travels from air into crown glass with an angle of incidence of 30 degrees, what will the angle of refraction be? What is the angle of deviation?

$n_i = 1$ $n_i \sin \angle i = n_r \sin \angle r$
$n_r = 1.523$ $(1) (\sin 30) = (1.523) (\sin r)$
$\angle i = 30$ $0.5 = (1.523) (\sin r)$
$\angle r = ?$ $\sin r = (0.5)/(1.523)$
$\angle d = ?$ $\sin r = 0.32830$
            $\angle r$ = 19 degrees
            $\angle d$ = i − r = 30 − 19 = 11 degrees

Example 2-17

Type A Calculator:

1* $\boxed{\times}$ 30 $\boxed{\text{sin}}$ $\boxed{\div}$ 1.523 $\boxed{=}$ $\boxed{\text{sin}^{\text{-1}}}$ The calculator should say 19.165.., which rounds to 19.

Type B Calculator:

1* $\boxed{\times}$ $\boxed{\text{sin}}$ 30 $\boxed{\div}$ 1.523 $\boxed{=}$ $\boxed{\text{sin}^{\text{-1}}}$ $\boxed{=}$ The calculator should say 19.165.., which rounds to 19.

---

*It is not necessary to punch in multiplication by 1. It is shown here in case there is a problem in which neither of the materials is air.

2-18. If a ray of light travels from crown glass into air with an angle of incidence of 30 degrees, what will the angle of refraction be? What is the angle of deviation?

$n_i = 1.523$	$n_i \sin \angle i = n_r \sin \angle r$
$n_r = 1$	$(1.523)(\sin 30) = (1)(\sin r)$
$\angle i = 30$	$(1.523)(0.5) = \sin r$
$\angle r = ?$	$\sin r = 0.7615$
$\angle d = ?$	$\angle r = \textbf{50 degrees}$
	$\angle d = i - r = 30 - 50 = \textbf{-20 degrees}$

Note: Because the ray is going from a more dense material to a less dense material, the angle of refraction is greater than the angle of incidence and the deviation is negative. (Look at the lower right side of the diagram on p. 29.)

Example 2-18

Type A Calculator:

1.523 $\boxed{\times}$ 30 $\boxed{\text{sin}}$ $\boxed{\div}$ 1* $\boxed{=}$ $\boxed{\text{sin}^{\text{-1}}}$ The calculator should say 49.5966.., which rounds to 50.

Type B Calculator:

1.523 $\boxed{\times}$ $\boxed{\text{sin}}$ 30 $\boxed{\div}$ 1* $\boxed{=}$ $\boxed{\text{sin}^{\text{-1}}}$ $\boxed{=}$ The calculator should say 49.5966.., which rounds to 50.

---

*It is not necessary to punch in division by 1. It is shown here in case there is a problem in which neither of the materials is air.

2-19. If a ray of light travels from an unknown material into air with an angle of refraction of 20 degrees and an angle of incidence of 13 degrees, what is the index of the material?

$n_i = ?$	$n_i \sin \angle i = n_r \sin \angle r$
$n_r = 1$	$(n_i)(\sin 13) = (1)(\sin 20)$
$\angle i = 13$	$(n_i)(0.22495) = 0.34202$
$\angle r = 20$	$n_i = (0.34202)/(0.22495)$
	$n_i = \textbf{1.52}$

Optical Formulas Tutorial

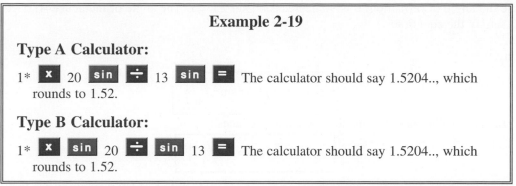

Example 2-19

Type A Calculator:

1* **x** 20 **sin** **÷** 13 **sin** **=** The calculator should say 1.5204.., which rounds to 1.52.

Type B Calculator:

1* **x** **sin** 20 **÷** **sin** 13 **=** The calculator should say 1.5204.., which rounds to 1.52.

*It is not necessary to punch in multiplication by 1. It is shown here in case there is a problem in which neither of the materials is air.

EXERCISES: (Round angles to whole angles, and round indices to two decimal places.)

20. If a ray of light travels from crown glass (n = 1.523) into air with an angle of incidence of 35 degrees, what is the angle of refraction?

21. If a ray of light travels from air into CR-39 (n = 1.498) with an angle of incidence of 28 degrees, what is the angle of refraction?

22. If a ray of light travels from CR-39 (n = 1.498) into air and emerges into the air with an angle of 45 degrees, what was the angle of incidence?

23. A ray of light travels from plate glass (n = 1.523) into water (n = 1.33). The angle of incidence is 15 degrees. What is the angle of refraction?

24. A researcher uses a light box to shine a thin line of light into a piece of unknown retracting material. The material is placed so that the light enters the unknown material at an angle of 45 degrees. If the angle of refraction is traced and measured to be 26 degrees, what is the index of refraction of the material? Round the index to two decimal places (three significant digits).

CRITICAL ANGLE

When light travels from a more dense material to a less dense material at just the right oblique angle, it is possible for the ray to emerge parallel to the surface of the refracting material.

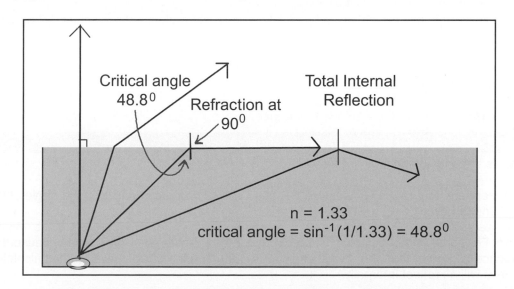

Critical angle 48.8^0

Refraction at 90^0

Total Internal Reflection

n = 1.33
critical angle = $\sin^{-1}(1/1.33) = 48.8^0$

In such a case the angle of refraction, r, is 90 degrees and sin $\angle r = 1$. The angle of incidence (i) necessary for this to occur will satisfy the equation:

$n_i \sin i = n_r$

$\sin i = n_r/n_i$

$$\text{critical angle} = \sin^{-1}\left(\frac{n_r}{n_i}\right)$$

When the ray is traveling into air, the above equation reduces to

$$\text{critical angle} = \sin^{-1}\left(\frac{1}{n}\right)$$

The angle that satisfies the equation is the **critical angle** of the **material of index n in air.** A ray that is incident at an angle greater than the critical angle will be reflected back into the incident material, or will be reflected internally. This is **total internal reflection.**

EXAMPLES:

2-20. What is the critical angle in air of water (n = 1.33)?

$\sin^{-1}(1/n) = \sin^{-1}(1/1.33)$

$\qquad = \sin^{-1} 0.75188$

$\qquad = 48.8 \text{ degrees}$

This means that if a beam of light traveling from water to air is at an angle to the surface that is greater than 49 degrees, the beam is reflected back into the water.

Example 2-20

Type A Calculator:

1 $\div$ 1.33 $=$ sin⁻¹ The calculator should say 48.75. . ., which rounds to 49.

Type B Calculator:

sin⁻¹ (1 $\div$ 1.33) $=$ The calculator should say 48.75. . ., which rounds to 49.

2-21. What is the critical angle in air of a diamond with n = 2.42?

$\sin^{-1}(1/n) = \sin^{-1}(1/2.42)$

$\qquad = \sin^{-1} 0.4132 = 24.4 \text{ degrees}$

A ray attempting to leave a diamond, n = 2.42, will reflect back into the diamond if the angle of incidence is greater than 24.4 degrees.

2-22. What is the critical angle of CR-39 in air?

$\sin^{-1}(1/n) = \sin^{-1}(1/1.498)$

$\qquad = \sin^{-1} 0.66756 = 41.9 \text{ degrees}$

$\sin i = 1/n = 1/1.498 = 0.66756; \ i = 41.9 \text{ degrees}$

EXERCISES: (Round angles to whole angles.)

25. What is the critical angle of flint glass in air? (n = 1.70)

26. What happens to a ray of light leaving CR-39 (n = 1.498) and entering air if the angle of incidence is: (Use Snell's Law.)
    a. 15 degrees?   b. 25 degrees?   c. 35 degrees?   d. 45 degrees?   e. 55 degrees?
    (**Note:** For some of the calculations the calculator will indicate an error. This is because the angle of incidence is greater than the critical angle for CR-39, and the error shown on the calculator indicates that the rays will all reflect internally.)

27. What is the critical angle of a diamond (n = 2.42) when it is immersed in water? (*Hint:* Use the first of the critical angle formulas.)

APPARENT DEPTH

When an observer (in air) is looking at an object that is not in air, the object appears to be displaced from its actual position. If a coin is placed at the bottom of a bowl of water, the coin appears to be closer than it actually is. To a fish swimming in a pond, a bug flying in the air above the water will look farther away than it is.

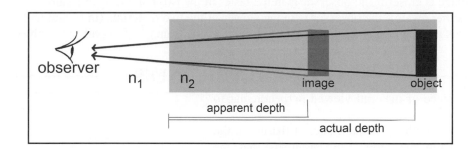

The approximate formula for the apparent depth of an object (the coin or the bug in the examples) is:

$$\text{Apparent depth} = \frac{n_1}{n_2} \text{ Actual depth}$$

where:
n_1 = index of the material the "observer" is in
n_2 = index of the material the object is in
(See diagram above.)

$$\text{Actual depth} = \frac{n_2}{n_1} \text{ Apparent depth}$$

EXAMPLES:

2-23. A fish is 55 cm (about 22 inches) away from the side of an aquarium. The observer is in air; the index of the water in the tank is 1.33. What is the apparent distance of the object from the side of the tank?
Apparent depth = (n_1/n_2) (actual depth)
$= (1/1.33)$ (55 cm)
$= 41.35 \ldots$
= 42 cm
Since there are two significant digits in 55 cm, the answer rounds to 42 cm.

2-24. A scuba diver looks up at a person watching over the side of a boat. The observer's face is 11 feet above the surface of the water. How far above the surface does the observer's face appear to be to the scuba diver?
Apparent depth = (n_1/n_2) (actual depth)
$= (1.33/1)$ (11 ft)[4]
$= 14.63$
= 15 ft
Since there are two significant digits in 11 ft, the answer rounds to 15 ft.

---

[4]It is not necessary to punch in division by 1. It is shown here in case there is a problem in which neither of the materials is air.

2-25. The bottom of a pool appears to be 6 feet below the surface of the water. How deep is the pool at that point? Use n = 1.33 for the index of the water in the pool.

Actual depth = (n^2/n^1) (apparent depth)

$\qquad$ = (1.33/1) (6 ft)[5]

$\qquad$ = 7.98

$\qquad$ **= 8 ft**

Why is the actual depth greater than the apparent depth?

Note that the image is closer if the observer is in the faster of the two materials (in Examples 2-23 and 2-25, air) and the image is farther away if the observer is in the slower of the two materials (in Example 2-24, water).

Also note that this is an approximation and assumes that the line from the observer to the object is perpendicular to the surface.

APPARENT THICKNESS

The thickness of a piece of material viewed perpendicular to one surface of the material is related to the apparent depth. Here the object is the "bottom" of the material (based on the observer viewing from the "top") and assumes that the observer is in air.

$$\text{apparent thickness} = \frac{\text{actual thickness}}{\text{n of the material}}$$

If an object is observed through several different media, the apparent depth is the sum of the apparent thickness of each layer.

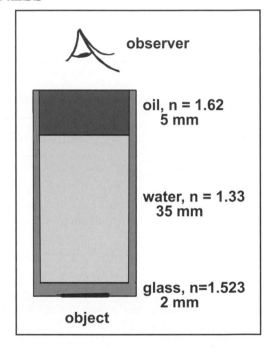

EXAMPLE:

2-26. If an object is under a glass containing a 5-mm layer of oil (n = 1.62) over 35 mm of water (n = 1.33), and if the thickness of the glass (n = 1.523) at the bottom of the container is 2 mm, the apparent depth of the object is the apparent thickness of oil + apparent thickness of water + apparent thickness of glass.

Apparent thickness = (5/1.62) + (35/1.33) + (2/1.523)

$\qquad$ = 3.09 + 23.32 + 1.31

$\qquad$ = 27.72

$\qquad$ = 28 mm

EXERCISES:

28. An object is imbedded in a 6-inch polycarbonate cube, n = 1.586. If the object is at the center of the cube, how far from each side does it appear to be?

29. A fish looks up at an insect flying above the water. If the insect is 8 inches above the water directly above the fish, how far above the water does the insect appear to be to the fish?

---

[5]It is not necessary to punch in division by 1. It is shown here in case there is a problem in which neither of the materials is air.

30. A small specimen is pressed under a glass slide (n = 1.523) that is 1 mm thick. The slide is in a carrier that has a 3.5 mm layer of oil, n = 1.62. How far from the top of the oil layer does the specimen appear to be?

LATERAL DISPLACEMENT

The angle of refraction and the angle of deviation can be used to determine how much a ray will be displaced when it goes through a material with flat parallel sides. The diagram below shows the relationship between the angles $\angle i$, $\angle r$, and $\angle d$, as described in the section on the Laws of Refraction, p. 26.

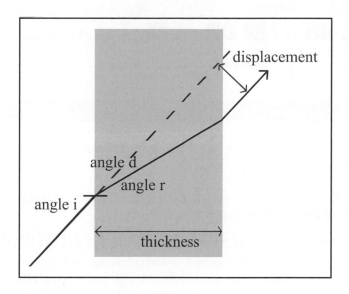

The amount that the ray is displaced depends on the angle at which the ray meets the interface with the new material and the thickness of the material. The formula for the lateral displacement of the ray is

$$\text{displacement} = \text{thickness} \left(\frac{\sin \angle d}{\cos \angle r} \right)$$

EXAMPLE:

2-27. A ray travels through a pane of glass, n = 1.523, that is 5.5 mm thick and has flat, parallel sides. The ray has an angle of incidence to the surface of 45. How much will the ray be displaced from its original position when it exits the pane of glass?

a. First we need to use Snell's Law on p. 29 to find the angle of refraction. Verify for yourself that the angle of refraction will be 27.7 degrees.

b. According to the angle formula on p. 26, the angle of deviation is 17.3.

c. Using the formula
displacement = (thickness)(sin $\angle d$)/(cos $\angle r$),
displacement = (5.5 mm)(sin 17.3)/(cos 27.7)
= (5.5)(0.2974)/(0.8854)
= 1.8 mm

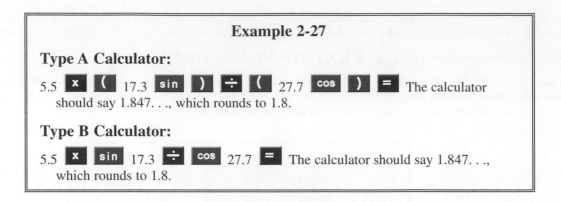

Example 2-27

Type A Calculator:

5.5 | x | | (| 17.3 | sin | |) | | ÷ | | (| 27.7 | cos | |) | | = | The calculator
should say 1.847. . ., which rounds to 1.8.

Type B Calculator:

5.5 | x | | sin | 17.3 | ÷ | | cos | 27.7 | = | The calculator should say 1.847. . .,
which rounds to 1.8.

EXERCISES:

31. A ray passes through a pane of lead glass with an angle of incidence of 36 degrees. The pane of glass is 10.5 mm thick. How much is the ray displaced from its original path? The glass has an index of refraction of 1.70.

32. How much will a ray be displaced when traveling through a tank of water that is 18 inches deep, if the angle of incidence of the ray is 50 degrees?

—————— DISPERSION AND ABBÉ NUMBER ——————

Visible light travels at about 186,000 miles/second in a vacuum. So do X rays, radio waves, and everything else in the electromagnetic spectrum. When a ray or wave enters any material traveling from a vacuum, it slows down. Different waves, however, will be slowed different amounts. An X ray will not travel at the same speed in crown glass, for example, as a ray from the infrared spectrum.

The same is true of the different wavelengths in the visible spectrum. Red waves of wavelength 660 nm will travel at a different speed in crown glass than blue waves of wavelength 460 nm. In the United States the index of refraction of a refracting material is measured for a particular yellow wavelength of 588 nm. The index of refraction for any particular material actually varies, however, depending on the wavelength of the light ray.

Shorter waves are slowed more than longer waves for all of our glasses lens materials. When white light (made up of all colors) passes through a lens, the blue waves slow more and therefore are refracted more than the red waves, and the light is broken down into its component colors. This is *dispersion*. Dispersion causes *chromatic aberrations.* The image formed by the blue rays is a different distance from the lens and has a different size than the image formed by the red rays, resulting in fringes of color around the images seen through the lens. In the eyecare professions the ability of a material to break white light into its component colors is measured by use of the *Abbé number* of the material. To compute the Abbé number, we need to know the index of refraction for several different wavelengths. The standard in the United States is to use $\lambda = 588$ nm for yellow, $\lambda = 486$ for blue, and $\lambda = 656$ for red.

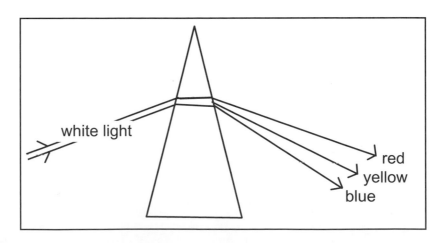

white light

red
yellow
blue

The greater the spread from red to blue, the higher the dispersive value of the material and the lower the Abbé value of the material.

The formula for the Abbé number is

$$\frac{n_{yellow} - 1}{n_{blue} - n_{red}}$$

The Abbé number is also called the **V-value,** the **nu value**, or the **constringence**. The Abbé number is the inverse of the **dispersive value** of the material.

EXAMPLE:

2-28. For a particular crown glass material $n_{yellow} = 1.5230$, $n_{blue} = 1.5293$, and $n_{red} = 1.5204$.[6] The Abbé number for this glass is

$$\frac{1.523 - 1}{1.5293 - 1.5204} = \frac{0.5230}{0.0089} = 583.76 = 59$$

In this case the index for red and the index for blue are relatively close together, so the denominator is relatively small and the Abbé number is relatively large. The higher the Abbé number, the lower the dispersive value for the material and the less the chromatic aberration of the lens.

ABBÉ NUMBERS FOR SOME COMMON OPHTHALMIC MATERIALS

Crown glass	59-61
CR-39	56-58
Barium crown	Low 50s
Trivex*	43-45
Flint	Low 30s
Polycarbonate	29-31

*Trivex is registered to PPG Industries. Technical information is from http://corporate.ppg.com/PPG/opticalprod/en/monomers/products/Properties.htm.

EXERCISE:

33. For a particular flint glass, $n_{yellow} = 1.7200$, $n_{blue} = 1.7378$, and $n_{red} = 1.7130$.[6] What is the Abbé number of the material? (Round to the nearest whole number.) What is the index of refraction of the material? **Note:** The denominator of this fraction is relatively large compared with the denominator of the Abbé value for crown glass. Because the indexes for red and blue are much further apart in this flint glass, the chromatic aberration for this material is much greater than for crown glass and the Abbé value for the material is smaller than the value for crown glass.

---

[6]The values for n are taken from Meyer-Arendt HR: *Introduction to Classical and Modern Optics,* ed 4, Englewood Cliffs, NJ, 1995, Prentice-Hall.

The questions preceded by an asterisk (*) are advanced questions. They are not likely to be on the ABO exam but might be on the ABOM exam or the COT exam.

The questions are not presented in the order of the subjects in the section. Some of the questions may require interpretation of the material in the section.

1. Lens one has an index of refraction of 1.498. Lens two has an index of refraction of 1.586. Which of the following is a true statement?
   a. The speed of light in lens one is the same as in lens two because the speed of light is constant.
   b. The speed of light is greater in lens one.
   c. The speed of light is greater in lens two.
   d. The speed of light remains the same in both lenses, but the ray is bent more in lens one.

2. Because of total internal reflection, when an optical fiber is bent, the light that entered the end of the fiber
   a. scatters but follows the curve of the optical fiber.
   b. bends evenly with the curve of the optical fiber.
   c. reflects internally in a series of straight line paths.
   d. tends to speed up, since it is in a vacuum.

3. A ray that passes obliquely through a pane of glass that has flat parallel sides will be
   a. displaced but not deviated.
   b. deviated but not displaced.
   c. both displaced and deviated.
   d. neither deviated nor displaced.

4. What is the speed of a ray of light when it travels through a material that has an index of refraction of 1.33?
   a. 147,000 meters per second
   b. 147,000 miles per second
   c. 140,000 meters per second
   d. 140,000 miles per second

5. What color light is transmitted by a piece of red CR-39 material?
   a. red
   b. green
   c. blue
   d. violet

6. When rays travel from the source,
   a. the rays near the source are parallel.
   b. the rays near the source diverge.
   c. the rays near the source converge.
   d. the rays near the source show no vergence.

7. The "normal" to a surface is
   a. an imaginary line that is parallel to the surface.
   b. an imaginary line that represents the path of the ray in the refracting material.
   c. an imaginary line that is perpendicular to the surface.
   d. an attribute of manufactured materials.

8. A _____ of light is a group of rays divergent from a single point on a light source.
   a. photon
   b. ray
   c. pencil
   d. beam

9. The angle of incidence
   a. is less than the angle of reflection.
   b. is greater than the angle of reflection.
   c. is equal to the angle of reflection.
   d. may be less than, greater than, or equal to the angle of reflection.

10. When light passes obliquely from one material to another, which of the following changes?
    a. speed
    b. direction
    c. wavelength
    d. all of the above

11. Which of the following electromagnetic waves are arranged in order of decreasing wave length?
    a. radar, infrared, X rays, visible, cosmic rays
    b. radio waves, infrared, visible, ultraviolet
    c. X rays, ultraviolet, visible, infrared, radar
    d. radio, ultraviolet, visible, infrared, X rays

12. When a light ray travels from air to glass at an angle greater than the critical angle,
    a. most of the light will be reflected but part will be refracted.
    b. most of the light will refract but part will be reflected.
    c. total reflection will occur.
    d. total transmission will occur.

13. Rays of light originating from a distance greater than 6 meters are considered to be
    a. a beam.
    b. diverging.
    c. converging.
    d. parallel.

14. Parallel light rays reflected from a flat smooth mirror will be
    a. diffused.
    b. parallel.
    c. diverging.
    d. converging.

15. "Visible light" is in the range of wavelengths approximately between
    a. 400 and 600 nm.
    b. 200 and 700 nm.
    c. 380 and 760 nm.
    d. 200 and 380 nm.

16. A perfectly black surface
    a. absorbs all light.
    b. reflects all light.
    c. absorbs black light.
    d. reflects black light.

17. From which of the following materials should you expect the greatest amount of chromatic aberration?
    a. Crown glass (Abbé = 59)
    b. Trivex* (Abbé = 44)
    c. Polycarbonate (Abbé = 31)
    d. Flint (Abbé = 35)

18. When a beam of light emerges from water into air, the speed of the light
    a. increases.
    b. remains the same.
    c. decreases.
    d. will vary with the density of the water.

19. The optical index of a transparent medium is a ratio of the speed of light in a vacuum to
    a. the speed of light in air.
    b. the index of refraction of the medium.
    c. the speed of light leaving the medium.
    d. the speed of light after refraction into the medium.

20. What is the speed of light in crown glass?
    a. 122,000 miles per second
    b. 125,000 miles per second
    c. 186,000 miles per second
    d. 100,000 miles per second

21. You decide to install solar collectors on your roof to help heat your home. If you want to maximize energy absorption, which of the following colors should the collectors be?
    a. white
    b. green
    c. blue
    d. black

22. When a ray of light travels from an optically dense material to an optically rare material at a small oblique angle,
    a. it bends toward the normal to the surface.
    b. it bends away from the normal to the surface.
    c. total internal reflection will occur.
    d. it travels undeviated from its original course.

23. Visible light, going from high frequency to low frequency, is
    a. red, orange, yellow, green, blue, violet.
    b. red, violet, blue, green, yellow, orange.
    c. violet, blue, green, yellow, orange, red.
    d. yellow, green, blue, violet, red, orange.

24. Which of the following best explains the change that occurs when light reflects from a surface?
    a. There is a change in speed.
    b. There is a change in wavelength.
    c. There is a change in frequency.
    d. None of these changes occur.

25. Which of the following is considered the smallest amount of light possible?
    a. photon
    b. ray
    c. pencil
    d. beam

26. The sun is located 93,000,000 miles from the earth. The length of time required for light to travel that distance is approximately
    a. 50 minutes.
    b. 2 minutes.
    c. 8 minutes.
    d. 8 hours.

27. To a scuba diver, a bird flying over the water will appear to be
    a. closer than it actually is.
    b. farther away than it actually is.
    c. in its actual position.
    d. diving.

28. What is the index of refraction for a medium if the speed of light through it is measured to be 1.6×10^8 meters/second?
    a. 1.498
    b. 1.523
    c. 1.66
    d. 1.88

29. When a light ray travels from glass to air at an angle greater than the critical angle,
    a. most of the light will be reflected but part will be refracted.
    b. most of the light will refract but part will be reflected.
    c. total reflection will occur.
    d. total transmission will occur.

30. A _____ of light is composed of all of the light originating from all the points on a light source.
    a. photon
    b. ray
    c. pencil
    d. beam

*Trivex is registered to PPG Industries. Technical information is from http://corporate.ppg.com/PPG/opticalprod/en/monomers/products/Properties.htm.

31. What is the speed of light in CR-39?
    a. 2.00×10^8 meters/second
    b. 2.00×10^{10} meters/second
    c. 3.00×10^8 meters/second
    d. 3.00×10^{10} meters/second

32. When you are looking at a person standing in a swimming pool, why do the legs appear to be shorter than they actually are?
    a. Because the light coming from the water is reflected.
    b. Because the light coming from the water is refracted.
    c. Because the light coming from the water is entering a material with lower index of refraction than air.
    d. Because the light coming from the water is demonstrating total internal reflection.

33. The reason that you see a red color when you look at a red rose is that
    a. red waves are refracted at the rose.
    b. red waves reflect from the rose and all other waves are absorbed.
    c. red waves are absorbed at the rose and all other waves are reflected.

34. A pencil of light travels 2.5 meters from its source to a screen. The vergence of the pencil of light at the screen is
    a. 6.25.
    b. 5.0.
    c. 2.5.
    d. 0.4.

35. What is the speed of light in Trivex?
    a. 1.96×10^8 meters/second
    b. 1.96×10^{10} meters/second
    c. 0.51×10^8 meters/second
    d. 0.51×10^{10} meters/second

36. A _____ is the path of a single photon of light.
    a. corpuscle
    b. ray
    c. pencil
    d. beam

37. A person is 10 feet in front of a plane (flat) mirror. The person's image is _____ behind the mirror.
    a. 5 feet
    b. 10 feet
    c. 15 feet
    d. 20 feet

38. An object imbedded in glass will appear to be
    a. closer than it actually is.
    b. farther away than it actually is.
    c. in its actual position.
    d. floating.

39. Green light passes from air to crown glass. What happens to the wavelength of the light?
    a. It remains the same.
    b. It changes direction.
    c. It decreases.
    d. It increases.

40. When is the vergence of a wavefront considered to be zero?
    a. When the wavefront encounters a material of greater index of refraction
    b. When the wavefront is parallel to the optical axis
    c. When the wavefront converges to the focal point
    d. When the distance from the source is optical infinity

41. A pencil of light falls on a screen that is 2 meters away from the source of the light. What is the vergence of the light at the screen?
    a. 2
    b. 1
    c. 0.5
    d. 0.25

42. An object is placed 1.5 feet from a plane (flat) mirror. The image formed by the mirror is _____ away from the object.
    a. 0.75 foot
    b. 1 foot
    c. 1.5 feet
    d. 3 feet

43. What is the speed of a ray of light when it travels through a material that has an index of refraction of 1.66?
    a. 112,000 miles per second
    b. 112,000 meters per second
    c. 181,000 miles per second
    d. 181,000 meters per second

44. The critical angle for a material is the angle beyond which all light within the material is
    a. refracted.
    b. reflected.
    c. refracted back into the incident material.
    d. bent toward the normal.

45. A ray passes from one material to a second material, with an angle of incidence that is larger than the angle of refraction.
    a. The ray is traveling from a "faster" material to a "slower" material.
    b. The ray will be absorbed by the material as heat.
    c. The ray is demonstrating total internal reflection.
    d. The ray is traveling from a "slower" material to a "faster" material.

46. What is the speed of light in crown glass?
    a. 1.97×10^8 meters/second
    b. 1.97×10^{10} meters/second
    c. 2.10×10^8 meters/second
    d. 2.10×10^{10} meters/second

47. When light enters air from water, the angle of refraction will be
    a. greater than the critical angle.
    b. greater than the angle of incidence.
    c. less than the angle of incidence.
    d. less than the critical angle.

48. When light travels from one material to another material,
    a. the frequency of the light changes.
    b. the wavelength of the light changes.
    c. both frequency and wavelength of the light change.
    d. only the speed of the light changes.

*49. What is luminous intensity?
    a. It is a measure of the focusing power of the source.
    b. It is a number specifying the strength of the light falling on a surface.
    c. It is a measure of the wavelength.
    d. It is the determination of the watts of light emitted from the source.

*50. If a ray of light travels from air to flint glass (n = 1.60) at an angle of 37 degrees, what is the angle of refraction into the glass?
    a. 22 degrees
    b. 25 degrees
    c. 35 degrees
    d. 41 degrees

*51. You are using a lamp that is 0.4 meter away and provides 25 lux of illumination on your workspace. What illumination will be provided if you move the lamp to 0.2 meter from the workspace?
    a. 50 lux
    b. 100 lux
    c. 250 lux
    d. 400 lux

*52. What is the critical angle for light rays passing from quartz (n = 1.54) into water (n = 1.33)?
    a. 31.3 degrees
    b. 45.0 degrees
    c. 51.4 degrees
    d. 59.7 degrees

*53. The wavelength of sodium light in air is 589 nm. What is its frequency?
    a. 1.47×10^{14} Hz
    b. 1.77×10^{14} Hz
    c. 1.96×10^{14} Hz
    d. 5.09×10^{14} Hz

*54. A fish is swimming 20 inches away from the side of an aquarium. How far inside the aquarium does the fish appear to be? The index of refraction of the water is 1.33.
    a. 15 inches
    b. 20 inches
    c. 27 inches
    d. 40 inches

*55. A pane of crown glass is 4 inches thick. A ray is incident on the pane of glass at an angle of 32 degrees. How much is the ray displaced from its incident path?
    a. 10.9 inches
    b. 2.3 inches
    c. 0.9 inch
    d. 0.4 inch

*56. A 6-inch cube of polycarbonate material (n = 1.586) will appear to be
    a. 9.5 inches thick.
    b. 7.2 inches thick.
    c. 6 inches thick.
    d. 3.8 inches thick.

*57. The wavelength of sodium light in air is 589 nm. What is its wavelength in water (n = 1.33)?
    a. 752 nm
    b. 589 nm
    c. 443 nm
    d. 227 nm

*58. A ray of light travels from water (n = 1.33) to air at an angle of 30 degrees. What is the angle of refraction?
    a. 19 degrees
    b. 22 degrees
    c. 35 degrees
    d. 42 degrees

*59. What is the critical angle for light rays passing into air from a material with n = 1.66?
    a. 37 degrees
    b. 28 degrees
    c. 22 degrees
    d. 25 degrees

*60. The vergence P of a pencil of light at a plane that is a distance of p meters from the source of the light is
    a. p^2.
    b. $1/p^2$.
    c. $1/p$.
    d. p.

SECTION III – LENSES

A *lens* is composed of a transparent material with two polished surfaces that is designed to change the direction of the incident light rays.

Parallel rays of light are said to have **no vergence** or **zero vergence**. Rays of light traveling toward each other are **converging**, or have **positive vergence**. Rays of light traveling away from each other are **diverging**, or have **negative vergence.** By convention, a distance measured in the direction of travel of the light ray will be positive, and a distance measured opposite the direction of travel of the light ray will be negative.

A lens that adds positive vergence to the incident rays is a **plus power** lens, and a lens that adds negative vergence to the incident rays is a **minus power** lens. The change in vergence caused by the lens is a result of several factors:

- Index of refraction of the lens material
- Index of refraction of the material around the lens
- Curvature of each of the two lens surfaces
- Thickness of the lens
- Surface that the light rays enter first
- Wavelength of the rays

The effect of each of these factors, except the wavelength of the rays, is considered at some point in this book. Because the different wavelengths give slightly different indices for any given refracting material, this last factor is actually taken into account when the index of refraction of the material is considered.

REFRACTION THROUGH A LENS

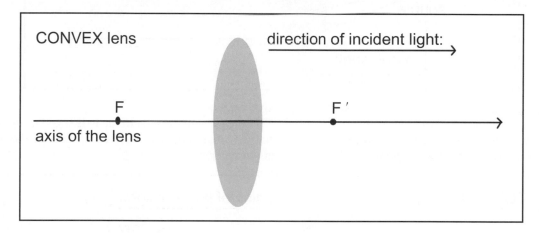

The **axis of a lens** is a ray or an imaginary line that is perpendicular to *both sides* of the lens. Because the ray is perpendicular to each side, Snell's Law tells us that it will not change direction when it enters and exits the lens. Therefore this ray travels through the lens without being deviated (no change in direction) and without being displaced (remains on the original path).

CONVEX LENS

A convex lens, also called a positive or plus power lens, adds positive vergence to the incident rays of light. The lens changes incident rays with zero vergence (parallel rays) to rays with positive vergence (converging rays).

Because the convex lens increases the vergence of the rays, it is a converging lens, has a positive focal length, and is a positive lens. The **secondary focal point** (F′) of the lens is the point where parallel incident rays cross the axis of the lens. The focal point is considered a **real** *focal point* because the rays *actually cross there*. This focal length is *positive* because the measurement is from the lens to the secondary focal point, which is in the direction of travel of the rays of light.

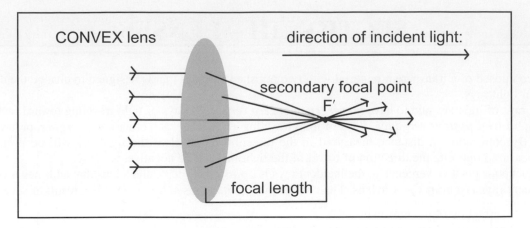

The ***primary focal point*** (F) is a point on the axis where the rays diverging from a light source would result in parallel rays when they exit from the lens.

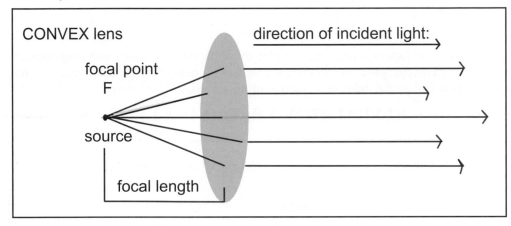

Converging incident rays will emerge with higher positive vergence.

Diverging incident rays will emerge having less negative vergence with respect to the axis (ray 1), zero vergence, or positive vergence with respect to the axis (ray 2). What the final vergence will be depends on the amount of divergence the rays have when they are incident on the lens surface.

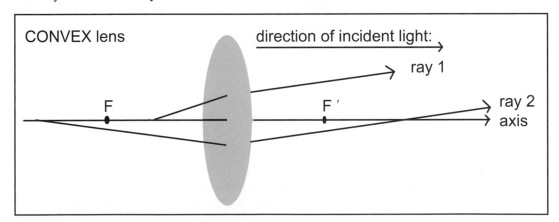

CONCAVE LENS

For the concave lens, also called a negative or minus power lens, incident rays with zero vergence are changed to rays with negative vergence; they are now diverging rays. Because this lens increases the divergence of the rays, it is a diverging lens and has a negative focal length. The ***secondary focal point*** (F′) of the lens is the point from which the rays would have emerged to have the observed amount of divergence. The focal point is considered a ***virtual*** *focal point* because the rays *did not actually emerge from there*. This focal length is **negative** because the measurement from the lens to the secondary focal point is to the left, or opposite the direction of travel for the ray.

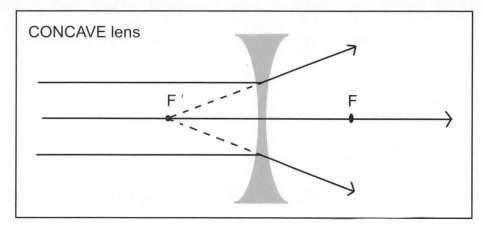

Rays that are converging toward the primary focal point (F) will emerge from the lens parallel to the axis. The primary focal length is measured from the primary focal point to the lens.

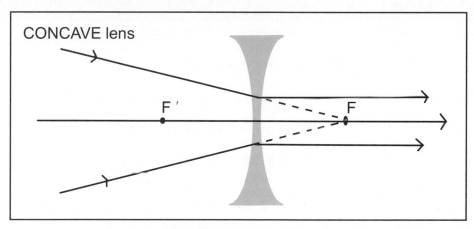

If the incident rays are already diverging, they will emerge with higher negative vergence. If the incident rays have positive vergence, they will emerge with either less positive vergence, zero vergence, or negative vergence.

—— FOCAL LENGTH FORMULA ——

The unit of measurement of the refractive power of a lens or a surface is the ***diopter***. The diopter was introduced by a French ophthalmologist, Monoyer, in 1872. The capital letter D stands for diopter in our optical formulas. When the lens is in air, the power of the lens in diopters is equal to the reciprocal of the focal length of the lens in meters.

$$D = \frac{1}{f_{meters}} = \frac{100}{f_{cm}} = \frac{1000}{f_{mm}} = \frac{39.37}{f_{inches}} \approx \frac{40}{f_{inches}}$$

where:
D = the power of the lens in diopters
f = the focal length of the lens in meters, centimeters, millimeters, or inches

EXAMPLES:

3-1. What is the dioptric power of a lens that has a focal length of +0.5 m?
D = 1/f = 1/0.5 = +2.00D

3-2. What is the dioptric power of a lens that brings parallel rays of light to a point focus 16 inches from the lens?
D = 39.37/f = 39.37/16 = +2.460D

Note: The conversion from meters to inches is 1 meter = 39.37 inches. Many people round this to 1 meter = 40 inches. This rounding is frequently acceptable. In this case the formula becomes D = 40/f, where f is in inches. When this approximation is used, the answer to Example 3-2 will be D = 40/16 = +2.50D.

When the lens power is known and the focal length is needed, the formula above can be converted to:

$$f_{meters} = \frac{1}{D} \quad \text{or} \quad f_{inches} = \frac{39.37}{D} \approx \frac{40}{D}$$

When a lens is in a material other than air, the formula becomes

$$D = \frac{n}{f_{meters}} \quad \text{or} \quad f_{meters} = \frac{n}{D} \quad \text{or} \quad f_{inches} = \frac{39.37n}{D}$$

where n = the index of the material surrounding the lens

EXAMPLE:

3-3. A lens has a focal length of 20 cm when it is in water. What is the dioptric power of the lens in water? (Index of water = 1.33.)

D = 1.33/0.20 = +6.65D

EXERCISES:

1. What is the dioptric power of a lens that has a focal length of +5 cm?

2. What is the focal length in inches of a lens of power +4.00D?

3. What is the focal length in meters, centimeters, millimeters, and inches of a –5.00D lens?

4. The eye contains a plus lens that is able to change shape. When the eye is at rest, the lens has an approximate power of +20D (in air). When the lens accommodates, the shape of the lens changes, adding plus power. If the eye at rest focuses at infinity, and if it can accommodate to focus on this page, which is probably about 40 cm away, the lens must add enough plus power to bring the focus from infinity to 40 cm. How much plus power must the crystalline lens inside the eye globe *add* to accommodate for reading?

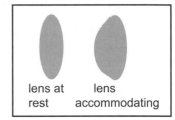

lens at   lens
rest   accommodating

5. A young child can focus from infinity to 10 cm away. How much plus power must this child's crystalline lens be able to add during accommodation for the distance of 10 cm?

6. A lens has a focal length of 8 inches. What is its dioptric power?

DIOPTERS

In practice, diopters are expressed in increments of one eighth of a diopter. All eighths are truncated to two decimal places. For example, one eighth is 0.125, but this is truncated (changed) to 0.12.

STANDARD DIOPTRIC INCREMENTS

0.12D (This is really 0.125, with the 5 truncated.)
0.25D
0.37D (This is really 0.375, with the 5 truncated.)
0.50D
0.62D (This is really 0.625, with the 5 truncated.)
0.75D
0.87D (This is really 0.875, with the 5 truncated.)
0.00D

A lens or surface will also have a sign to show whether it is a converging (+) or a diverging (–) lens or surface.

In the exercises in this book, if we are referring to a lens that might actually be ordered or made, we will change the dioptric values to one of these decimal increments. In many calculations the end result will be an effective power, and then we will not change the answer to eighths because the result of the exercise would not necessarily be a lens that a person would wear.

LENS SURFACES

Three types of surface are used in lens design. These are *plano*, *convex*, and *concave*.

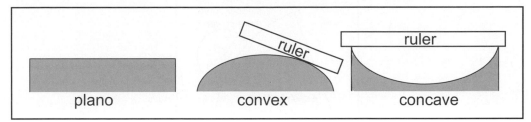

PLANO SURFACE

- The surface is flat.
- The surface does not change the vergence of incident light.
- The surface has zero power.
- The surface has an infinitely large radius of curvature.
- Abbreviate as pl.

CONVEX SURFACE

- The surface bulges.
- A flat edge placed on the surface will rock, since it touches at only one point.
- The surface increases the vergence of incident light. It converges parallel incident light rays.
- The surface has plus power.
- Abbreviate as CX.

CONCAVE SURFACE

- The surface is hollow.
- A flat edge placed on the surface will not rock, since it touches at two places.
- The surface decreases the vergence of incident light. It diverges parallel incident light rays.
- The surface has minus power.
- Abbreviate as CC.

LENS TYPES

Lens surfaces can be combined in different ways to give different lens types. Lenses are classified as either *flat* or *bent*. They are also classified by their surface combinations.

A *bent* lens is a lens that has one convex surface and one concave surface.

A *flat* lens is a lens that is not bent. It can have one flat surface combined with either one concave or one convex surface. It can have two concave surfaces, or it can have two convex surfaces. All of these lenses are examples of flat lens designs. If a lens does not have one convex surface and one concave surface, it is a flat design.

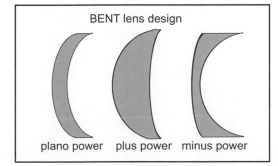

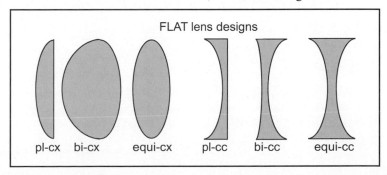

RADIUS OF CURVATURE

A surface must be curved for it to alter the vergence of the light striking it. A surface with a long radius of curvature will be a relatively flat surface, so the change in vergence will be small. A surface with a short radius of curvature will have a relatively steep surface, so the change in vergence will be large.

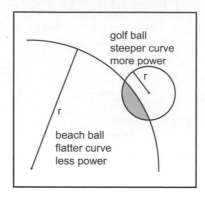

The amount of vergence change caused by a lens surface also depends on the refractive index of the material from which it is made. The dioptric power of a lens surface can be determined by use of the surface power formula.

SURFACE POWER FORMULA

$$D = \frac{n_r - n_i}{r}$$

where:
D = the power of the surface in diopters
n_r = the refractive index of the refracting side of the surface
n_i = the refractive index of the incident side of the surface
r = the radius of curvature of the surface in meters

For our purposes air is usually on one side of the surface. Air has a refractive index of 1. Therefore the formula is more often written as:

$$D = \frac{n_r - 1}{r}$$

We will ignore whether the light is entering or leaving the lens when it is refracted by this surface. Using 1 – n for the numerator when the light leaves a lens surface (traveling back into air) changes the sign of the resulting surface power and requires that we discuss the sign of r. We will leave the discussion of the sign of r until Section VII. For now we will determine the sign of the surface power from the description of the lens or the lens surface.

EXAMPLE:

3-4. What is the dioptric power of a crown glass (n = 1.523) surface with a radius of curvature of 35 cm?
(*Note:* The radius in the formula is in meters, so 35 cm = 0.35 m.)
D = (1/523 – 1)/(0.35) = 1.49D

Example 3-4

Type A Calculator:

(1.523 – 1) * ÷ 0.35 = The calculator should say 1.49.

Type B Calculator:

(1.523 – 1) * ÷ 0.35 = The calculator should say 1.49.

---

*You may do 1.523 – 1 = 0.523 in your head and just punch in the 0.523. In this case you do not need the (and) keys.

The surface power formula can be rearranged to find the radius of curvature of a surface:

$$r = \frac{n-1}{D}$$

EXAMPLE:

3-5. What is the radius of curvature in millimeters of a +5.00D surface made of crown glass (n = 1.523)?
D = +5.00D
n = 1.523   r = (1.523 – 1)/(5) = 0.1046 m = 104.6 mm

EXERCISES: (Round diopter answers to two decimal places and the radius to whole millimeters.)

7. What is the power of a convex surface made from CR-39 (n = 1.498) if the radius of curvature is 5 cm?

8. What is the power of a concave surface made from Trivex[1] (n = 1.53) if the radius of curvature is 0.33 meter?

9. A surface is to be created from polycarbonate (n = 1.586) with a power of +3.75D. What is the radius of curvature of the tool used to finish the surface?

10. A tool used to create a concave lens surface has a radius of curvature of 25 mm.
    a. What power will the surface have if it is made from crown glass, n = 1.523?
    b. What power will the surface have if it is made from a high-index glass with an index of 1.70?
    c. A pad with a thickness of 2 mm is placed on the tool before the surface is completed, changing the radius of curvature of the tool to 27 mm. Now what power will each of the surfaces in a and b have?

11. The back (or concave) surface of a contact lens has a radius of curvature of 7.72 mm. If the material of the contact lens has an index of refraction of 1.47, what is the dioptric power of the surface of the lens?

12. A contact lens modification tool is used to flatten the surface of the contact lens in Exercise 11.
    a. Will flattening the surface make the radius longer or shorter? Which of the following would be flatter: 7.76 mm or 7.68 mm?
    b. What is the new surface power of the contact lens using the choice in part a?

---

[1]Trivex is a trademark of PPG. Technical information is from http://corporate.ppg.com/PPG/opticalprod/en/monomers/products/Properties.htm.

NOMINAL POWER FORMULA

The nominal power of a lens is the combined power of its front and back surfaces. We normally refer to the convex surface on a bent (or *meniscus*) lens as the front surface. The nominal power formula disregards the thickness of the lens and is sometimes referred to as the ***thin lens formula.***

$$D_N = D_1 + D_2$$

or

$$D_1 = D_N - D_2$$

or

$$D_2 = D_N - D_1$$

where:
D_N is the nominal power of the lens in diopters
D_1 is the front surface power in diopters
D_2 is the back surface power in diopters

Since this formula disregards the thickness of the lens, it gives an approximate power. This approximation formula loses accuracy for powers over +4.00. The formula also loses accuracy for lenses that are ground thicker than normal.

EXAMPLES:

3-6. If the front surface power is +6.00D and the back surface power is –10.00D, the lens has a nominal power of +6.00 + (–10.00) = –4.00D.
Note: Historically, a bent lens with a front surface power of +6.00D or a back surface power of –6.00D was called a *meniscus* lens. Now we refer to *any* bent lens as a ***meniscus*** lens, and a bent lens with one surface of +/– 6.00D as a ***true meniscus*** lens or a ***Meniscus*** lens.

3-7. A lens has a front surface power of +1.00D and a back surface power of –8.25D. What is its nominal power[2]?
$D_N = D_1 + D_2 = (+1.00) + (-8.25) = -7.25D$

3-8. If a lens has a nominal power of +3.50 and a front surface of +9.25, what is its back surface power[2]?
$D_2 = D_N - D_1 = (+3.50) - (+9.25) = -5.75D$

3-9. A lens power of –3.12 is required. The back surface will be –8.75. What is the front surface power[2]?
$D_1 = D_N - D_2 = (-3.12) - (-8.75) = +5.63 = +5.62D$ when converted to one-eighth diopter steps
Note: The –3.12 is really –3.125, so the answer is really +5.625, which we convert to one-eighth diopter steps by dropping the 5.

---

[2]See Section I pp. 1-3 for addition and subtraction of signed numbers and pp. 4-6 for use of the calculator with signed numbers.

Optical Formulas Tutorial

Look at the following drawings and determine the power of each lens. Describe each lens, stating whether is *bent* or *flat,* and name the lens type, such as *bi-convex* or *equi-concave, meniscus,* and so on.

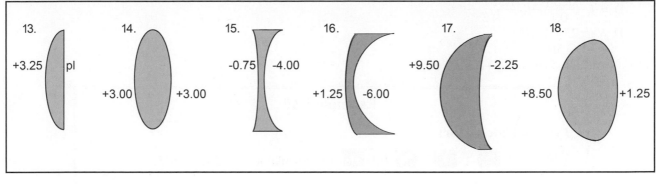

	13.	14.	15.	16.	17.	18.
Nominal power	_____	_____	_____	_____	_____	_____
Flat/bent	_____	_____	_____	_____	_____	_____
Lens type	_____	_____	_____	_____	_____	_____

19. What is the nominal power of an equi-convex lens in which both surface powers are +2.37D?

20. What is the front surface power of a +4.00D lens if it has a back surface power of −3.62D?

21. What is the back surface power of a −3.00D lens if it has a front surface power of +2.25D?

22. What is the front surface power of a +3.75D lens if it has a back surface power of −1.25D? (This lens was historically called a ***periscopic*** lens. This bent lens design had a front surface power of +1.25D for all minus lenses and a back surface power of −1.25D for all plus lenses.)

23. If I need a lens with an Rx of +3.00D and I am given a lens blank with a front surface of +9.00, what power curve would I need to create on the back of the lens?

LENSMAKER'S EQUATION

The nominal power of a lens is given by the formula $D_N = D_1 + D_2$. This formula does not take into account the lens material or its curvature. A lensmaker makes a lens by producing curves on the front and back surfaces of the lens.

$$D_N = \pm \frac{n-1}{r_1} \pm \frac{n-1}{r_2}$$

where:

D_N = the nominal power of the lens in diopters
n = the refractive index of the lens material
r_1 = the radius of curvature of the front surface in meters
r_2 = the radius of curvature of the back surface in meters

Note: For each fraction, + is used when the surface is convex and − is used when the surface is concave. This way we do not have to consider whether r is positive or negative, nor do we have to consider the order of (n − 1) and (1 − n).

EXAMPLE:

3-10. What is the power of a crown glass (n = 1.523) meniscus lens made with a front surface curve of 10 cm and an ocular or back surface curve of radius 20 cm?

D = ?

n = 1.523

r_1 = 10 cm = 0.1 m

r_2 = 2 cm = 0.2 m

$$D = +\frac{1.523 - 1}{0.1} - \frac{1.523 - 1}{0.2}$$

D = +5.23 − 2.615

  = +2.615D,

    which changes to **+2.62D**

Example 3-10

Type A Calculator:

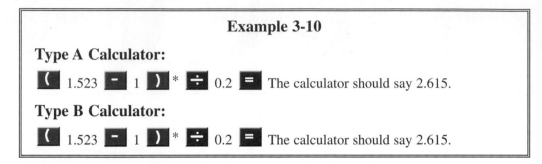

(1.523 − 1) * ÷ 0.2 = The calculator should say 2.615.

Type B Calculator:

(1.523 − 1) * ÷ 0.2 = The calculator should say 2.615.

Note: The front surface of a **meniscus** lens is convex (and therefore has plus power), and the back surface is concave (and therefore has minus power). Therefore the sign of the first fraction is + and the sign of the second fraction is −.

This sign convention would not be used in a physics text. For now we will consider the result of each surface calculation to be negative if the surface is concave and positive if the surface is convex. We will explore the signs further in Section VII when we discuss thick lenses.

EXERCISES: (Change dioptric powers to the nearest one-eighth diopter.)

24. What is the dioptric power of a crown glass (n = 1.523) bi-concave lens with radii of curvature of 247 mm and 149 mm?

25. What is the dioptric power of a meniscus CR-39 (n = 1.498) lens that has a front surface curve of radius 40 cm and a back surface curve of radius 16 cm? (Do you remember the old name for this style of lens?)

26. If a high-index lens with an index of refraction of 1.60 has a convex surface made on a tool with a radius of curvature of 8 cm and a concave surface made on a tool with a radius of curvature of 15 cm, what is the resulting power of the lens? What would the lens power have been if the material had been CR-39 (n = 1.498)?

CYLINDERS AND COMPOUND LENSES

Up to this point we have been talking about spherical surfaces. Every point on a spherical surface is an equal distance from a particular point called the center of the sphere. This distance is the radius of curvature of the surface.

Now we consider lenses made with one or more surfaces that do not have a single center of curvature. Consider what a football or a doughnut looks like. The surface of a doughnut is a **toric surface**. If a doughnut lying flat on a surface is cut horizontally, the result is circles. If the doughnut is cut vertically, the result is circles. However, the horizontal circles are different size circles from the vertical circles, so the horizontal curvature is different from the vertical curvature. When we look at the surface of the doughnut lying flat on a table, or at the football shown on p. 53, the **horizontal meridian** or direction is less curved than the **vertical meridian** or direction. If the football or doughnut is held at some other direction, the meridian of most curvature and of least curvature will have some orientation other than horizontal and vertical. If the football is standing up on one end, the flatter curve is vertical and the steeper curve is horizontal. If the doughnut is leaning sideways against its box, the flatter curve will be at some other angle but the steeper curve will still be perpendicular (at 90 degrees) to it.

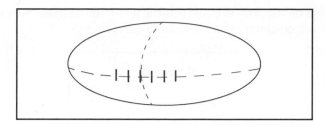

A toric surface is considered to be a spherical design, even though the surface is not a cut from a sphere, because the curve of the two major directions is a circle.

Next we consider a *cylindrical surface*. A can is a cylinder. In the diagram below, the can has straight sides horizontally and round sides vertically.

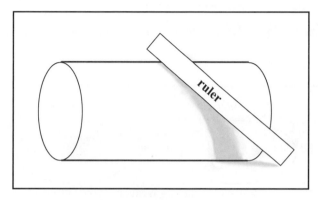

A ruler does not rock when placed, or meridian, of the surface. Therefore a cylindrical surface is one with no power in one direction and maximum power 90 degrees away. The direction having no curvature is referred to as the *axis of the cylinder*. The can shown here has a horizontal axis.

Placed in a different direction, or meridian, the ruler does rock. It rocks the most 90 degrees away from the axis of the cylinder.

A *compound lens*, or a *spherocylindrical lens,* is a lens with at least one toric surface. For glasses lenses a spherocylindrical lens has one toric surface and one spherical surface. We can think of the spherocylindrical lens as a spherical lens sandwiched with a cylindrical lens that has no power in one direction and the cylinder power in the other direction.

─────────────────── **LENS MERIDIANS** ───────────────────

Look at the diagrams of some lenses seen from the front and from the side. Each lens has a place where the lens is the thickest and a place where the lens is the thinnest. In plus lenses the thickest place is called the optical center of the lens. In a minus lens the thinnest place is called the optical center of the lens. In each case the optical center of the lens is the point in the lens where a ray of light will pass through the lens without changing direction. This occurs because at that one point the sides of the lens are parallel to each other.

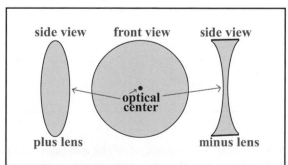

An imaginary line on the lens surface that goes from one edge of the lens to the other edge, passing through the optical center of the lens, is called a *meridian*. Drawing meridians is like cutting the lens up into pie wedges. A meridian can be in any direction on the lens. A circle is made up of 360 degrees. We choose to start at the right side of the circle and have the degrees go counterclockwise around the circle.

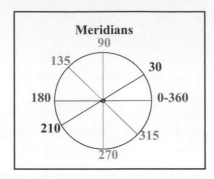

When you are facing a person wearing glasses, the meridians run counterclockwise from the right side of the lens to the left side of the lens, regardless of which lens you are looking at. For now, you can ignore degrees in the bottom of the lens.

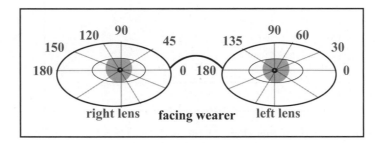

We call the 0- to 180-degree meridian the 180 meridian.

OPTICAL CROSS

An optical cross is a graphical representation of the power of a lens, showing the power in the two major meridians on the lens. On a lens the two major meridians are always 90 degrees apart.

A SPHERE

The first lens shown here is a +1.00 DS, or +1.00 diopter sphere. On every meridian of the lens the power is +1.00. The two lines that are perpendicular to each other become the diagram or *optical cross* of the lens.

The optical cross for a sphere shows any two meridians, since all meridians have the same power, and it indicates that the two major meridians have the power of +1.00.

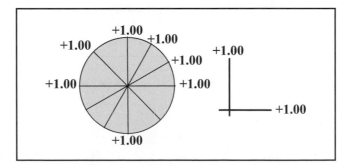

A CYLINDER

In this example, pl is the *sphere power*, +2.00 is the *amount of the cylinder,* and 180 is the *axis of the sphere*, also called the *axis of the prescription.* The lens cross shows that the meridian of the pl power is 180. The lens cross has to show only one axis, since the other is understood to be 90 degrees away. Therefore only the 180 or the 90 is needed. Or, no axis at all might be shown if the orientation of the cylinder is not yet determined.

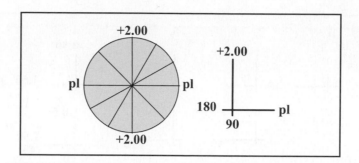

A TORIC LENS

We can think of the *toric lens* as a sandwich of a sphere lens, in this example the +1.00, and a cylindrical lens, in this case having pl on the 180 and +2.00 on the 90th meridian. In this example +1.00 is the *sphere power*, +2.00 is the *amount of the cylinder*, and 180 is the *axis of the sphere*, also called the *axis of the prescription*. The toric lens is also called a *spherocylindrical* lens or a *compound lens*. A toric lens has varying "powers" on each of its meridians. The sphere power alone is present along the axis of the lens, and the sphere and cylinder powers combined are present 90 degrees away from the axis of the lens.

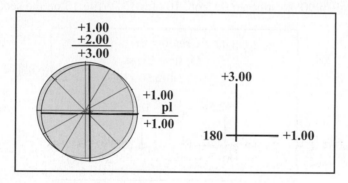

Rx NOTATION

The Rx has three entries: sphere power, cylinder amount, and axis of the sphere power. In the example above:

- The **sphere power** is +1.00 because that is the power everywhere on the lens in the "sandwich."
- The **cylinder amount** is the difference between the two major powers on the lens.
- The **axis of the Rx** is the meridian where the sphere power is in effect: it is where the cylinder power is 0.

——— PUTTING THE Rx ON THE OPTICAL CROSS ———

EXAMPLES:

3-11. On the optical cross at the top of p. 56, diagram the Rx −1.50 +1.00 ×045.
1. Draw two lines 90 degrees from each other. They can be in the approximate orientation of the axis of the Rx, or they can be horizontal and vertical.
2. Label the axis. Put the axis of the Rx on the end of one line.
3. Put the sphere power on the axis line, since the sphere power alone is present along the axis of the prescription. The sphere power of +1.50 and the axis of 45 go on the same line.
4. Add the sphere and cylinder amounts together, and put the resulting total power on the line 90 degrees away from the axis of the prescription: +1.50 + (+1.00) = −0.50. The power of −0.50 goes on the second line.
5. Add or subtract 90 from the axis, and put this number on the second line. The degree used must be between 0 and 180. Therefore, to find the second meridian, if the axis is 90 or less, add 90; if the axis is greater than 90, subtract 90. Since 45 is less than 90, the second meridian is 45 + 90 = 135.

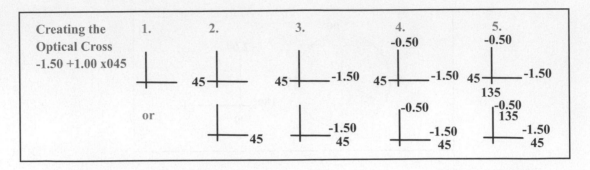

Creating the Optical Cross
-1.50 +1.00 x045

3-12. On the optical cross below, diagram +2.50 –2.50 ×103.
1. Draw two lines 90 degrees from each other.
2. Label the axis. Put the axis of the Rx, 103, on the end of one line.
3. Put the sphere power on the axis line, since the sphere power alone is present along the axis of the prescription. The +2.50 and the 103 are paired on the same line.
4. Add the sphere and cylinder amounts together, and put the resulting total power on the line 90 degrees away from the axis of the prescription. +2.50 + (–2.50) = 0 or pl, so the pl goes with the 13 meridian.
5. The axis is greater than 90, so subtract 90 from 103 for 13. Write 13 on the second line.

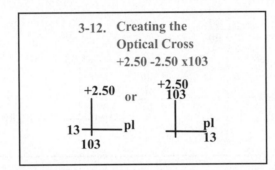

3-12. Creating the Optical Cross +2.50 -2.50 x103

DIAGRAMMING AN Rx ON THE OPTICAL CROSS

1. Draw lines 90 degrees from each other.
2. Put the axis of the Rx on one line.
3. Put the sphere power of the Rx on the same line. *Note*: **The sphere power and the axis of the Rx go together.**
4. Add the sphere power and the cylinder amount together, and put the result on the second line.
5. Change the axis of the Rx by 90 and put it on the second line.

EXERCISES:

Put the following prescriptions on an optical cross.
27. +3.50D

28. –1.00 –1.00 ×180

29. +0.50 –2.00 ×030

30. –1.00 +1.00 ×080

31. –6.50 –0.50 ×022

32. +4.25 –1.75 ×136

TAKING THE Rx FROM THE OPTICAL CROSS

There are three ways that a prescription can be written, so there are three ways in which it can be taken from the optical cross:

- Minus cylinder form: the most common form for opticians in the United States
- Plus cylinder form: used by many refractionists
- Cross cylinder form: used by some physicians outside the United States

The optical cross represents the powers on the lens and the meridians where they are found. This is a graphic representation of the powers that would be found when a lensmeter (also known as lensmeter, vertometer, or focimeter) is used to determine the prescription of the lens. The procedure shown here is what you do when determining the Rx of a lens using the lensmeter.

Use the number line below to determine the sphere power in the examples that follow.

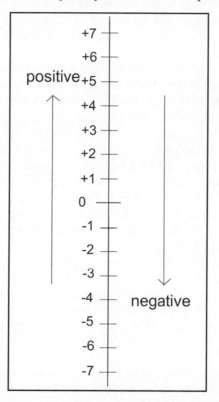

MINUS CYLINDER FORM

EXAMPLES:

3-13. Using the optical cross illustrated at right below, write the Rx in minus cylinder form.

  1. Sphere power: Take the most plus or the least minus power on the optical cross as the sphere power. If the number line above is used, the sphere power is the power that is highest up on the line. Since +3.00 is higher on the number line than +2.00, we start with **+3.00 for the sphere power.**

  2. Axis: The meridian of the power selected for the sphere will be the axis for the Rx. We used +3.00 for the sphere power, and it is combined with the axis 90 on the optical cross, so the **axis of the Rx is 90.**

  3. Cylinder amount: The *difference* between the powers in the two meridians gives the cylinder amount. The cylinder amount is found by subtracting the sphere power from the power on the other meridian, that is, the power not used in step 1 minus the power used: +2.00 – (+3.00) = –1.00D. Using the number line, we start at the sphere power and determine how far and in what direction we have to go to arrive at the

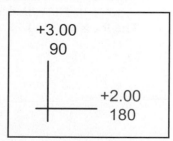

second power. Starting at +3.00 on the number line, we travel down, in the negative direction, 1.00 to get to +2.00. **The cylinder amount is –1.00.** **The Rx is +3.00 –1.00 ×090.**

3-14. Using the optical cross at right, write the Rx in minus cylinder form.

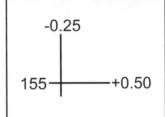

1. Sphere power: Take the most plus or the least minus power on the optical cross as the sphere power. If the number line above is used, the sphere power is the power that is highest on the line. Because –1.25 is higher on the number line than –2.25, we start with **–1.25 for the sphere power.**
2. Axis: The meridian of the power selected for the sphere will be the axis for the Rx. We used –1.25 for the sphere power, and it is combined with the axis 55 on the optical cross, so the **axis of the Rx is 55.**
3. Cylinder amount: The *difference* between the powers in the two meridians gives the cylinder amount. The cylinder amount is found by subtracting the sphere power from the power on the other meridian, that is, the power not used in step 1 minus the power used: –2.25 – (–1.25) = –1.00. Using the number line, we start at the sphere power and determine how far and in what direction we have to go to arrive at the second power. Starting at –1.25 on the number line, we travel down, in the negative direction, 1.00 to get to –2.25. **The cylinder amount is –1.00.**

The Rx is –1.25 –1.00 ×055.

3-15. Using the optical cross at right, write the Rx in minus cylinder form.

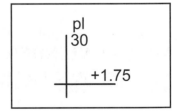

1. Sphere power: Take the most plus or the least minus power on the optical cross as the sphere power. Since +0.50 is the most plus or least minus, or the highest on the number line, **+0.50 is the sphere power.**
2. Axis: The meridian of the power selected for the sphere will be the axis for the Rx. The meridian of 155 is paired with the power of +0.50 on the optical cross, so the **axis of the Rx is 155.**
3. Cylinder amount: The *difference* between the powers in the two meridians gives the cylinder amount. 0.25 – (+50) = –0.7. Using the number line, we start at the sphere power and determine how far and in what direction we have to go to arrive at the second power. Starting at +0.50 on the number line, we travel down, in the negative direction, 0.75 to get to –0.25. **The cylinder amount is –0.75.**

The Rx is +0.50 –0.75 ×155.

3-16. Using the optical cross at right, write the Rx in minus cylinder form.
1. Sphere power: +1.75 is the most plus or least minus, or the highest on the number line. Therefore **+1.75 is the sphere power.**
2. Axis: The sphere power of +1.75 is not paired with an axis on the diagram. We know, however, that the two meridians are 90 degrees apart. Since 30 is less than 90, we add 90 to 30 for a meridian of 120. The sphere power of +1.75 is paired with the meridian of 120, so the **axis of the Rx is 120.**
3. Cylinder amount: pl means 0. Therefore +1.75 – (0) = –1.75. Using the number line, we start at +1.75 and go in the negative direction 1.75 to get to 0. **The cylinder amount is –1.75.**

The Rx is +1.75 –1.75 ×120.

1. Choose the power that is most plus or least minus. This is the power that is highest on the number line or on the lensmeter power drum. This is the sphere power.
2. Choose the meridian that is paired with the sphere power for the axis. *Note*: **The sphere power and the axis of the Rx go together.**
3. Enter the power that you did *not* use in step 1 in your calculator, and subtract the power that you *did* use. This is the cylinder amount.

PLUS CYLINDER FORM

EXAMPLES:

3-17. Using the optical cross to the right, write the Rx in plus cylinder form.
1. Sphere power: Take the least plus or the most minus power on the optical cross as the sphere power: +2.00D. This is the power that is the lower of the two on the number line.
2. Axis: The meridian of the power selected for the sphere will be the axis for the Rx: ×180.
3. Cylinder amount: The *difference* between the powers in the two meridians gives the cylinder power. This is found by subtracting the sphere power from the power on the other meridian, that is, the power not used in step 1 minus the power used: +3.00 − (+2.00) = +1.00D.

The Rx is +2.00 +1.00 ×180.

```
        +3.00
        90
                    +2.00
                    180
```

Note: The cylinder amount represents how far the second power is from the first power. In the minus cylinder example the cylinder was the result of moving from +3.00 to +2.00. In the plus cylinder example we moved from +2.00 to +3.00.

Note: If you have been using a lensmeter, you will recognize the number line as the power drum. Writing the Rx from the optical cross is the same technique that you use when **neutralizing** glasses. **Neutralizing a lens** means determining the prescription of the lens.

3-18. Using the optical cross at right, write the Rx in plus cylinder form.
1. Sphere power: Take the least plus or the most minus power on the optical cross as the sphere power:
   −2.25. This is the power that is the lower of the two on the number line.
2. Axis: The meridian of the power selected for the sphere will be the axis for the Rx: ×145.
3. Cylinder amount: The *difference* between the powers in the two meridians gives the cylinder power. This is the power not used in step 1 minus the power used: −1.25 − (−2.25) = +1.00D.

The Rx is −2.25 +1.00 ×145.

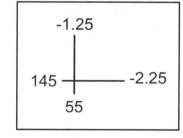

3-19. Using the optical cross at right, write the Rx in plus cylinder form.
1. Sphere power: Take the least plus or the most minus power on the optical cross as the sphere power: −0.25. This is the power that is the lower of the two on the number line.
2. Axis: The meridian of the power selected for the sphere will be the axis for the Rx. In this diagram the axis for the power of −0.25 is not present, but we know that it is 90 degrees from the one that is present. Since155 is more than 90, we subtract 90 from it; 155 − 90 = 65, so the axis is 65.

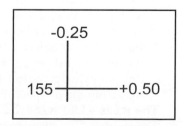

3. Cylinder amount: The *difference* between the powers in the two meridians gives the cylinder power. This is the power not used in step 1 minus the power used. Thus +0.50 – (–0.25) = +0.75
The Rx is –0.25 +0.75 ×065.

3-20. Using the optical cross at right, write the Rx in plus cylinder form.
  1. Sphere power: Take the least plus or the most minus power on the optical cross as the sphere power: pl. This is the power that is the lower of the two on the number line.
  2. Axis: The meridian of the power selected for the sphere will be the axis for the Rx: × 30.
  3. Cylinder amount: The *difference* between the powers in the two meridians gives the cylinder power. This is the power not used in step 1 minus the power used. +1.75 – (0) = +1.75.
  The Rx is pl +1.75 ×030.

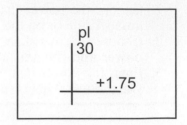

WRITING THE Rx FROM THE OPTICAL CROSS IN PLUS CYLINDER FORM

1. Choose the power that is least plus or most minus. This is the power that is lowest on the number line or on the power drum. This is the sphere power.
2. Choose the meridian that is paired with the sphere power for the axis. *Note*: **The sphere power and the axis of the Rx go together.**
3. Enter the power that you did *not* use in step 1 in your calculator, and subtract the power that you *did* use. This is the cylinder amount.

EXERCISES:

Write each Rx first in minus cylinder form and then in plus cylinder form.

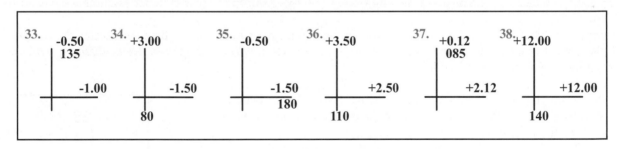

	33.	34.	35.	36.	37.	38.
Minus cylinder form:	_____	_____	_____	_____	_____	_____
Plus cylinder form:	_____	_____	_____	_____	_____	_____

CROSS CYLINDER FORM

An alternative way to correct for a compound astigmatic error is to use two cylinders at right angles (90 degrees) to each other. The cross cylinders represent the powers on a toric surface. Remember, a cylinder has *plano power on its axis* and plus or minus power 90 degrees from its axis.
  1. First cylinder: Select a power on one meridian, and assign it the axis from the other meridian: +3.00 ×180.
  2. Second cylinder: Select the power on the other meridian, and assign it the axis from the first meridian: +2.00 ×090.
  The Rx is +3.00 ×180 ◯ +2.00 ×090.
  The symbol ◯ means *combined with*.

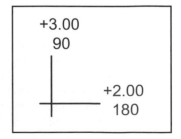

A cylinder has one plano side. An example of a plus cylinder is pl +5.00 ×180. When referring to a true cylinder, we can write that same Rx as +5.00 ×180 because the pl is *assumed* to be there. Even more precise is +5.00 DC ×180. Whenever an Rx is in the form ***power × axis***, there is an assumed pl in front of the power. Thus −3.50 ×125 means pl −3.50 ×125. This is why, in this notation, *the axis goes with the assumed pl, not the power.*

3-21.   Write the Rx shown at right in cross cylinder form.
1. Choose either power. Combine it with the opposite axis: **–1.25 ×145.**
2. Choose the other power. Combine it with the other axis: **–2.25 ×055.**
The answer is **–1.25 ×145 ◯ –2.25 ×055.**

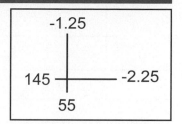

3-22.   Write the Rx shown at right in cross cylinder form.
1. Choose either power. Combine it with the opposite axis: **–0.25 ×155.**
2. Choose the other power. Combine it with the other axis: **+0.50 ×065.**
The answer is **–0.25 ×155 ◯ +0.50 ×065.**

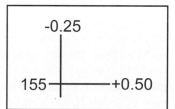

3-23.   Write the Rx shown at right in cross cylinder form.
1. Choose either power. Combine it with the opposite axis: **+1.75 ×030.**
2. Choose the other power. Combine it with the other axis: **pl ×120,**
     which means zero power. This part is therefore unnecessary.
The answer is **+1.75 ×030.**
Note: Since cross cylinder notation assumes a pl in front of each part of the Rx, +1.75 ×030 means pl +1.75 ×030. So, because the lens is in fact a cylinder (pl or zero power on one of the two major meridians), the cross cylinder notation describes this lens completely with just the one element.

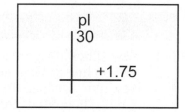

Having discussed cross cylinder form, we will now discuss how to put a cross cylinder prescription on the optical cross:

1. Place one of the axes on the optical cross diagram. Place the other cylinder power with this axis.
2. Place the remaining cylinder power with the remaining axis.

3-24.   Place the prescription +10.00 ×023 ◯ +7.50 ×113 on the optical cross.

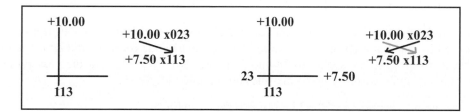

Write each Rx in cross cylinder form.

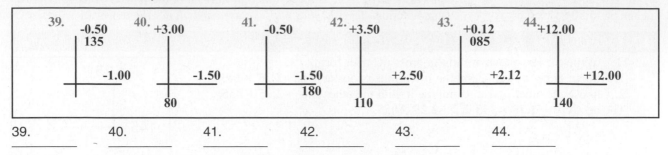

39. _____ 40. _____ 41. _____ 42. _____ 43. _____ 44. _____

FLAT TRANSPOSITION

Some physicians write prescriptions in plus cylinder form, and others write prescriptions in minus cylinder form. The equipment dictates the format the physician uses to write the Rx. Some phoropters use plus cylinder lenses, whereas others use minus cylinder lenses.

Modern lenses are made in minus cylinder form, which means that the toric surface is the concave surface. Lenses made in plus cylinder form would have the toric surface on the convex side. The prescriber who writes the Rx in plus cylinder form does not intend that the lenses be made in that form unless a note on the Rx specifically requests plus cylinder. If the prescription arrives in plus cylinder form, it may have to be rewritten. We call this process flat transposition.

RULES FOR FLAT TRANSPOSITION

1. New sphere: Algebraically add the sphere power and the cylinder amount.
2. New cylinder: Change the sign of the cylinder amount.
3. New axis: Change the axis by 90 degrees. If the axis is less than 90 degrees, add 90. If the axis is more than 90 degrees, subtract 90.

EXAMPLES:

3-25. Transpose the prescription +2.00 +1.00 ×180 to minus cylinder form.
1. New sphere power: Algebraically add the original sphere and cylinder powers.
   (+2.00) + (+1.00) = +3.00
2. New cylinder amount: Change the sign of the original cylinder amount.
   +1.00 becomes −1.00
3. New axis power: Add 90 degrees to the original axis if it is 90 degrees or lower. Subtract 90 degrees from the original axis if it is greater than 90 degrees.
   180 − 90 = 090
Transposed Rx: +3.00 −1.00 ×090.

Look back at Examples 3-13 and 3-17. The identical optical crosses resulted in two prescriptions, but in each case the lens that was used to create the Rx was the same. The plus and minus forms of the Rx do not change the lens itself. Look at your answers to Exercises 33 to 38 and demonstrate to yourself that the plus cylinder form can be derived from the minus cylinder form by using the rules above, and vice versa.

3-26. Transpose the prescription −3.50 +2.00 ×020 to minus cylinder.
1. New sphere: (−3.50) + (+2.00) = −1.50D
2. New cylinder: +2.00 becomes −2.00D
3. Axis: 020 + 90 = 110
The transposed Rx is −1.50 −2.00 ×110.

Check the answer by placing both prescriptions on an optical cross. They are identical. We have not changed the Rx; we have only changed the way it was written.

45. Transpose the following prescriptions into minus cylinder form.
    a. −0.50 +1.50 ×030   _____
    b. +1.00 +3.00 ×135   _____
    c. −2.37 +1.50 ×070   _____

46. Transpose the following prescriptions into plus cylinder form.
    a. +2.00 −3.00 ×060   _____
    b. −1.00 −0.75 ×140   _____
    c. −1.62 −1.75 ×065   _____

CROSS CYLINDER TRANSPOSITION

To determine the cross cylinder form of a prescription, either:

1. Put the prescription on an optical cross, and then remove it in cross cylinder form, or
2. Flat transpose the prescription, and then cross connect the spheres and the axes

For example, what is the cross cylinder version of the Rx −1.00 +1.50 ×110?

Rx:	−1.00 +1.50 ×110
Transposing gives:	+0.50 −1.50 ×020
Cross connecting spheres:	−1.00 +1.50 ×110

+0.50 −1.50 ×020

The Rx becomes: −1.00 ×020 ⊃ +0.50 ×110

47. Rewrite the following prescriptions as cross cylinders.
    a. −1.00 +2.00 ×090   _____
    b. +2.50 −3.62 ×130   _____
    c. +1.00 −1.50 ×096   _____

48. Rewrite the following cross cylinder prescriptions in minus cylinder form. (The optical cross may be helpful.)
    a. −1.00 ×110 ⊃ +2.00 ×020   _____
    b. +3.25 ×080 ⊃ +1.00 ×170   _____
    c. +10.50 ×013 ⊃ +9.50 ×103   _____

HAND NEUTRALIZATION

The term *neutralization* originated from the way the power of a lens used to be determined. When you are looking at the image of the edge of a surface through a lens as the lens is moved, either the edge appears to move in the same direction as the lens movement, or the edge appears to move in the opposite direction from the lens movement.

A plus lens shows *against movement*. If you hold a plus lens about an inch above an edge and move the lens to the right, the *image* of the edge seen through the lens will move to the left. The movement that you are looking at is the image of the edge with respect to the actual edge.

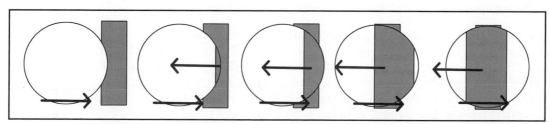

A minus lens shows ***with movement***. If you hold a minus lens about an inch above an edge and move the lens to the right, the *image* of the edge seen through the lens will move to the right. You are looking at the movement of the image of the edge compared with the actual position of the edge behind the lens.

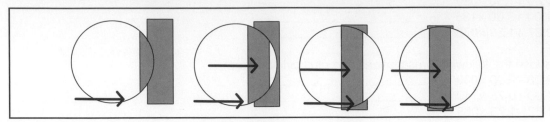

A plano lens shows no movement, or ***neutral movement***.

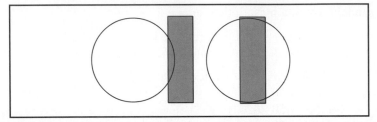

If we hold together two lenses with equal amounts of power but opposite signs, they will *neutralize* each other's movement. If we can neutralize the movement of an unknown lens with a +5.00D lens, the unknown lens must be a −5.00D lens.

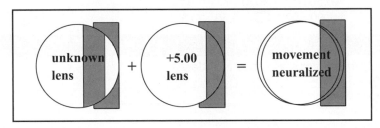

If we can neutralize the movement in only one direction with the +5.00D lens, but in the other direction we need a +6.00D lens, the power in the first meridian is −5.00D and the power in the second meridian is −6.00D.

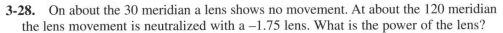
EXAMPLES:

3-27. In the horizontal meridian, a lens is hand-neutralized with a +1.00D lens, and in the vertical meridian the movement is neutralized with an *additional* +2.00D lens. What is the power of the lens?
   1. Horizontal is the 180-degree meridian. Neutralization by a +1.00D lens means a power of −1.00D in this meridian in the unknown lens. Therefore one leg of the optical cross is −1.00 at 180.
   2. Vertical is the 90-degree meridian. Neutralization by adding +2.00D to the +1.00D already used means that it took +3.00D to neutralize the movement. The power on the 90-degree meridian is −3.00D in the unknown lens. Thus −3.00 at 90 goes on the other leg of the optical cross.
   3. The optical cross is shown diagrammed at right.
   4. Removing the Rx from the optical cross gives an Rx of −1.00 −2.00 ×180, or −3.00 +2.00 ×090.

   Note: The *additional* +2.00 lens gave the amount of the cylinder.

3-28. On about the 30 meridian a lens shows no movement. At about the 120 meridian the lens movement is neutralized with a −1.75 lens. What is the power of the lens?
   1. On the 30 meridian there is plano power, so pl goes on one leg of the optical cross with the meridian of 30.
   2. On the optical cross a power of +1.75 goes with the meridian of 120.
   3. The optical cross is diagrammed at right.
   4. Removing the Rx from the optical cross gives an Rx of pl +1.75 ×030, or +1.75 −1.75 ×120.

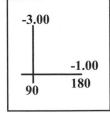

49. A lens is hand neutralized and is found to show no horizontal motion when a −4.00D lens is used and no vertical motion when *just* a −1.00D lens is used. What is the power of the lens?

50. A lens is hand-neutralized and is found to show no horizontal motion when a +4.00D lens is used and no vertical motion when a +2.00D lens is *added* to the +4.00. What is the power of the lens?

51. A lens is hand neutralized and is found to show no horizontal motion when a +2.50D lens is used and no vertical motion when *just* a −1.00D lens is used. What is the power of the lens?

52. A lens is hand neutralized and is found to show no motion at about the 45-degree meridian when a −1.00D lens is used and no motion at about the 135-degree meridian when *an additional* −0.50D lens is included. What is the power of the lens?

53. Find a plus spherical lens and a minus spherical lens of equal and opposite powers, and try looking at the way they neutralize movement.

PRESCRIPTION NOTATION

PRESCRIPTION NOTATION

SPHERE NOTATION
- Sign must be + or −.
- Value under +/−1.00D should have leading zero.
- Decimals are expressed to two places, and are in truncated eighths: 0.12, 0.25, 0.37, 0.50, 0.62, 0.75, 0.87, and 0.00.
- A sphere power of 0.00 is written pl.
- D or DS may be used on non-compound prescriptions; it is usually not entered for compound prescriptions.

CYLINDER NOTATION
- Sign must be + or −.
- Value under +/−1.00D should have a leading zero.
- Decimals are expressed to two places and are in truncated eighths: 0.12, 0.25, 0.37, 0.50, 0.62, 0.75, 0.87, and 0.00.
- A cylinder power of 0.00 is not entered. Spherical prescriptions use only the sphere power.
- D or DC is usually not entered.

AXIS NOTATION
- Axis should be written with three digits: 001, 015, 155, and so on.
- Axis is from 001 to 180. An axis of 000 is 180. Subtract 180 from any axis over 180. (This may happen occasionally as the result of a calculation.)
- The degree sign is not written.

EXAMPLES:

		Corrected:
3-29.	+5.00 −0.00 ×020 is a sphere with a zero cylinder power:	+5.00, or +5.00 DS.
3-30.	+5.00 −.5 ×145 needs the cylinder rewritten as −0.50:	+5.00 −0.50 ×145.
3-31.	+5.00 −0.50 ×225 needs the axis rewritten as 045:	+5.00 −0.50 ×045.
3-32.	+5.00 −1.32 ×050 needs the cylinder rounded to −1.37:	+5.00 −1.37 ×050.
3-33.	0.00 −3.00 ×100 needs the sphere power rewritten pl:	pl −3.00 ×100.

3-34. pl −3.00 ×100° needs the degree sign dropped: pl −3.00 ×100.

3-35. 5.00 −0.50 ×013 requires determining the sign of the sphere; you may *not* assume the sign to be +.   *Call the refractionist.*

3-36. pl −3.00 ×45 needs the axis rewritten as 045:   pl −3.00 ×045.

EXERCISES:

Decide what is wrong with the following (if anything) and correct it.

54. +8.5 −1.00 ×15

55. 3.50 +1.50 ×135

56. −.37 −1.50 ×188

57. −1.37 +2.00 ×115

58. +3.80 −0.00 ×132

59. +0.00 +0.62 ×10°

60. +2.25 +2.12 ×011

61. −3.00 0.75 ×15

62. pl −0.87 ×136

63. +4.37 DS

64. −7.55

65. +.67 −.67 ×10

66. −3.125 +3.125 ×067

67. −1.11 −0.03 ×015

68. +0.50 DS −0.50 DC ×210°

69. +20.50 −8.50 ×045

Note: Your employer and the OD or MD or refractionist who writes the prescriptions that you fill may write an Rx any way they choose. **The above rules are *only* for *us*.**

—————————— CIRCLE OF LEAST CONFUSION ——————————

A spherical lens, having the same curvature in all meridians, brings the image of a distant point source to a point focus.

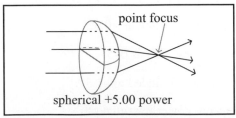

A cylindrical lens is a lens that has one flat or plano side. A cylindrical lens brings the image of a distant point source to a line focus.

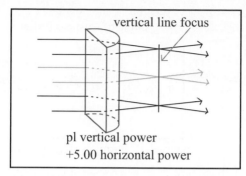

As you can see from the cross cylinder notation, a spherocylinder lens can also be thought of as two cylindrical lenses sandwiched together. When we showed the prescription in cross cylinder form, we were writing the prescription as two cylinders back to back. The spherocylinder lens brings the image of a distant point source to two line foci, one for each cylinder, instead of one point focus.

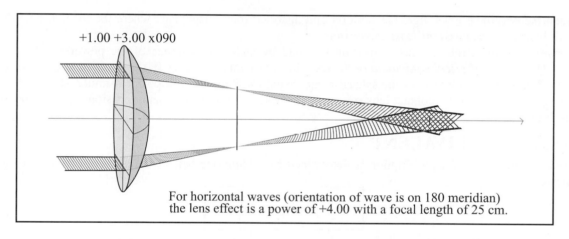

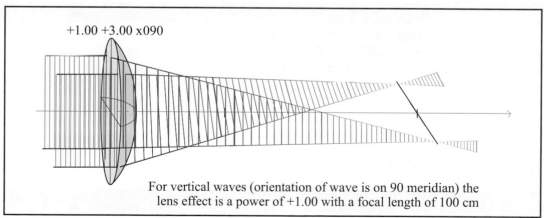

The interval between the two focal lines in a compound lens is called the ***interval of Sturm***. The length of the interval of Sturm is an indication of the length of the ***astigmatic interval.*** The interval of Sturm for a prescription is the difference between the focal lengths of the major meridian powers. The ***toricity*** of a surface is the difference between the two radii of curvature of the toric surface. The cylinder amount in the Rx notation is a way of judging the relative toricity of a lens, or comparing the astigmatic intervals of two lenses. The Rx +5.00 –4.00 ×090 has a much longer astigmatic interval than does the Rx +5.00 –0.50 ×090.

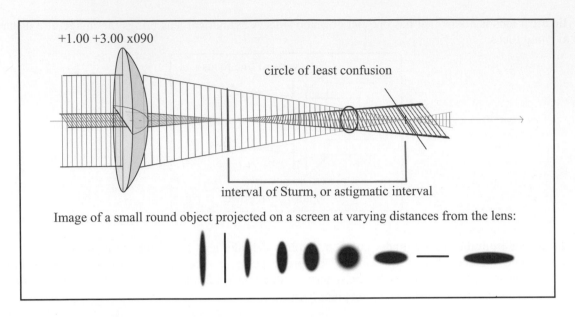

+1.00 +3.00 x090

circle of least confusion

interval of Sturm, or astigmatic interval

Image of a small round object projected on a screen at varying distances from the lens:

Between the two focal lines, light has a blurry and distorted focus. The plane where the focus has no distortion (but is still blurry) is the *circle of least confusion*.

The position of the circle of least confusion is found by taking the average of the powers in the two major meridians. This is the *spherical equivalent* of the Rx. The approximate distance of the circle of least confusion from the lens can be determined by use of the spherical equivalent for D in the focal power formula, D = 1/f. We use the spherical equivalent for initial contact lens selection, for base curve selection, and occasionally for approximating power or thickness.

SPHERICAL EQUIVALENT

The spherical equivalent of a prescription is determined by adding one half of the amount of the cylinder to the sphere power.

$$D_{sph.eq.} = \frac{D_{cyl}}{2} + D_{sphere}$$

EXAMPLES:

3-37. What is the spherical equivalent of the Rx −2.00 −1.00 ×090?
1. One half of the cylinder is (−1.00)/2 = −0.50.
2. Add this amount to the sphere power: (−0.50) + −2.00 = −2.50.
The spherical equivalent is −2.50D.

3-38. What is the spherical equivalent of the Rx +4.00 −3.00 ×125?
(−3.00)/2 + (+4.00) = (−1.50) + (+4.00) = **+2.50D.**

3-39. What is the spherical equivalent of the Rx −5.25D?
Answer: **−5.25D.**

EXERCISES: (Round to hundredths of a diopter.)

Determine the spherical equivalent for the following prescriptions.

70. −1.00 −0.50 ×090   _____

71. pl −2.00 ×170   _____

72. +2.00 −3.00 ×025   _____

73. −1.25 +1.25 ×160   _____

74. +1.00 +2.00 ×060   _____

75. −0.50 +1.50 ×030   _____

76. +1.00 +3.00 ×135   _____

77. −2.37 +1.50 ×070   _____

78. −1.00 −0.75 ×140   _____

79. −1.62 −1.75 ×065   _____

REFRACTIVE ERRORS

An *emmetropic eye* is an eye that, without accommodating, brings parallel incident light rays to a point focus on the retina. No correction is needed.

An *ametropic* eye is an eye that, without accommodating, does not bring parallel incident light rays to a point focus on the retina. Correction is needed to bring the distant focus to the retina.

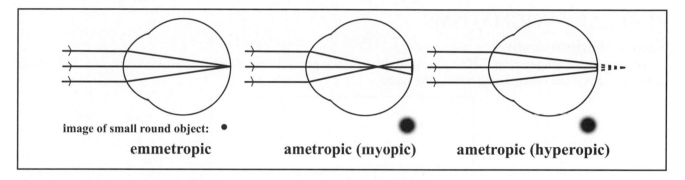

image of small round object: ●

emmetropic   **ametropic (myopic)**   **ametropic (hyperopic)**

TYPES OF AMETROPIA

Hyperopia or Farsightedness

In *hyperopia* parallel rays of light come to a point focus behind the retina. In *axial hyperopia* the eye appears to be *too short*. In *refractive hyperopia* the refractive surfaces of the eye appear to be *too flat*, or the eye has too little plus power.

For correction, hyperopia requires a plus lens to add more power to the eye system, increasing the convergence of the light rays and bringing parallel incident light rays to a point focus on the retina.

Since the retina absorbs light, the focus never actually falls behind the retina. In the case of all of the types of hyperopia discussed here, when we say the focus is behind the retina, we mean that the vergence is such that the focus would form behind the retina if the light continued to that point.

In all cases of ametropia, when the focus is not on the retina, a blurred image forms on the retina. How blurred the image is depends on how far the focal plane is (or would be) from the retina.

Myopia or Nearsightedness

In *myopia* parallel rays of light come to a point focus in front of the retina. In *axial myopia* the eye appears to be *too long*. In *refractive myopia* the refractive surfaces of the eye appear to be *too steep*, or the eye has too much plus power.

For correction, myopia requires a minus lens to reduce the convergence of the light rays, bringing parallel incident light rays to a point focus on the retina.

Astigmatism

In *astigmatism* parallel rays of light do not come to a point focus on the retina. Instead, there are two line foci, corresponding to the maximum and minimum powers in the eye system. Almost all astigmatism is *refractive*. Astigmatism is usually the result of a toric cornea or of a toric or tilted crystalline lens.

In *regular astigmatism* the rays of light form two focal lines at 90 degrees from each other. This condition is corrected by use of compound or spherocylinder lenses.

In *irregular astigmatism* the light rays form many focal lines or form focal lines not at 90 degrees to each other. A damaged or irregular cornea usually causes irregular astigmatism. This condition cannot be corrected with spherocylindrical lenses. It usually requires the creation of a new optical surface. The new surface may be a contact lens or a corneal transplant.

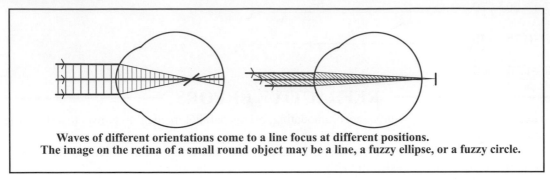

Waves of different orientations come to a line focus at different positions.
The image on the retina of a small round object may be a line, a fuzzy ellipse, or a fuzzy circle.

REGULAR ASTIGMATISMS

Simple Astigmatism

Simple hyperopic astigmatism **(SHA)** is a condition in which parallel rays of light come to two line foci, one falling on the retina and the other falling behind the retina.

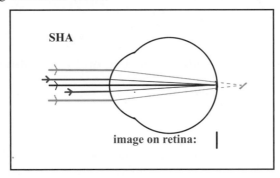

An example of a prescription that corrects for SHA is pl +2.00 ×180, which can be transposed to +2.00 –2.00 ×090. The major meridian powers of this Rx are pl and +2.00. One power (the pl) indicates that the refraction in that meridian requires no correction. The other power (the +2.00) indicates that the refraction in that meridian is hyperopic.

Simple myopic astigmatism **(SMA)** is a condition in which parallel rays of light come to two line foci, one falling on the retina and the other falling in front of the retina.

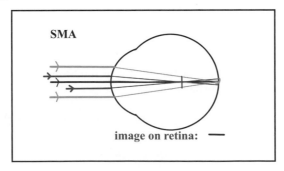

An example of a prescription that corrects for SMA is pl –2.00 ×090, which can be transposed to –2.00 +2.00 ×080. The major meridian powers of this Rx are pl and –2.00. One power (the pl) indicates that the refraction in that meridian requires no correction. The other power (the –2.00) indicates that the refraction in that meridian is myopic.

Compound Astigmatism

***Compound hyperopic astigmatism* (CHA)** is a condition in which parallel rays of light come to two line foci, both of which fall behind the retina.

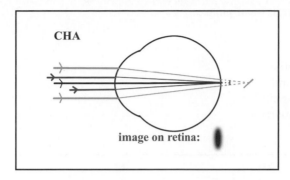

An example of a prescription that corrects for CHA is +1.00 +2.00 ×180, which can be transposed to +3.00 −2.00 ×090. The major meridian powers of this Rx are +1.00 and +2.00. Both of these powers indicate that the refraction in their respective meridians is hyperopic.

***Compound myopic astigmatism* (CMA)** is a condition in which parallel rays of light come to two line foci, both of which fall in front of the retina.

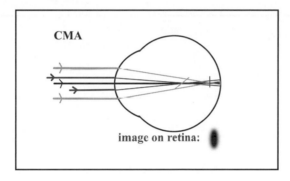

An example of a prescription that corrects for CMA is −1.00 −2.00 ×090, which can be transposed to −3.00 +2.00 ×180. The major meridian powers of this Rx are −1.00 and −2.00. Both of these powers indicate that the refraction in their respective meridians is myopic.

Mixed Astigmatism

***Mixed astigmatism* (MA)** is a condition in which parallel rays of light come to two line foci, one falling in front of the retina and the other falling behind the retina.

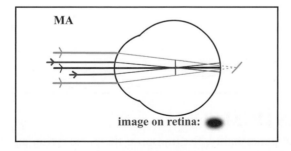

An example of a prescription that corrects for MA is +1.00 −1.50 ×090, which can be transposed to −0.50 +1.50 ×180. The major meridian powers of this Rx are +1.00 and −0.50. One power (the +1.00) indicates that the refraction in that meridian is hyperopic. The other power (the −0.50) indicates that the refraction in that meridian is myopic.

Determine the refractive error illustrated by the following diagrams. The diagrams do not show the rays of light. If there are two short lines, they represent the location of the two major focal planes. If there is one small circle, it represents the location of the single focal plane.

H: Hyperopia
M: Myopia
SHA: Simple hyperopic astigmatism
SMA: Simple myopic astigmatism
CHA: Compound hyperopic astigmatism
CMA: Compound myopic astigmatism
MA: Mixed astigmatism

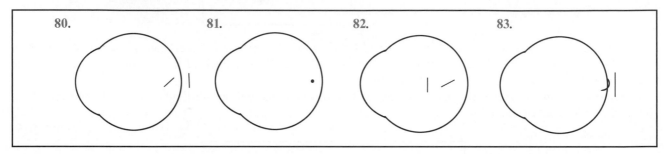

80. _____

81. _____

82. _____

83. _____

84. _____

85. _____

86. _____

87. _____

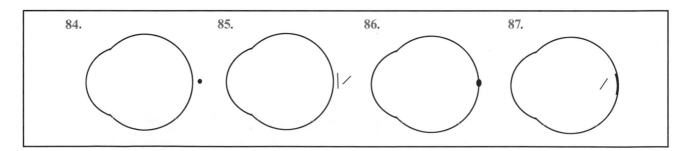

EVALUATING THE ASTIGMATISM

To determine the wearer's visual abnormality, flat transpose the prescription and then consider the powers in the major meridians.

EVALUATING THE ASTIGMATISM

POWER IN MAJOR MERIDIANS	REFRACTIVE ERROR
pl +	Simple hyperopic astigmatism (SHA)
pl −	Simple myopic astigmatism (SMA)
+ + (unequal power)	Compound hyperopic astigmatism (CHA)
− −	Compound myopic astigmatism (CMA)
+ −	Mixed astigmatism (MA)

EXAMPLE:

3-40. For an Rx +3.00 −1.00 ×135, flat transposition gives +2.00 +1.00 ×045. The two major powers (+3.00 and +2.00) are both +. Therefore the prescription corrects for CHA.

EXERCISES:

Determine the nature of the refractive error for the following prescriptions.

88. −1.00 −0.50 ×090 _____

89. pl −2.00 ×170 _____

90. +2.00 −3.00 ×025 _____

91. −1.25 +1.25 ×160 _____

92. +1.00 +2.00 ×060 _____

93. −0.50 +1.50 ×030 _____

94. +1.00 +3.00 ×135 _____

95. −2.37 +1.50 ×070 _____

96. +2.00 −0.75 ×140 _____

97. +1.62 −1.62 ×065 _____

———————— WITH AND AGAINST THE RULE ASTIGMATISM ————————

Astigmatism is said to be ***with the rule astigmatism*** if the steepest meridian of the cornea or the crystalline lens is near the vertical meridian. In this case the correction requires using a minus cylinder with the axis near the 180 meridian or a plus cylinder with the axis near the 90 meridian.

For example, the Rx +3.00 −3.00 ×180 has a correction of +3.00 on the 180 or horizontal meridian and no correction on the 90 meridian. Since the cornea is steeper (or has more plus power) on the 90 meridian, the extra plus power on the 180 meridian of the glasses lens will result in equal power in all meridians.

Astigmatism is said to be ***against the rule astigmatism*** when the steepest meridian of the cornea or the crystalline lens is near the horizontal meridian. In this case the correction requires use of a minus cylinder with the axis near the 90 meridian or a plus cylinder with the axis near the 180 meridian. An Rx that corrects for against the rule astigmatism might look like +3.00 −1.00 ×085. In this case more plus power is required near the 90 meridian than near the 180 meridian to correct both major meridian powers.

Astigmatism is said to be ***oblique astigmatism*** if the steepest meridian is more than 30 degrees away from the horizontal or the vertical meridians. Examples of this are the prescriptions −2.00 +1.00 ×055 and +1.50 −0.50 ×132.

When contact lenses are being fitted, an instrument called the ***keratometer*** is used to determine the curvature near the center of the cornea. The readings are written in diopters and are typically called the "K readings." An example of a K reading is 44.00 @ 180 and 45.00 @ 90. This K reading indicates that on the horizontal meridian the cornea has a dioptric power (in air) of +44.00D and on the vertical meridian it has a dioptric power of +45.00D. Therefore the vertical meridian is steeper than the horizontal meridian and the astigmatism (assuming the crystalline lens is spherical) is with the rule. If the power of +44.00 gives a focus on the retina for this particular eye, the horizontal meridian does not require any correction but the vertical meridian requires a correction of −1.00D. Thus the Rx for this eye would be pl −1.00 ×180.

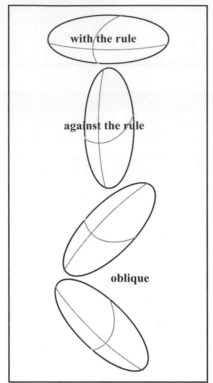

Many auto refractors now indicate the K readings along with the Rx.

To determine whether an Rx corrects for with the rule or against the rule astigmatism, look at the written prescription and the sign and axis of the cylinder.

WITH THE RULE, AGAINST THE RULE, AND OBLIQUE ASTIGMATISM

WITH THE RULE (WR) ASTIGMATISM
Minus cylinder form, axis within 30 degrees of the 180 meridian, *or*
Plus cylinder form, axis within 30 degrees of the 90 meridian
AGAINST THE RULE (AR) ASTIGMATISM
Minus cylinder form, axis within 30 degrees of the 90 meridian, *or*
Plus cylinder form, axis within 30 degrees of the 180 meridian
OBLIQUE (O) ASTIGMATISM
Cylinder axis from 31 to 59 degrees, *or*
Cylinder axis from 121 to 149 degrees

You may find it easier to remember the peacock's tail, which requires that the Rx be in *minus cylinder form.*

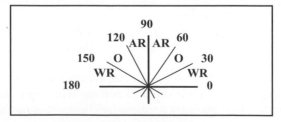

Optical Formulas Tutorial

Note: The term "with the rule" comes from the fact that the majority of astigmatic people have the steepest meridian on the vertical direction of the cornea.

EXAMPLES:

3-41. +3.00 −1.00 ×050   Oblique

3-42. +3.00 −1.00 ×155   With the rule

3-43. +3.00 +1.00 ×003   Against the rule

3-44. +3.00 +1.00 ×130   Oblique

EXERCISES:

Determine whether the following prescriptions correct for with the rule, against the rule, or oblique astigmatism.

98. −1.00 −1.00 ×180   _____

99. −0.50 −2.00 ×050   _____

100. −0.50 +2.00 ×080   _____

101. +0.75 − 1.50 ×110   _____

102. +2.00 +0.50 ×090   _____

103. −1.25 −0.75 ×130   _____

104. +1.00 +3.00 ×115   _____

105. −2.37 +1.50 ×070   _____

106. −1.00 +0.75 ×140   _____

107. −1.62 −1.75 ×065   _____

POWER IN OBLIQUE MERIDIANS

We learned that a cylinder exerts all of its power 90 degrees from its axis and exerts no power along its axis. The approximate power of a lens in any particular meridian varies between the powers in the two major meridians.

In optics, we often need to know the approximate power of a lens in a meridian other than its axis. For example, this information is needed when determining how much prism has been created when the pupillary distance is incorrect, when finding how much to move the lens in order to include prescribed prism, or in determining the amount of vertical imbalance in a pair of bifocals. All these subjects are covered in this book.

To find the approximate power of a lens in any meridian on the lens, use the ***oblique meridian formula:***

$$D_T = (\sin a)^2 \, D_C + D_S$$

where:
D_T = total power in the desired meridian
a = angle between the axis in the Rx and the meridian we want
D_C = power of the cylinder in the Rx
D_S = power of the sphere in the Rx

Look at the diagram on p. 68. The powers of the two major meridians are the two distances at which light is brought to a line focus. A piece of film between these two distances would show a blurred and distorted image, not a sharp line image. When the lensmeter is used, two powers give clearly focused lines and the powers between result in blurred images. Although we routinely refer to the "power" on a meridian other than the axis of the Rx, keep in mind that the lens does not *actually* have that power at that meridian.

As an alternative to using the formula, memorize the following:

- A cylinder exerts 100% of its power 90 degrees from its axis.
- A cylinder exerts 75% of its power 60 degrees from its axis.
- A cylinder exerts 50% of its power 45 degrees from its axis.
- A cylinder exerts 25% of its power 30 degrees from its axis.
- A cylinder exerts 0% of its power on axis.

Below is a step-by-step process to determine the power on the desired meridian:

1. Find the difference between the axis of the Rx and the meridian required. The order in which you subtract does not matter. Make sure you punch the ▢ so the calculator does the subtraction.

2. Punch the **sin** key (and then the ▢ for Type B calculators).

3. Punch the $\mathbf{x^2}$ key (and then the ▢ for Type B calculators). This intermediate number is the **percent of the cylinder** in decimal form that will be in effect at the required meridian.

4. Multiply times the amount of the cylinder. This intermediate number is the **amount of the cylinder** that will be in effect at the required meridian.

5. Add the result to the sphere power.

EXAMPLES:

3-45. What is the approximate total power along the vertical (90) meridian for the Rx −1.00 −2.00 ×060?

$D_T = ?$ $D_T = (\sin a)^2 D_C + D_S$
$D_S = -1.00D$ $D_T = [\sin (90 - 60)]^2 (-2.00) + (-1.00)$
$D_C = -2.00D$ $D_T = (0.25) (-2.00) + (-1.00)$
$a = 90 - 60 = 30$ $D_T = (-0.50) + (-1.00)$
$\mathbf{D_T = -1.50D}$

Alternatively, the desired meridian is 30 degrees from the axis of the Rx. The cylinder exerts 25% of its power 30 degrees away; 25% of −2.00D is −0.50. Adding −0.50 to the sphere power of −1.00 gives −1.50D.

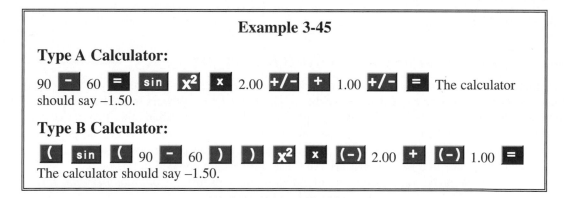

Example 3-45

Type A Calculator:

90 **−** 60 **=** **sin** $\mathbf{x^2}$ **x** 2.00 **+/−** **+** 1.00 **+/−** **=** The calculator should say −1.50.

Type B Calculator:

(**sin** **(** 90 **−** 60 **)** **)** $\mathbf{x^2}$ **x** **(−)** 2.00 **+** **(−)** 1.00 **=**
The calculator should say −1.50.

3-46. What is the approximate total power on the horizontal meridian for the Rx +2.25 −1.00 ×060?
180 − 60 = 120; or 60 to 0 is 60. Using either 60 or 120 for the angle α will give the correct result.
$\mathbf{D_T} = (\sin 60)^2 (-1.00) + (+2.25)$
    $= (0.75) (-1.00) + (+2.25)$
    $= (-0.75) + (+2.25)$
    $\mathbf{= +1.50D}$
Or, 75% of the cylinder is in effect 60 degrees from the axis; 75% of −1.00 is −0.75; +2.25 −0.75 is +1.50D.

3-47. What is the approximate total power of a −4.50 −2.50 ×125 lens on the horizontal meridian?
180 − 125 = 55 degrees

$D_T = (\sin 55)^2 (-2.50) + (-4.50)$
 $= (0.67)(-2.50) + (-4.50)$
 $= (-1.68) + (-4.50)$
 $= \mathbf{-6.18D}$

The shortcut is not usable in this case, but do check what the answer should be close to by noticing that 55 degrees is close to 60 degrees, so just under 75% of the cylinder is in effect, which comes to –1.87 DC. The total at 60 degrees away would be –6.37D. Our answer is just a little less than that, which is what we would expect.

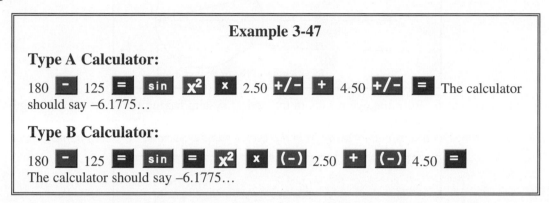

In Appendix 5 is a table with a key that can be memorized for finding the approximate power on a meridian in 5-degree increments. This table may be useful when a calculator is not available.

Note: We round the answers to this formula to two decimal places, not to one-eighth diopter steps. This is an intermediate formula; the answer to it will be used in another formula, so extra rounding now will bring in errors later. This is not a power that will be recorded in a wearer's records or ordered from a laboratory.

Note: This is a common but simplistic concept used for calculating prism, which will be covered in Section IV of this text. The approximate "power" on a meridian other than the major meridian (either the axis of the Rx or the meridian that is 90 degrees from the axis of the meridian) is useful only for prism calculations.

EXERCISES: (Round to hundredths of a diopter.)

108. What is the approximate total power in the horizontal meridian for the Rx
 –2.00 +3.00 ×045?

109. What is the approximate total power in the vertical meridian for the Rx
 –4.00 –2.00 ×180?

110. What is the approximate total power in the 140-degree meridian for the Rx
 +3.00 –1.00 ×080?

111. How much *cylinder power* is in effect along the 35-degree meridian in the Rx
 –2.50 +4.00 ×065?

112. What is the approximate total power on the 180 meridian of the Rx
 +6.00 –1.50 ×112?

113. What is the approximate total power on the 90 meridian for the Rx
 –10.25 +3.50 ×62?

———— VERTEX DISTANCE AND EFFECTIVE POWER ————

In any optical system, a lens effectively gains in plus power as it moves away from the rest of the system. This effective gain in plus power is the basis for focusable camera lenses. A plus lens placed in front of an eye becomes part of an optical system. The plus lens will *effectively* become stronger as it moves away from the eye because the total power of the lens plus the eye becomes stronger. The plus lens will *effectively* become weaker as it moves toward the eye because the total power of the lens plus the eye becomes weaker. Even though the lens itself does not change, the ***effective power*** of the lens changes based on its distance from the eye.

In the diagram below the plus lens is the correct power and distance away from the eye to focus parallel incident light rays on the retina. The focal length of the *optical system consisting of lens plus eye* is exactly the distance from the lens to the retina.

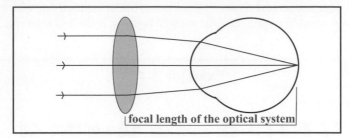

The same lens moved away from the eye results in the optical system having too short a focal length. The lens has *effectively* gained plus power. The effective power of the lens *with respect to the optical system comprising lens plus eye* is now too strong. *As a lens moves away from the eye, it gains plus power or loses minus power.*

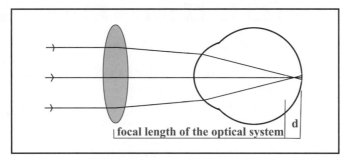

The same lens moved toward the eye results in the optical system having too long a focal length. The lens has *effectively* lost plus power. The effective power of the lens *with respect to the optical system comprising lens and eye* is now too weak. *As a lens moves toward the eye, it loses plus power or gains minus power.*

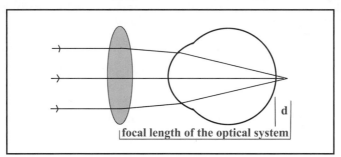

Similarly, the effective power of a minus lens will decrease as it is moved away from the eye. The minus lens is gaining plus, thus decreasing its effective power. As the minus lens moves toward the eye, it loses plus power, which effectively makes it a stronger minus lens.

The vertex distance is an indication of how far the ocular (or back) side of the lens is from the corneal apex. This is measured with a distometer.

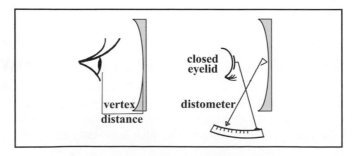

EFFECTIVE POWER

The effective power formula is

$$D_E = \frac{D_L}{1 + dD_L}$$

where:

D_E = new effective power
D_L = original lens power
d = change in vertex distance in meters

If the lens is moved toward the eye, d is positive. If the lens is moved away from the eye, d is negative. (We try to get people to choose glasses that will sit close to the eye, since this almost always improves the optics of the lens with respect to the eye. A good way to remember the sign of d is that closer is good—that is, positive.)

EXAMPLES:

3-48. The Rx reads OD –6.00D, refracted VD 10 mm. The glasses fit at 13 mm. If no adjustment is made to the prescription, what is the effective power of the –6.00D lens?

$d = -3$ mm $= -0.003$ meters (negative because the lens is moving away)

$$D_E = \frac{D_L}{1 + dD_L}$$

$$= \frac{-6.00}{1 + (-0.003)(-6.00)}$$

$$= \frac{-6.00}{1.018}$$

$$D_E = -5.89D$$

Example 3-48, Exact

Type A Calculator:

6.00 [+/-] [÷] [( ] 1 [+] 0.003 [+/-] [x] 6.00 [+/-] [ )] [=] The calculator should say –5.8939...

Type B Calculator:

[(-)] 6.00 [÷] [( ] 1 [+] [(-)] 0.003 [x] [(-)] 6.00 [ )] [=] The calculator should say –5.8939...

Many people use a formula that approximates the change in power.

$$\text{Change in power} = \frac{dD^2}{1000}$$

where d is measured in millimeters. In Example 3-48, this gives $(3)(6.00)^2/1000 = 0.108 = 0.11D$ change. Since the lens is a minus lens moving away from the wearer's eye, the lens gains plus power or loses minus power and the effective power is approximately $-6.00 + 0.11 = -5.89$.

Example 3-48, Approximate

Type A Calculator:

3 [x] 6.00 [x^2] [÷] 1000 [=] The calculator should say 0.108.

Type B Calculator:

3 [x] 6.00 [x^2] [÷] 1000 [=] The calculator should say 0.108.

3-49. The Rx reads OD +15.00D, refracted VD 14 mm. The wearer is to be fitted with contact lenses, vertex distance = 0 mm. If the fitter starts with a +15.00 contact lens, what effective power will the wearer experience?
d = 14 mm – 0 mm = 14 mm = +0.014 meters (positive because the lens is moving toward the eye)

$$D_E = \frac{D_L}{1 + dD_L} = \frac{+15.00}{1 + (+0.014)(+15.00)} = \frac{+15.00}{1.21}$$

D_E = +12.40D

In this example the approximation formula for the change in power is $dD^2/1000 = (14)(15)^2/1000 = 3.15D$ change in power. The lens is a plus lens moving toward the eye; thus it loses in plus power. The effective power is +15.00 –3.15 = +11.85D. This is not a very good approximation of the actual answer. The approximation formula is useful only for small vertex distance changes or low lens powers.

When calculating effective power for a toric lens, calculate the powers in the major meridians separately and then convert back to Rx notation. The optical cross is a good tool to use for this.

3-50. The Rx reads OD balance, OS –9.00 –2.50 ×154, refracted at 10 mm. The glasses fit at 8 mm. If no adjustment is made to the left lens prescription, what effective power will the wearer experience?
The powers in the major meridians are –9.00D and –11.50D. The lens is moving 2 mm toward the eye, so d = +2 mm = +0.002 m.
The effective power on the 154 meridian is:

$$D_E = \frac{D_L}{1 + dD_L} = \frac{-9.00}{1 + (+0.002)(-9.00)} = \frac{-9.00}{0.982}$$

D_E on the 154 meridian = –9.16D
The effective power on the 064 meridian is:

$$D_E = \frac{D_L}{1 + dD_L} = \frac{-11.50}{1 + (+0.002)(-11.50)} = \frac{-11.50}{0.977}$$

D_2 on the 064 meridian = –11.77D
Use the optical cross to see what is happening:

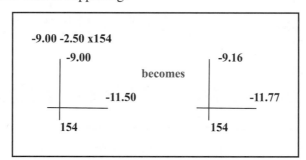

Removing the effective powers from the optical cross, the effective prescription is **–9.16 –2.61 ×154.**
Notice that if you performed the calculations on the –2.50 cylinder instead of the actual power in the 064 meridian, the effective cylinder amount would appear to be –2.51 rather than –2.61. This answer would underestimate the effect of moving the lens without compensating for the power change.

When determining the *actual effective power,* do not change to one-eighth diopter steps. Round to two decimal places. This is the power that the wearer will "see" if the Rx is made as written, based on where the glasses will sit on the face. This is an academic exercise and will not be used for anything. We are *not* going to order or make this lens, so we do not round the answer to one-eighth diopter steps.

EXERCISES: (Round to hundredths of a diopter.)

114. The Rx is OD –5.00D refracted at 10 mm VD
    OS –6.50D
What are the effective powers if this person is fitted with contact lenses of these powers? Current vertex distance is 0 mm.

Redo this exercise using the approximation formula. Note that because the power is "low," the approximation formula works for this example.

115. The Rx is OD +5.00 +2.00 ×090 refracted at 8 mm
     OS +6.00 +2.50 ×145

What is the effective power of the lenses if the glasses made of this prescription are worn with a vertex distance of 14 mm?

Note: Powers in the major meridians in the OD are +5.00D and +7.00D. Use the formula to find the effective power in each of these meridians, then convert back to the Rx notation. You may wish to use the optical cross. What are the major meridian powers in the OS?

Note: In this case the sphere amount becomes stronger, since it is a plus lens moving away from the face. At the same time the cylinder amount became stronger as well. If the cylinder amount changes, it will change in the same direction that the sphere changes. As a general rule, the cylinder amount will change if it is 2.00D or more and the cylinder amount will not change if it is 1.00D or less. If the cylinder amount is between 1.00D and 2.00D, it will change for (1) large VD changes or (2) high prescriptions.

COMPENSATED POWER

For high-power prescriptions that will be worn at a vertex distance other than the refracted distance, we must determine what power lens to order so that the wearer will be looking through the power intended by the prescriber. This is the *compensated* or *recomputed* power.

Three methods are used to calculate the power that should be ordered to compensate for worn vertex distance:

- Step-by-step method
- Full formula method
- Approximate formula method

STEP-BY-STEP METHOD

1. The diagrams on p. 78 show that the prescribed lens plus the eye globe gives a focal length that results in corrected vision. The lens with power D has a focal length of f = 1/D. (The fact that the eye changes this focal length for the eye and lens system does not need to be considered here.) If the Rx calls for +10.00 DS, for example, the lens-only focal length is:

$$f = 1/10 = 0.1 \text{ meter} = 100 \text{ mm}$$

2. The change in vertex distance changes the total focal length of the desired lens plus the eye system. When the lens is moved away from the eye, the focal length found in step 1 will increase by that difference. If the lens is moved toward the eye, the focal length found in step 1 will decrease by that difference. For the +10.00D lens, if the refracted vertex distance is 12 mm and the worn vertex distance is 9 mm, the lens is moved 3 mm toward the eye and the desired lens focal length would be:

$$100 - 3 = 97 \text{ mm}$$

3. The compensated power is found by use of the formula for focal length again, this time D = 1/f. In the example used here the desired focal length is 97 mm = 0.097 m, so the lens to be ordered is:

$$D = 1/f = 1/0.097 = +10.31 \text{ DS}$$

This answer is rounded to either +10.25 or +10.37 DS when the prescription is ordered from the laboratory and recorded in the refractionist's records.

FULL FORMULA METHOD

The compensated power formula is

$$D_C = \frac{D_L}{1 - dD_L}$$

where:

D_C = compensated power (what will be ordered)
D_L = original lens power
d = change in vertex distance in meters

If the lens is moved toward the eye, d is positive. If the lens is moved away from the eye, d is negative. The answer when this formula is used will be identical to the answer obtained by the step-by-step method.

EXAMPLES:

3-51. The Rx reads OD –6.00D, refracted VD 10 mm. The glasses fit at 13 mm. What power lens should be ordered so that the wearer will be looking through the power intended by the refractionist?

$$D_C = \frac{D_L}{1 - dD_L}$$

$$= \frac{-6.00}{1 - (-0.003)(-6.00)}$$

$$= \frac{-6.00}{0.982}$$

$D_E = -6.11D$ (order –6.12D)

Example 3-51, Exact

Type A Calculator:

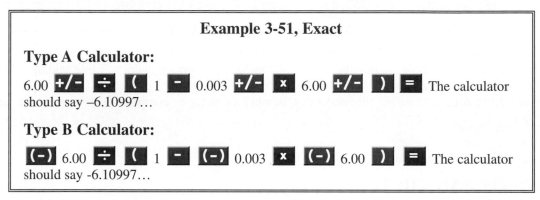

6.00 +/– ÷ (1 – 0.003 +/– × 6.00 +/–) = The calculator should say –6.10997…

Type B Calculator:

(–) 6.00 ÷ (1 – (–) 0.003 × (–) 6.00) = The calculator should say -6.10997…

Try the approximation formula change = dD^2/1000, where d is in mm. The result is (3)(6.00)^2/1000 = 0.108 = 0.11D. Since the lens is negative and is moving away from the eye, a stronger lens would be ordered, so the result is –6.00 – 0.11 = – 6.11D. Order –6.12D.

Example 3-51, Approximate

Type A Calculator:

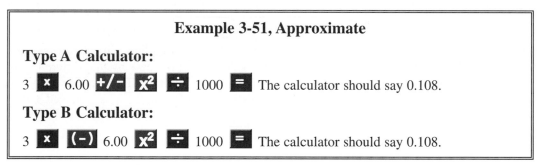

3 × 6.00 +/– x² ÷ 1000 = The calculator should say 0.108.

Type B Calculator:

3 × (–) 6.00 x² ÷ 1000 = The calculator should say 0.108.

When the step-by-step method is used:
f = 1/D = 1/(–6.00) = –0.16666 = –167 mm
The lens moves 3 mm away from the face, so the focal length must be longer. The new focal length is –0.1666 – 166.7 mm –(–3 mm) = –163.7 mm = 0.1637 meters.
New D = 1/f = 1/(0.164) = –6.11, which will be rounded to –6.12.

3-52. The Rx reads OS –9.00 –2.50 ×154, refracted at 10 mm. The glasses fit at 8 mm. What power lens should be ordered so that the wearer will be looking through the power intended by the refractionist? The powers in the major meridians are –9.00D and –11.50D. The lens is moving 2 mm toward the eye, so d = +2 mm = +0.002 m.
The compensated power on the 154 meridian is:

$$D_C = \frac{D_L}{1 - dD_L} = \frac{-9.00}{1 - (+0.002)(-9.00)} = \frac{-9.00}{1.018}$$

D_C on the 154 meridian = –8.84D

The compensated power on the 064 meridian is:

$$D_C = \frac{D_L}{1 - dD_L} = \frac{-11.50}{1 - (+0.002)(-11.50)} = \frac{-11.50}{1.023}$$

D_C on the 064 meridian = –11.24D

Using the optical cross to see what is happening:

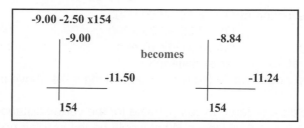

When the compensated powers are removed from the optical cross, the prescription becomes –8.84 –2.40 ×154, which changes to **–8.87 –2.37 ×154.** Notice that if you performed the calculations on the –2.50 cylinder rather than the actual power in the 064 meridian, the effective cylinder amount would appear to be –2.49 rather than –2.40 and would round to –2.50 cylinder. Using this answer would result in a prescription with too much cylinder power.

WHAT YOU REALLY NEED TO KNOW FOR COMPENSATED POWER

	LENS MOVES:	
	AWAY FROM EYE	**TOWARD EYE**
Plus lens	Order weaker lens	Order stronger lens
Minus lens	Order stronger lens	Order weaker lens

Note: The compensated power is changed to eighths of a diopter, but the effective power is not. The effective power is what the wearer is *actually seeing* if the lenses are ordered without compensation. The compensated power *will be made in the laboratory.* We change to eighths when we are actually going to order or make the lens. If the answer is halfway between two 1/8D increments, change to the next weaker 1/8D.

Note: When adjusting the prescription for vertex distance changes, in most states the optician may order a lens power that is compensated for worn vertex distance and therefore is different from the prescription written by the refractionist. It is good policy to call the refractionist and request permission to order the compensated power. The compensated power should be communicated so that it may be recorded in the wearer's records. When contact lenses are being fitted, permission from the refractionist is unnecessary because calculating compensating power is part of the contact lens fitting procedure.

APPROXIMATE FORMULA METHOD

As noted previously, the approximation formula is

$$\text{Change in power} = \frac{dD^2}{1000}$$

where *d is measured in mm.* For the example in the step-by-step method, the +10.00 lens is moved 3 mm closer to the eye. The approximate change is $(3)(10)^2/1000 = 0.30$ diopters. A plus lens moved toward the eye must be ordered as stronger, so the change in power of 0.30D would be added to the original lens power of +10.00, giving a compensated power of +10.30. The power rounded to one-eighth diopter steps would again be +10.25 or +10.37.

EXERCISES: (Change answers to eighths of a diopter.)

116. The Rx is OD –5.00D refracted at 10 mm VD
        OS –6.50D

    If the Rx is to be dispensed as contact lenses, what contact lens powers would you use to *start* the fitting? (Contact lenses have a vertex distance of 0.)

117. The Rx is OD +5.00 +2.00 ×090 refracted at 8 mm
OS +6.00 +2.50 ×145
What lens powers would be ordered for glasses that are to be worn with a vertex distance of 14 mm?

118. Demonstrate for yourself that the compensated power formula gives the same answer as the step-by-step method for a +10.00 DS lens moved 3 mm toward the eye.

119. A myope receives a prescription of OD −6.50 −2.00 ×090
OS −8.25 −0.25 ×090
refracted VD 10 mm
The glasses chosen are at 13 mm vertex distance.
  a. Through what effective power would the wearer be looking if the above prescription were ordered as is?
  b. What prescription could be ordered to compensate for the vertex distance?
  c. The wearer decided to try contact lenses. What would be the *starting point* for the lens power? (Change the answers to the nearest 0.25D. In an actual fitting situation the result would be adjusted based on what is available in this power range in the contact lens series of choice.)
  d. The wearer's daughter wants her mother to have "nice, big, stylish frames" that fit at 17 mm vertex distance. What power would be ordered for these glasses?

BACK AND FRONT VERTEX POWER

The nominal power of a lens is the sum of the two surface powers. When a lens is thick, the nominal power is not accurate. If the surface powers are substantially different from each other, the order of the surfaces, as well as the thickness of the lens, will affect the power of the lens.

The **back vertex power** is the power measured at the back of the ophthalmic lens, is what the wearer sees, and is what is normally measured in the lensmeter. In a meniscus lens having one convex side and one concave side, we consider the front of the lens to be the convex side of the lens.

The formula for the *back vertex power* of the lens is

$$D_B = \frac{D_1}{1 - \left(\frac{t}{n}\right)D_1} + D_2$$

where:
D_1 = front surface power
D_2 = back surface power
t = thickness between the front and back vertices of the lens, in meters
n = index of refraction for the lens material

Note: The back vertex of the lens is the point where the axis of the lens intersects the back surface of the lens. The focal length based on this definition of back vertex power is the distance from the back vertex of the lens to the secondary focal point.

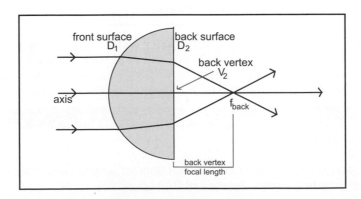

Optical Formulas Tutorial

The *front vertex power*, also called the *neutralizing power*, is the power found when the ray is incident first on the back side of the lens. Contact lens manufacturers use the front vertex power. For contact lenses it is listed as the *FVP*. To measure the front vertex power in the lensmeter, place the lens with the front surface toward the lens stop rather than the back surface. For a bifocal lens we use the difference between the distance and near front vertex powers to determine the add power of the segment when it is molded or fused to the front surface of the lens.

The formula for the *front vertex power* of the lens is

$$D_F = \frac{D_2}{1 - \left(\frac{t}{n}\right)D_2} + D_1$$

where:

D_1 = front surface power
D_2 = back surface power
t = thickness between the front and back vertices of the lens, in meters
n = index of refraction for the lens material

Note: The front vertex of the lens is the point where the axis of the lens intersects the front surface of the lens. The focal length based on this definition of front vertex power is the distance from the front vertex of the lens to the first focal point.

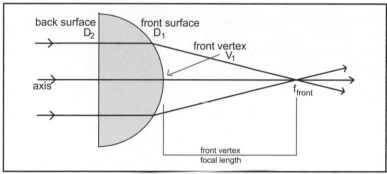

The diagrams above show that for the back vertex power the ray enters D_1 first, travels the thickness of the lens, and exits D_2. The thickness of the lens becomes important after the ray enters the front surface of the lens, so the back vertex power formula adjusts the power of the front surface. Similarly, the front vertex power formula adjusts the power of the back surface. The *equivalent power* of the lens is determined by use of the formula

$$D = D_1 + D_2 - (t/n)D_1D_2$$

The equivalent power is actually the way to locate the principal planes for a thick lens. This is discussed in Section VI. A variation on the equivalent power formula is sometimes used for an *approximation* of the back and front vertex powers:

$$D_B \approx D_1 + D_2 + (t/n)(D_1)^2$$
$$D_F \approx D_1 + D_2 + (t/n)(D_2)^2$$

EXAMPLE:

3-53. Find the front and back vertex powers of a thick lens made of CR-39 (n = 1.498) with surface curves of +12.00 and –3.00 and a center thickness of 14 mm.

$$D_B = \frac{D_1}{1 - \left(\frac{t}{n}\right)D_1} + D_2$$

$$= \frac{+12.00}{1 - \left(\frac{0.014}{1.498}\right)(+12.00)} + (-3.00)$$

$$= \frac{+12.00}{0.8879} - 3.00$$

$$= +13.52 - 3.00$$

$$\mathbf{D_B = +10.52D}$$

Example 3-53, Back Vertex Power

Type A Calculator:

$(\quad 12.00 \quad \div \quad (\quad 1 \quad - \quad (\quad 0.014 \quad \div \quad 1.498 \quad \times \quad 12.00 \quad) \quad) \quad) \quad + \quad 3.00 \quad +/- \quad =$

The calculator should say 10.5157…

Type B Calculator:

$(\quad 12.00 \quad \div \quad (\quad (\quad 1 \quad - \quad (\quad 0.014 \quad \div \quad 1.498 \quad \times \quad 12.00 \quad) \quad) \quad) \quad + \quad (-) \quad 3.00$

$=$ The calculator should say 10.5157.

$$D_F = \frac{D_2}{1 - \left(\frac{t}{n}\right)D_2} + D_1$$

$$= \frac{-3.00}{1 - \left(\frac{0.014}{1.498}\right)(-3.00)} + (+12.00)$$

$$= \frac{-3.00}{1.0280} + 12.00$$

$$= -2.92 + 12.00$$

$$\mathbf{D_F = +9.08D}$$

Approximation formula:

$D_B \approx D_1 + D_2 + (t/n)(D_1)^2$
  $= +12.00 + (-3.00) + (0.014/1.498)(+12.00)^2$

$\mathbf{D_B} \approx +9.00 + 1.35 = \mathbf{+10.35D}$

$D_F \approx D_1 + D_2 + (t/n)(D_2)^2$
  $= +12.00 + (-3.00) + (0.014/1.498)(-3.00)^2$

$\mathbf{D_F} \approx +9.00 + 0.08 = \mathbf{+9.08D}$

Note: The lens will read +10.52 in the lensmeter, and this is what the wearer will experience (ignoring vertex distance). The front and back vertex powers are not changed to one-eighth diopter steps because they are actual powers: they will not be ordered from a laboratory or noted in the wearer's records.

EXERCISES: (Round to hundredths of a diopter.)

What are the nominal power, back vertex power, and front vertex power of the following lenses?

120. $D_1 = +6.50$
  $D_2 = -6.50$
  $t = 2$ mm
  $n = 1.50$

121. $D_1 = +10.25$
  $D_2 = -5.25$
  $t = 6$ mm
  $n = 1.60$

122. $D_1 = +12.50$
  $D_2 = -2.50$
  $t = 9$ mm
  $n = 1.586$

The questions with an asterisk (*) in front of the question number are advanced questions. They are not likely to be on the ABO exam but might be on the ABOM exam or the COT exam.

The questions are not presented in the order of the subjects in the section. Some questions cannot be answered directly from the text and will require thought.

1. When the path of light is drawn through a lens, the primary focal point of a converging lens is
   a. to the right of the lens.
   b. to the left of the lens.
   c. at the point where the rays actually emerge from the lens.
   d. at the point where the incident ray enters the lens.

2. During a refraction the desired lens power is determined to be +10.00 with a vertex distance of 14 mm. The optician selects a frame that positions the back surface of the lens 9 mm from the cornea. The compensated lens power would be:
   a. +9.50.
   b. +10.00.
   c. +10.50.
   d. +11.00.

3. An optical cross has a power of +3.12 on the 017 meridian and +1.37 on the 107 meridian. One of the possible ways to write the prescription of this lens is
   a. +4.50 +1.75 ×017.
   b. +1.37 +1.75 ×107.
   c. +3.12 −1.75 ×107.
   d. +1.37 −1.75 ×017.

4. The power on the horizontal meridian of the Rx −3.00 −2.50 ×125 is
   a. −4.68.
   b. −5.50.
   c. −3.52.
   d. −4.25.

5. The lens diagrammed below is a(n) _____ lens.
   a. equi-convex
   b. equi-concave
   c. plano-convex
   d. plano-concave

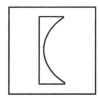

6. Calculate the total power in the 060 meridian for the prescription −4.37 −1.00 ×060.
   a. −5.37D
   b. −5.12D
   c. −4.87D
   d. −4.37D

7. The Rx −3.50 +1.00 ×110 is an example of
   a. simple myopic astigmatism.
   b. mixed astigmatism.
   c. presbyopic astigmatism.
   d. compound myopic astigmatism.

8. What is the focal length of a +4.75D lens?
   a. 2.1 m
   b. 2.1 cm
   c. 21 mm
   d. 8.3 inches

9. The spherical equivalent of the prescription +2.00 −0.50 ×175 is:
   a. +2.00D.
   b. +1.75D.
   c. +1.50D.
   d. +1.25D.

10. A person with myopia has a best distance focus at 25 cm. What approximate lens power is required to allow the person to focus at "infinity"?
    a. −2.25D
    b. −4.25D
    c. −4.00D
    d. −5.00D

11. When a person is reading at 50 cm, how much accommodation is required?
    a. +5.00D
    b. +4.00D
    c. +3.00D
    d. +2.00D

12. An individual has been wearing a pair of eyeglasses (+12.00 sph OU) with adjustable pads for several months. The initial vertex distance was 12 mm. The person returns complaining that the vision is now worse than when the eyeglasses were first fit. Which of the following would be your first course of action?
    a. Because of the decreased vision, refer the person back to the refractionist.
    b. Redo the lenses and match the original base curves.
    c. Recheck the vertex distance and adjust the frame back to a vertex distance of 12 mm.
    d. Remake the lenses.

13. What is the dioptric power difference for the following prescription?
OD +0.75
OS –0.50
   a. 0.25D
   b. 0.75D
   c. 1.25D
   d. 1.50D
14. The spherical equivalent of the prescription –1.75 –1.50 ×065 is:
   a. –1.75D.
   b. –2.25D.
   c. –2.50D.
   d. –3.00D.
15. What is the dioptric power difference for the following prescription?
OD –0.37
OS +0.25
   a. 0.25D
   b. 0.62D
   c. 0.87D
   d. 1.00D
16. Which of the following principles describes how lenses work?
   a. vergence
   b. refraction
   c. reflection
   d. dispersion
17. When a plus lens is moved away from the eye, its effective power:
   a. increases.
   b. decreases.
   c. does not change.
   d. creates prism.
18. A lens shape containing one convex surface and one concave surface is called a(n) _____ lens.
   a. equi-convex
   b. bi-convex
   c. flat
   d. meniscus
19. When rays diverge on leaving a lens, the image of the object
   a. is a virtual image.
   b. is a real image.
   c. forms at the primary focal point of the lens.
   d. does not exist.
20. An incident ray traveling parallel to the axis of a convex lens impacts the lens at a distance from the midpoint. When emerging from the lens, the ray will travel obliquely to the axis of the lens
   a. until it crosses the axis behind the focal point.
   b. and never cross the axis.
   c. and cross at the focal point.
   d. and form a virtual image at the focal point.

21. The lens diagrammed below is a(n) _____ lens.
   a. equi-convex
   b. equi-concave
   c. bi-concave
   d. bi-convex

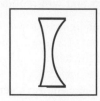

22. The focal length of a +3.75D sphere is:
   a. 21 cm.
   b. 27 cm.
   c. 36 cm.
   d. 57 cm.
23. Using a standard lens clock, you measure the lens front surface power as +4.00D and the back surface as –8.00D. The nominal power of this lens is:
   a. +4.00D.
   b. –4.00D.
   c. +12.00D.
   d. –12.00D.
24. If the front surface power is +3.00D, what back surface power would be used to create a –7.00D lens?
   a. –7.00D
   b. +7.00D
   c. –4.00D
   d. –10.00D
25. A +5.00D lens has a focal length of 20 cm. The object being viewed is located at infinity. Using the standard drawing, the image is formed
   a. at infinity.
   b. at 20 feet.
   c. 20 cm to the right of the lens.
   d. 20 cm to the left of the lens.
26. Transpose the prescription –1.87 +0.62 ×163.
   a. –1.25 –0.62 ×073
   b. –2.50 –0.62 ×073
   c. –1.25 –0.62 ×063
   d. –2.50 –0.62 ×063
27. A convex surface made from a material with an index of refraction of 1.523 has a radius of curvature of 10 cm. What is the surface power?
   a. –1.50
   b. +1.50
   c. +5.23
   d. –5.23

28. On a converging meniscus lens
    a. the back vertex power is always stronger than the front vertex power.
    b. the back vertex power is always weaker than the front vertex power.
    c. the nominal power is stronger than either of the front or back vertex powers.
    d. the stronger vertex power depends on whether or not the lenses are made in corrected curve form.

29. Which of the following statements best describes the power of a cylinder along its axis?
    a. There is no cylinder power in effect along the cylinder axis.
    b. The full power of the cylinder is in effect along the cylinder axis.
    c. Only half the cylinder power is in effect along the axis.
    d. Three-quarters of the cylinder power is in effect along the axis.

30. If a lens has a flat front surface and a concave back surface, it has _____ power.
    a. no
    b. minus
    c. plus
    d. converging

31. The lens diagrammed below is a(n) _____ lens.
    a. equi-convex
    b. bi-convex
    c. flat
    d. meniscus

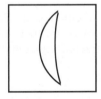

32. An optical cross has a power of –2.00 at the 157 meridian and +0.25 at the 067 meridian. The prescription of this lens is:
    a. +0.25 –2.25 ×157
    b. –2.00 +2.25 ×067
    c. –2.00 +0.25 ×067
    d. +0.25 –2.25 ×067

33. A person with presbyopia complains about difficulties reading at 20 inches with a +2.50 add. Of the following, which is the first potential explanation to discuss?
    a. The power is not strong enough to bring the image into focus at this distance.
    b. A +2.50 add is best used at 40 inches.
    c. A +2.50 add is appropriate for this distance. The patient should be reexamined.
    d. The focal length of a +2.50 add is approximately 16 inches.

34. Lenses form images by:
    a. always converging light.
    b. always diverging light.
    c. diffracting light.
    d. refracting light.

35. The prescription +0.87 –0.87 ×125 indicates a refractive error known as:
    a. simple hyperopic astigmatism.
    b. compound hyperopic astigmatism.
    c. simple myopic astigmatism.
    d. compound myopic astigmatism.

36. A lens is to be made with a power of –5.25. If the front surface is chosen to be +2.25, what is the nominal back surface power?
    a. –7.50
    b. –6.00
    c. –3.00
    d. +3.00

37. Plus lenses will show _____ movement.
    a. with
    b. against
    c. scissors
    d. no

38. When wearing strong plus lenses, the wearer is experiencing
    a. corrected curve power.
    b. nominal power.
    c. front vertex power.
    d. back vertex power.

39. When the path of light is drawn through a lens, the primary focal point of a diverging lens is
    a. to the right of the lens.
    b. to the left of the lens.
    c. at the point where the rays actually emerge from the lens.
    d. at the point where the incident ray enters the lens.

40. The prescription +1.25 –1.00 ×090 indicates a refractive error known as
    a. simple hyperopic astigmatism.
    b. compound hyperopic astigmatism.
    c. simple myopic astigmatism.
    d. compound myopic astigmatism.

41. If you hold a magnifying glass 40 mm away from a combustible material and the small point of light coming through the lens burns an area, the power of the lens in diopters is
    a. +0.25D.
    b. +2.50D.
    c. +25.00D.
    d. +250D.

42. The prescription +0.50 −0.75 × 045 indicates a refractive error known as
    a. hyperopia.
    b. compound hyperopic astigmatism.
    c. mixed astigmatism.
    d. compound myopic astigmatism.
43. When a high minus powered lens is moved closer to the eye, the compensated power must
    a. be increased.
    b. be decreased.
    c. remain the same.
    d. change the cylinder axis.
44. The prescription +1.00 +0.25 ×180 is an example of
    a. with the rule astigmatism.
    b. against the rule astigmatism.
    c. mixed astigmatism.
    d. axial hyperopia.
45. Which of the following lenses contains no power in the 90-degree meridian?
    a. −2.50 +2.50 ×180
    b. −2.50 +2.50 ×090
    c. −2.50 +2.50 ×045
    d. −2.50 +2.50 ×135
46. Given the Rx −0.75 +1.50 ×005, how much of the +1.50 cylinder is in effect at axis 140?
    a. +0.50D
    b. +0.75D
    c. +1.00D
    d. +1.50D
47. What is the approximate total power in the vertical meridian for the prescription +3.62 −1.50 ×057?
    a. +2.87D
    b. +3.18D
    c. +3.58D
    d. +3.60D
48. A virtual image is
    a. an image in which no light rays pass through the image.
    b. always formed by a convex lens.
    c. an image that results from converging rays.
    d. formed when light rays meet at the image.
49. Calculate the dioptric power difference in the vertical meridian for the following prescription:
    OD −2.00 −1.00 ×030
    OS −1.00 −1.00 ×120
    a. 1.00D
    b. 1.25D
    c. 1.50D
    d. 1.75D
50. Transpose the prescription +1.25 −0.37 ×041.
    a. +0.87 +0.37 ×151
    b. +1.62 +0.37 ×151
    c. +1.12 +0.37 ×131
    d. +0.87 +0.37 ×131

51. Which of the following instruments is used to determine vertex distance?
    a. lens caliper
    b. distometer
    c. millimeter rule
    d. lensmeter
52. _____ lenses are thicker in the middle than the edges.
    a. Equi-convex
    b. Equi-concave
    c. Bi-concave
    d. Plano-concave
53. OD −12.00 −2.50 ×135
    OS −11.00 −2.00 ×045
    The refracted distance is 14 mm, and the eyeglasses fit at a vertex distance of 10 mm. Using the above prescription, calculate the compensated power of the lenses that would be ordered.
    a. OD −11.50 −2.25 ×135
       OS −10.50 −1.87 ×045
    b. OD −12.62 −2.75 ×135
       OS −11.50 −2.25 ×045
    c. OD −12.62 −2.50 ×135
       OS −11.50 −2.00 ×045
    d. OD −11.50 −2.50 ×135
       OS −10.50 −2.00 ×045
54. Minus lenses will show _____ movement.
    a. with
    b. against
    c. scissors
    d. no
55. Using the prescription OU −9.00D, calculate the compensated power for beginning a contact lens fitting if the refracted vertex distance is 12 mm.
    a. −9.87D
    b. −9.50D
    c. −8.75D
    d. −8.00D
56. Spherocylindrical (compound) ophthalmic lenses usually have
    a. spherical surfaces only.
    b. cylindrical surfaces only.
    c. one cylindrical surface and one spherical surface.
    d. all of the above.
57. When glasses are placed in the lensmeter in the normal position, with the back or concave surface toward the lens stop and the front or convex surface toward the optician, the lensmeter reading will give the
    a. back vertex power.
    b. front vertex power.
    c. nominal power.
    d. corrected curve power.

*58. A plastic bi-concave lens has an index of refraction of 1.50. The radii of curvature of the surfaces are 25 cm and 22 cm. What is the focal length of the lens?
   a. 4.3 cm
   b. 7.8 cm
   c. 14.5 cm
   d. 23.4 cm

*59. A patient brings you a prescription written in the following form:
OU −1.25 × 85 ⊃ −0.75 ×175
What is the prescription in minus cylinder form?
   a. −1.25 −0.50 ×175
   b. −1.25 −0.75 ×175
   c. −0.75 −0.50 ×175
   d. −0.75 −0.50 ×085

*60. When a lens is being hand neutralized, no movement of the image occurs on the horizontal meridian when the lens is combined with a −1.75D lens and no movement of the image occurs on the vertical meridian with an added −1.50 lens. The Rx of the unknown lens is
   a. +1.75 +1.50 ×180.
   b. +1.75 +3.25 ×180.
   c. −1.75 −1.50 ×180.
   d. +1.75 −1.50 ×180.

*61. A lens made from Trivex (n = 1.53) has a front surface power of +8.25, a back surface power of −4.25, and a thickness of 5.5 mm. The back vertex power of this lens is
   a. +3.76D
   b. +4.00D.
   c. +4.06D.
   d. +4.25D.

*62. For the Rx +2.00 −1.00 ×090 the circle of least confusion is located at
   a. 33.3 cm.
   b. 50.0 cm.
   c. 66.7 cm.
   d. 100 cm.

*63. The prescription +1.75 +0.75 ×140 may also be written as
   a. +2.50 ×140 ⊃ +1.75 ×050.
   b. +2.50 ×050 ⊃ +1.75 ×140.
   c. +1.75 ×140 ⊃ +0.75 ×050.
   d. +1.75 ×050 ⊃ +0.75 ×140.

*64. The image movement on the 45 meridian of an unknown lens is neutralized when it is sandwiched with a +0.50 lens. When the same lens is sandwiched with only a −0.75 lens, the movement is neutralized on the 135 meridian. The Rx of the unknown lens is
   a. +0.75 −1.25 ×045.
   b. +0.50 −0.75 ×045.
   c. −0.50 +0.75 ×045.
   d. −0.50 +1.25 ×045.

*65. Which of the following best describes against the rule astigmatism?
   a. The astigmatism may be corrected by placement of a minus cylinder at 180 degrees.
   b. The astigmatism may be corrected by placement of a minus cylinder at 90 degrees.
   c. Against the rule astigmatism is easier to correct with contact lenses.
   d. Against the rule astigmatism is always associated with the most common type of astigmatism.

*66. A lens made from a 1.66 index plastic has a center thickness of 4.8 mm, a front surface power of +12.25D, and a back surface power of −4.75D. When the lens is placed in the normal position in the lensmeter, it will show a power of about
   a. +6.50D.
   b. +7.50D.
   c. +8.00D.
   d. +12.75D.

*67. Which of the following is a false statement?
   a. The interval of Sturm is formed by a sphero-cylinder lens.
   b. The interval of Sturm is located at the focal plane nearest the lens.
   c. Images at the distance of the circle of least confusion are undistorted.
   d. The circle of least confusion is located in the interval of Sturm.

SECTION IV – PRISMS

PRISM DEFINITIONS

A prism is formed by two flat surfaces inclined at an angle to one another. We usually think of a prism as a transparent wedge.

A prism has a base and an apex. The angle made at the apex is called the *apical angle,* the *apex angle,* the *refracting angle,* or the *prism angle*. Any of these terms may be used.

A prism has no focal power. A prism deviates the light passing through it but does not change its vergence. Light passing through a prism undergoes refraction at both surfaces and exits refracted or *deviated* toward the base.

When a beam of light passes through a prism, the three Ds occur: *dispersion, displacement,* and *deviation*.

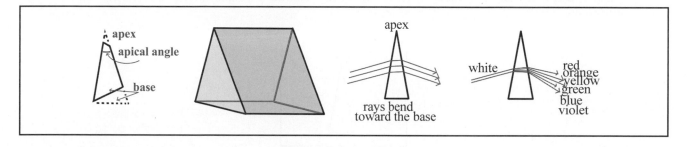

DISPERSION OF LIGHT BY A PRISM

Dispersion is defined as the breaking up of white light into its component or *spectral* colors. Different wavelengths of white light travel at the same speed in air but travel at different speeds in other materials.

Red light travels faster than violet light in transparent materials other than air. When a ray of light enters a prism, each of its component colors is refracted a different amount at each of the prism's surfaces. The blue end of the spectrum is refracted more than the red end because the blue waves are slowed more than the red waves. Use the name **ROY G. BIV** to help remember the colors from longest wavelength and least refraction to shortest wavelength and most refraction.

OBJECT DISPLACEMENT BY A PRISM

An object viewed through a prism appears to be in a different place than if viewed without the prism. The object always appears to be *displaced* toward the apex of the prism.

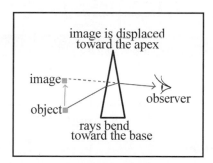

Because the image seen through the prism is displaced toward the apex, the eye turns toward the apex to view the image. An eye can be made to turn up, down, in, or out by placement of a prism in front of it. A *relieving* or *therapeutic* prism is placed in front of an eye with a weak or paralyzed muscle to displace the image in the same direction that the eye turns. In this case the base of the prism is placed over the weak muscle, sending the image in the same direction that the eye is turning. An *adverse prism* or *exercising prism* is placed with the apex over the weak muscle to make it work harder. This technique may be used during eye exercises designed to strengthen the weak muscle.

The human eye is sensitive to small amounts of prism. Unwanted or unintentional prism will result in discomfort for the wearer.

─── PRISM POWER ───

There are four different prism power units:

- Apical or refracting angle (discussed above)
- Deviating angle
- Centrad
- Prism diopter (the unit used by the optical industry and defined in ANSI Z80.1–1995)

DEVIATING ANGLE

The *deviating angle* is similar to the angle of deviation used when we discussed refraction in Section III. The deviating angle, $\angle d$, is the angle formed by the emerging ray with the path that the ray would have taken had the prism not been present.

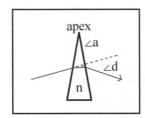

The deviating angle is related to the apical angle, $\angle a$, by the approximation formula

$$\angle d = \angle a \,(n - 1)$$

where:
$\angle d$ = deviating angle
$\angle a$ = apical angle
n = index of refraction of the prism material

This formula is an approximation for small $\angle a$ and $\angle d$ and is most accurate when the incident ray is close to perpendicular to the prism.

The formula can be rewritten as

$$\angle a = \frac{\angle d}{(n - 1)}$$

EXAMPLES:

4-1. A prism made of crown glass (n = 1.523) has an apical angle of 5 degrees. What is the angle of deviation?
$\angle d = 5 \,(1.523 - 1) = 5 \times 0.523 = 2.6$ degrees

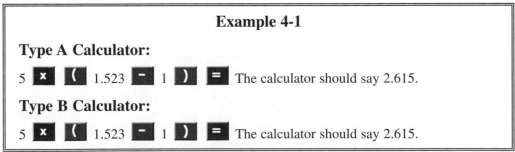

Note: Since you probably do not need the calculator to help you subtract 1 from n, you may just multiply 5×0.523 without the parenthesis.

4-2. A crown glass prism is needed that will change the path of incoming light rays by 12 degrees. What apical angle does the prism need?

$\angle$a = 12/(1.523 – 1) = 12/0.523 = 22.9 degrees

EXERCISES: (Round angles to the nearest one tenth.)

1. What is the approximate angle of deviation for a flint glass (n = 1.70) prism with an apical angle of 17 degrees?

2. A prism deviates light by 18 degrees and is made of CR-39 (n = 1.498). What is the apical angle of the prism?

3. A prism with a 10.0-degree apical angle deviates incident light by 6.0 degrees. What is the index of refraction of the prism material?

CENTRAD

The *centrad* measures the amount that a prism displaces an image. When we look at an object and then move a prism in front of our eyes, the image of the object "jumps" or moves a certain amount. How far the image appears to move depends on how far the object is from the prism and how strong the prism is.

When the prism displaces the image, the distance that the image moves can be traced out on a circle in which the radius is the distance between the object and the prism. The radian is a measurement for angles used instead of degrees by scientists and mathematicians. A centrad is one one-hundredth of a radian. If radians are used to measure the angle of deviation, $\angle$d, a one-centrad deviation for an object that is one meter from the prism would be equivalent to the image moving one one-hundredth of a meter *on the circumference of a circle.*

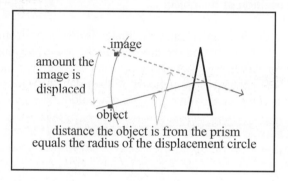

The centrad is the most accurate measurement of displacement and is used for very strong prisms. It is denoted by an inverted triangle ∇.

PRISM DIOPTER

The prism diopter is denoted by the Greek letter delta (Δ). This unit of prism measurement, proposed by C.F. Prentice in 1888, is the prism unit used in the ophthalmic laboratory. The prism diopter is actually an approximation of the centrad. It is close enough to the centrad for our purposes, as long as we are dealing with prisms that have a deviation of less than about 10 degrees or an apical angle of less than about 15 degrees.

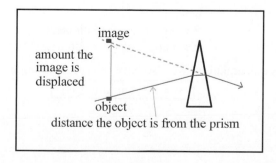

A prism diopter produces a displacement of 1 unit (along a straight line) at a distance of 100 units. In more common usage, a prism diopter produces an image displacement of 1 centimeter at an object distance of 1 meter. The difference between the prism diopter and the centrad is that the centrad measures the distance along the arc of a circle instead of along a straight line.

$$\text{prism diopter} = \frac{\text{displacement in centimeters}}{\text{distance in meters}}$$

EXAMPLE:

4-3. What is the power of a prism that produces a 2-cm displacement when the object is 3 m away?

$P^\Delta = \text{displacement (cm)/distance (m)} = 2/3 = 0.67^\Delta$

The formula may be rewritten to find either distance of object or displacement of image:

$$\text{displacement in centimeters} = \text{prism diopters} \times \text{distance in meters}$$

$$\text{distance in meters} = \frac{\text{displacement in centimeters}}{\text{prism diopters}}$$

EXAMPLE:

4-4. How much and in what direction will an object be displaced when viewed through a 3^Δ prism held base down 2 meters from the object?

$\text{displacement in centimeters} = \text{prism diopters} \times \text{distance in meters}$
$= 3 \times 2 = 6 \text{ cm}$

Since the prism is being held base down and the object is displaced toward the apex, the image will appear to be 6 cm higher than the position of the object.

Note: In the definition of prism diopter the distance the image is displaced from the object is a straight line. For weak prisms this distance is very close to equal to the distance on the arc of the circle discussed for the centrad. For weak prisms (less than 10^Δ) or for small apical angles (less than 15 degrees) the prism diopter is an acceptable measurement. For strong prisms the centrad is more accurate than the prism diopter. *For strong prisms the prism diopter overestimates the power of the prism.* Thus a 20^Δ prism would be weaker than a 20∇ prism.

EXERCISES:

4. What power prism would displace an object to the left by 2 cm when viewed through a prism that is 2 m away from the object?

5. How much displacement would a 2-diopter prism held base up cause in an object 4 m from the prism?

6. A 2-diopter prism makes an object viewed through it appear to be displaced 3 cm lower than it is. How far is the object from the prism, and what is its base direction?

RELATIONSHIP BETWEEN PRISM DEFINITIONS

The prism diopter is related to the angle of deviation and the apical angle. The approximate relationship for the deviating angle and prism diopter is

$$P = 100 \tan \angle d$$

where:
P = power in prism diopters
$\angle d$ = angle of deviation

Substituting $\angle d = a(n - 1)$ into this equation, we also have the approximation

$$P = 100 \tan [a(n - 1)]$$

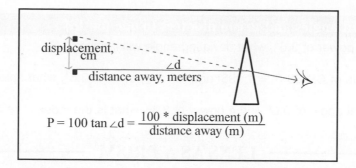

$$P = 100 \tan \angle d = \frac{100 * \text{displacement (m)}}{\text{distance away (m)}}$$

EXAMPLES:

4-5. What is the power in prism diopters of a crown glass (n = 1.523) prism having an apical angle of 5 degrees?

    a. $\angle d = a(n - 1)$
         $= 5(1.523 - 1)$
         $= 5(0.523)$
         $= 2.615°$

    b. $P = 100 \tan \angle d$
         $= 100 \tan 2.615$
         $= 100(0.04567...)$
         $= 4.6^\Delta$

or:

    $P = 100 \tan [a(n - 1)]$
       $= 100 \tan [5(1.523 - 1)]$
       $= 100 \tan [2.615]$
       $= 4.6^\Delta$

Example 4-5

Type A Calculator:

100 [x] [(] 5 [x] .523 [)] [tan] [=] The calculator should say 4.567...

Type B Calculator:

100 [x] [tan] [(] 5 [x] .523 [)] [=] The calculator should say 4.567...

4-6. What apical angle would be needed for a prism that will be made of polycarbonate (n = 1.586) and have a power of 6^Δ?

    a. $P = 100 \tan \angle d$
      $\tan \angle d = P/100$
          $= 6/100$
          $= 0.06$ (now use the $\tan^{-1}$ key)
      $\angle d = 3.4°$

    b. $\angle d = a(n - 1)$
      $3.4 = a(1.586 - 1)$
      $a = 3.4/0.586$
         $= 5.8°$

7. If a prism is to have a power of 3.5$^\Delta$, what deviating angle will it have?

8. If a prism is to be made of CR-39 (n = 1.498) and have a power of 3.5$^\Delta$, what apical angle should it have?

9. If a prism has an apical angle of 8.0° and a power of 8.4$^\Delta$, what is the index of refraction of the material from which it is made?

LENS AS A PRISM

A lens can be drawn as a set of prisms. Plus lenses act like stacked prisms with their bases toward the center of the lens. Minus lenses act like stacked prisms with their apices toward the center of the lens and their bases toward the edges of the lens.

The power of any lens is the result of the prismatic effect created by the incline of the surfaces with respect to each other at any particular point on the lens. We can think of the lens as if it were a series of different power prisms stacked on top of one another. Take a look at the "stacked prisms" in the diagrams below.

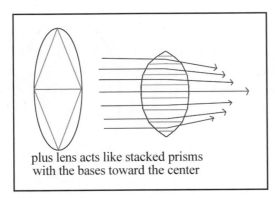

plus lens acts like stacked prisms with the bases toward the center

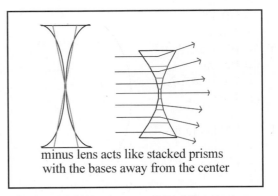

minus lens acts like stacked prisms with the bases away from the center

At the center of the lens the sides are parallel, there is no prism power, and the ray (or axis) is not bent or deviated. A ray traveling through the lens at any other point on the lens is bent or deviated based on the incline of the sides at that point. The farther from the center of the lens, the more the sides are inclined with respect to each other and the more the ray is deviated.

IMAGE MOVEMENT

Objects viewed through the center of a lens will not be displaced, since there is no prism present at the center of the lens. Objects viewed through points other than the center will be displaced toward the apex of the prism. In a plus lens the object is displaced away from the optical center. In a minus lens the object is displaced toward the optical center.

As a plus lens is moved down, an object viewed through the lens will be displaced upward toward the apex of the prism created by the lens. This is called *against movement* or *against motion.* The speed of the against movement is greater for a high-power plus lens than for a low-power plus lens.

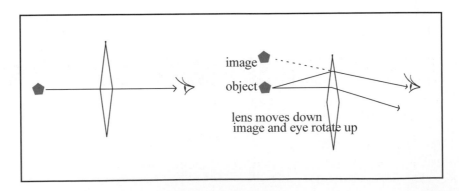

image

object

lens moves down
image and eye rotate up

Optical Formulas Tutorial

As a minus lens is moved down, an object viewed through the lens will be displaced down toward the apex of the prism created by the lens. This is called *with movement* or *with motion.* The speed of the with movement is greater for a high-power minus lens than for a low-power minus lens.

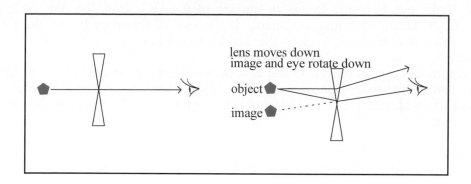

PRENTICE'S LAW

The amount of prismatic effect a person experiences when looking through a particular point on a lens depends on how far the point is from the optical center of the lens. This amount can be approximated by means of *Prentice's Law,* one of the most commonly used formulas in ophthalmic optics.

$$P = \frac{dD}{10} \text{ or } P = cD$$

where:

P = the prism power in prism diopters
d = the distance from the optical center in mm
c = the distance from the optical center in cm
D = the dioptric power of the lens

This formula may be solved for any of its variables:

$$d = \frac{10P}{D} \text{ or } c = \frac{P}{D}$$

or

$$D = \frac{10P}{d} \text{ or } D = \frac{P}{c}$$

Several forms of Prentice's Law are in use. This book uses the form that calls for d, the distance from the optical center in millimeters, because that is how the distance is most commonly measured in the ophthalmic laboratory and dispensary.

Note: This formula loses accuracy for low-power lenses.

Note: Ignore the sign (+ or –) of the power when using Prentice's Law.

STEPS TO SOLVING PRISM PROBLEMS

1. Determine the meridian that the observer or eye is on with respect to the lens OC.
2. Determine the lens power on that meridian.
3. Use Prentice's Law with the power from step 2 and the millimeter decentration from the problem. Ignore the sign of the power.
4. Determine the base direction using one of the three methods in the box on p. 100.

DETERMINING BASE DIRECTION

OPTION 1
1. PLUS LENS: Draw a diamond shape. If the eye is above or below the OC, draw the diamond vertically. If the eye is to the inside or outside of the OC, draw the diamond horizontally. MINUS LENS: Draw an hourglass shape. If the eye is above or below the OC, draw the hourglass vertically. If the eye is to the inside or outside of the OC, draw the hourglass horizontally.
2. Indicate where the eye is based on the description in the problem: either at the top or the bottom, or toward the bridge or away from the bridge, with respect to the OC.
3. Note where the widest part of the diamond or hourglass is with respect to the eye. That is the base direction.

OPTION 2
1. Draw a circle.
2. Draw a large X for the OC, and draw an N for the nasal side of the lens.
3. Draw an eye in the position in the lens that the problem indicates.
4. PLUS LENS: Draw a diamond with the wide part where the OC is and with one of the triangles over the eye. MINUS LENS: Draw an hourglass with the narrow part where the OC is and with one of the triangles over the eye.
5. Note where the widest part of the diamond or hourglass is with respect to the eye. That is the base direction.

OPTION 3
1. Answer the question: With respect to the eye, where is the OC? Up, down, in, or out?
2. PLUS lens: The answer to number 1 is where the base is. MINUS lens: The base is opposite the answer to number 1.

EXAMPLES:

4-7. What is the prismatic effect at a point 2 mm from the optical center of a +3.00D lens?

$$P = \frac{d \times D}{10} = \frac{2 \times 3}{10} = \frac{6}{10} = 0.6^\Delta$$

When recording a prism amount, we must also state the direction of the prism base relative to the wearer's eye. A point above the optical center of a plus lens will give a base-down effect, since the base of a plus lens is at the optical center, which is below the direction of gaze. A point above the optical center of a minus lens will give a base-up effect, since the base of a minus lens is away from the optical center.

4-8. What is the prismatic effect 2 mm above the optical center of a +5.00D lens?

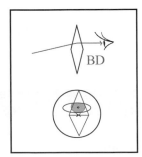

$$P = \frac{2 \times 5}{10} = \frac{10}{10} = 1.0^\Delta$$

The answer is written **1.0$^\Delta$ BD** (base down).

(In Option 3 for determining base direction [in the previous box] the person is looking above the OC. Therefore the OC is down. OC down, plus lens, base down.)

4-9. What is the prismatic effect of looking through a point 3 mm above the optical center of the Rx −3.00 −2.00 ×030?

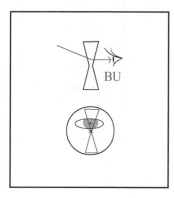

The wearer is looking above the OC. Therefore we need the power of the lens in the vertical or 90-degree meridian. To determine the *approximate* power on the 90th meridian, we need the oblique meridian formula, pp. 75 to 77 in Section III. The axis is 30; we need 90, so we need the amount of cylinder in effect 60 degrees from the axis. Looking back at p. 76, we see that 75% of the cylinder is in effect 60 degrees from the axis of the prescription. So the power on the vertical meridian is about −3.00 −1.50 = −4.50D.
Now use Prentice's Law:

$$P = \frac{d \times D}{10} = \frac{3 \times 4.50}{10} = \frac{13.50}{10} = 1.4^\Delta$$

The answer is about **1.4$^\Delta$ BU** (base up).
(In Option 3 for determining base direction the person is looking above the OC. Therefore the OC is down. OC down, minus lens, base up.)

Note: Always specify an amount and if possible a base direction when performing calculations involving prism.

4-10. How much prism is present 4 mm on the nasal side of the OC for the Rx +2.50 −1.00 ×010?

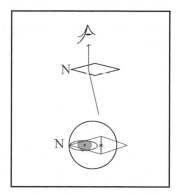

We need the power on the 180th meridian. We use the oblique meridian formula to determine that the approximate power on the 180 is +2.47.

$$P = \frac{d \times D}{10} = \frac{4 \times 2.47}{10} = \frac{9.88}{10} = 1.0^\Delta$$

The answer is about **1.0$^\Delta$ BO** (base out).
(In Option 3 for determining base direction the person is looking through the lens on the nasal side of the OC. Therefore the OC is out. OC out, plus lens, base out.)

4-11. The Rx is –5.50 –2.25 ×130. The OC is decentered out with respect to the eye. If the OC is 6 mm from the desired position, what is the prism effect?

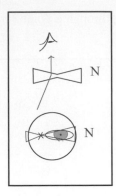

We need the power on the 180th meridian. The oblique meridian formula shows that the approximate power on the 180 is –6.82.

$$P = \frac{d \times D}{10} = \frac{6 \times 6.82}{10} = \frac{40.922}{10} = 4.092^\Delta = 4.1^\Delta$$

The answer is about **4.1$^\Delta$ BI** (base in).
(In Option 3 for determining base direction the person is looking on the nasal side of the OC. Therefore the OC is out. OC out, minus lens, base in.)

Note: The concept of having an approximate "power" on a meridian other than the major meridian (either the axis of the Rx or the meridian that is 90 degrees from the axis of the meridian) is useful only for prism calculations. When the prism present at a point not on one of the two major meridians is being determined, the induced prism will have both a horizontal and a vertical component. The process shown here gives a useful approximation for the prism. A more complete discussion of determining the horizontal and vertical components of the prism present at a point not on the major meridian is given in Brooks and Borish: *System for Ophthalmic Dispensing,* ed 2, p 434. Current laboratory computers make the more accurate calculations.

EXERCISES: (Round the answers to one-tenth prism diopter.)

10. How much prism does a wearer experience when looking 2 mm below the optical center of a +4.00D lens?

11. What approximate prism would a person experience looking 4 mm out on the horizontal meridian from the center of the Rx –0.50 +2.00 ×030?

12. Approximately how much prism would a person experience when looking through a point 5 mm toward the nasal side of a –1.00 +4.00 ×075 lens?

13. What is the prismatic effect 5 mm above the optical center of a –5.50D lens?

———— DETERMINING OVERALL PRISMATIC EFFECTS ————

When the wearer is looking through any point other than the optical centers of the lenses, the induced prism may have two possible effects. One effect results from both eyes rotating the same amount and in the same direction; the other effect results from the eyes rotating different amounts or in different directions.

Causing the eyes to rotate the same amount in the same direction may cause the wearer to experience distortion. Causing the eyes to rotate different amounts or in different directions will cause, at best, discomfort. (This is sometimes diagnosed as the optical catch-all *asthenopia,* which means visual discomfort regardless of cause.) With enough difference between the eyes, *diplopia,* or *double vision,* occurs. The wearer may unconsciously *suppress* the vision in one eye to relieve the discomfort that results from diplopia. The disassociation of the eyes that causes diplopia may result in asthenopia. Many things can cause sudden onset of diplopia. Incorrectly made glasses is one possible cause.

When prism is induced in each lens of a pair of glasses, we need to determine whether the prisms will cancel each other or compound each other. In canceling situations the eyes are rotating in the same direction. For example, base-up rotates the eye down (toward the apex). So base-up in both lenses will rotate both eyes down and is ***canceling***. Base-in in the right lens rotates the right eye out, to the right. Base-in in the left lens rotates the left eye out, to the left. So base-in in both lenses rotates the eyes in opposite directions and is ***compounding***.

CANCELING AND COMPOUNDING SITUATIONS

CANCELING SITUATIONS
Base up and base up
Base down and base down
Base in and base out
COMPOUNDING SITUATIONS
Base up and base down
Base in and base in
Base out and base out

In canceling situations, first subtract the smaller prism amount from the larger prism amount. Then assign the prism base direction to the lens originally having the larger prism amount. In compounding situations, add the two prism amounts together to give the total effect.

Following are some examples[1]:

RE	LE	EFFECT	RESULTING EFFECT
2^Δ BU	3^Δ BU	Canceling	1^Δ BU LE
2^Δ BU	3^Δ BD	Compounding	5^Δ BU RE or 5^Δ BD LE
2^Δ BI	2^Δ BO	Canceling	No imbalance

EXAMPLE:

4-12. A wearer complains of headaches when using new glasses. On checking, you find that the lenses have been made with a 70-mm distance between the optical centers, whereas the wearer's pupillary distance (PD) is 66 mm. For an Rx of OU +3.00 +2.00 ×060, how much prism is the wearer experiencing? Do the glasses meet ANSI standards?

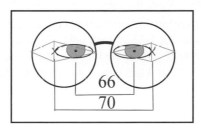

The OCs are on the horizontal meridian, so we first find the approximate power on the 180th meridian by using the oblique meridian formula.

180th meridian power = +4.50D

The PRP[2] distance of the glasses is off by 4 mm. We make the assumption that this error is split evenly at 2 mm for each lens. (If the wearer is present or if a monocular PD has been recorded, we would not make that assumption.) Using Prentice's Law,

$$P = \frac{d \times D}{10} = \frac{2 \times 4.50}{10} = \frac{9.00}{10} = 0.9^\Delta$$

---

[1]RE and OD mean right eye or right lens. LE and OS mean left eye or left lens. OU means both eyes or both lenses.
[2]PRP means prism reference point, the point on the lens where the prism amount is what is indicated on the Rx. MRP means major reference point and is the same as the PRP. When no prism is prescribed, the PRP and MRP are the OC, or optical center.

The lenses are plus lenses, so the base is where the optical center is. Since the glasses' PD is too big, the optical centers are out. Therefore each lens has about 0.9^Δ BO, which is compounding, and the wearer is experiencing a total of about **1.8^Δ BO**.

The glasses do not meet ANSI standards. The tolerance for horizontal prism is glasses PRP within 2.5 mm of the wearer's PD, or a total of up to 0.66^Δ of unprescribed prism.

STEPS FOR SOLVING PRP DISTANCE ERROR, ANSI STANDARDS PROBLEMS

1. Determine if the PRPs are incorrect by 2.5 mm or less. If they are, the glasses meet ANSI standards.
2. Determine the power on the 180th meridian for each lens.
3. Determine the amount that each PRP is off.
4. Use Prentice's Law to determine the prism and base direction induced in each lens.
5. Combine the prisms from the two lenses. If the total is 0.66^Δ or less, the glasses meet ANSI standards.

ANSI STANDARDS FOR PRISM: Z80.1-1999

For *a single unmounted lens* the position where the amount of prism prescribed occurs must be within 1 mm of the intended position. If the position of the correct amount of prism is off by more than 1 mm, there must be no more than $1/3^\Delta$ error in prism at the point that should have been the prism reference point (PRP). The prism tolerance must be met whether prism is prescribed or not. If prism is not prescribed, the prescribed prism is 0 and there must be no more than $1/3^\Delta$ of prism at the PRP.

In *a mounted pair of lenses* the distance between the PRPs must be within 2.5 mm of the requested PD, or horizontal prism error may total no more than $2/3^\Delta$. Vertical imbalance must be no more than $1/3^\Delta$, or the heights may differ by no more than 1 mm. The 2.5 mm rule does not apply to progressive addition lenses; they must be positioned within 1 mm of the requested position, both vertically and horizontally, and each lens individually must have no more than $1/3^\Delta$ at the PRP. Prism thinning is considered prescribed prism for this tolerance test. In other styles of multifocal lenses the heights of the segments may differ by no more than 1 mm unless unequal monocular heights were specified.

The correct method of determining whether the difference between the PRPs is in tolerance is to locate and dot the position of correct prism in each lens.

1. If the distance between these dots is within 2.5 mm of the requested PD, the glasses are within ANSI tolerance.
2. If the distance is greater than 2.5 mm, dot $1/3^\Delta$ in each lens and remeasure. If the actual OC measurement was more than the PD and the new dots are less than the PD, the glasses are within ANSI tolerance (or if the actual OC measurement was less than the PD and the new dots are more than the PD, the glasses are within ANSI tolerance).

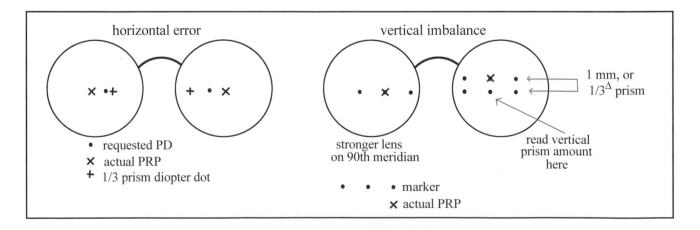

For vertical imbalance, center the *stronger* of the two lenses (on the 90th meridian) in the lensmeter and dot. Move to the weaker lens without changing the height of the glasses in the lensmeter. Read the amount of prism at this point. If the amount is less than $1/3^\Delta$, the glasses are within ANSI tolerance. If not, dot the lens, move the glasses up or down until the correct amount of prism is present, and redot. If the dots are within 1 mm, the glasses are within ANSI tolerance.

EXAMPLE:

4-13. A person has an Rx of:
OD −1.00 −1.00 ×045
OS −0.50 −1.00 ×135
The glasses received for this person have an OC of 72 mm rather than the requested 66 mm. How much prism will the person experience if the glasses are dispensed, and are they within ANSI tolerance?

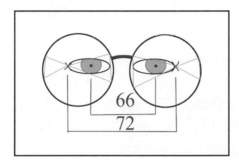

OD power on the horizontal meridian is about −1.50D (sphere + 50% cylinder).
OS power on the horizontal meridian is about −1.00D (sphere + 50% cylinder).
Each lens is off by 3 mm. Using Prentice's Law,
OD

$$P = \frac{d \times D}{10} = \frac{3 \times 1.50}{10} = \frac{4.50}{10} = 0.45^\Delta \text{ BI}$$

OS

$$P = \frac{d \times D}{10} = \frac{3 \times 1.00}{10} = \frac{3.00}{10} = 0.3^\Delta \text{ BI}$$

The lenses are minus lenses, and the optical centers are out. Since the base direction for minus lenses is opposite the direction of the optical centers, the base direction is in. Total prismatic effect is about **0.8^Δ BI.** *The glasses do not meet ANSI standards.*

Note: The use of calculations does not duplicate the results of the lensmeter test. There are two reasons for this:

1. Using the sine-squared method to calculate meridian power is inaccurate and does not take the vertical shift of the induced prism into account. The oblique meridian formula calculation on the 180 meridian is most accurate when the axis of the Rx is at 180 or 90 degrees.
2. In an anisometropic Rx (significant difference between the two lenses) the calculation of the distribution of the induced prism between the lenses will not duplicate the results of using the lensmeter. EXAMPLE:
OD +0.25
OS +3.00
Wearer's PD is 60, glasses DBC is 70. (Each lens is 5 mm too wide.)
   a. Using the calculations without monocular measurements, we get right lens-induced prism of 0.125^ BO and left lens-induced prism of 1.5^ BO for a total of 1.625^ unwanted prism, and the glasses fail.

b. Using the lensmeter test described in the ANSI standards, we get the following results:

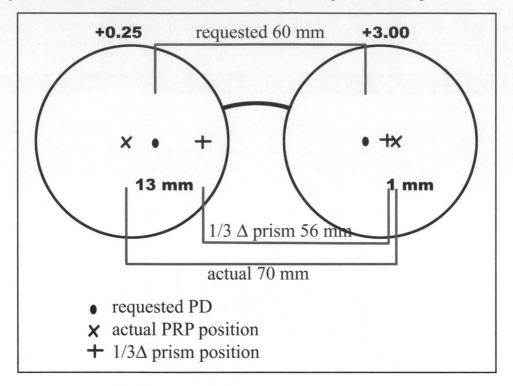

+0.25 requested 60 mm **+3.00**

✗ • + • +✗

13 mm **1 mm**

1/3 Δ prism 56 mm

actual 70 mm

• requested PD
✗ actual PRP position
+ 1/3Δ prism position

When this method is used, the glasses pass the standard for horizontal PRP placement. Because of this method, a prescription with no (plano) power (and no ground-in unwanted prism present on the 180 meridian) will always pass the standard regardless of the power of the second lens.

Note: The lensmeter test is described in the ANSI Z80.1 standards and is used to make the decision to pass or fail the glasses.

Note: When the 2.5 mm rule is applied, all of the 2.5 mm may apply to one lens. Thus, if the measurements are monocular, if one lens has the PRP placed correctly and the other does not, the incorrect lens may be off by 2.5 mm.

EXERCISES: (Round prism amount to the nearest one tenth.)

14. About how much prism would a wearer experience if the following prescription was made to an OC distance of 72 mm instead of 68 mm as requested? Do the glasses meet ANSI standards?
Rx OD −0.50 −4.00 ×060   OS +3.00 −4.00 ×030

15. What approximate prism would a wearer experience if the following prescription was made to a PRP distance of 70 mm rather than 66 mm as requested? Do the glasses meet ANSI standards?
Rx OD −0.50 DS with 5△ BU   OS +1.00 −4.00 ×030

16. About how much prism would a wearer experience if the following prescription was made to a PRP distance of 63 mm rather than 61 mm as requested? Do the glasses meet ANSI standards?
Rx OD −10.50 −4.00 ×060   OS −13.00 −4.00 ×030

17. On final inspection, a pair of +12.50 OU aphakic glasses shows 1 mm of vertical imbalance: the OD optical center is 1 mm higher than the OS optical center. According to ANSI standards, these glasses are dispensable. How much vertical prism will the glasses have if the wearer's eyes are level?

18. The wearer's reading PD is 66 mm, and the OC distance of pre-made reading glasses is 60 mm. If the Rx is +1.00 OU, how much prism is in effect? If you dispensed these glasses to fill an Rx of +1.00 OU, would they meet ANSI standards? How much prism would be in effect if the Rx and pre-made reading glasses were +2.50 OU?

SPLITTING PRISM

Occasionally a prescription shows prism in just one lens. To balance the weight of the lenses and improve the cosmetic effect of the prism, you may *split the prism* between the two lenses. In this case, divide the amount of the prism in half. Assign one half with the base direction requested in the lens where it was prescribed. Assign the other half of the prism amount to the other lens with the base in the *compounding* direction.

Before ordering, always contact the refractionist and request permission to split the prism. There will be instances in which the prescriber will not want this process to be done.

EXAMPLES:

4-14. Given the prescription OD pl 5^Δ BU; OS pl, how should the prism be split to even the weight of the glasses?
Split the prisms in half, 2.5^Δ OU. Place 2.5^Δ BU in the right lens and 2.5^Δ BD in the left lens. (BU and BD compound each other.) This results in 5^Δ of vertical imbalance, with the right eye rotating down as the original Rx indicated.
Order the Rx: OD pl 2.5^Δ BU
OS pl 2.5^Δ BD

4-15. Given the prescription: OD pl 5^Δ BU
OS pl 3^Δ BI
how could the prism be split to even the weight and thickness of the glasses?
The vertical prism would be split 2.5D BU in the right lens and 2.5D BD in the left lens.
The horizontal prism would be split 1.5^Δ BI OU. The result would be:
OD pl 2.5^Δ BU & 1.5^Δ BI
OS pl 2.5^Δ BD & 1.5^Δ BI
A discussion of the method for locating this prism in the lensmeter appears on pp. 120 to 125.

You may want to split the prism unequally in an effort to equalize weight and thickness if the prescriptions in the right and left lenses are very different. This will require determining the edge thickness for the lens and the prism. These thickness formulas are in Section V.

EXERCISES:

In Exercises 19 to 22, if the refractionist indicated that splitting the prism is acceptable, what prism would you order?
19. OD +2.50 DS 3^Δ BU
OS +2.50 DS

20. OD −5.00
OS −5.00 4^Δ BI

21. OD −1.00 −1.00 ×180 3^Δ BO
OS −1.00 −1.00 ×180

22. OD +1.50 −0.50 ×090
OS +1.00 5^Δ BD

EXCESSIVE OR UNWANTED PRISM

Even when the PRP distance of the completed glasses is correct, the wearer may still indicate that something "seems" or "feels" wrong. The reason could be optical centers that are offset equal amounts, resulting in equal amounts of prism in each lens that cancel each other. For example, if the optical centers are 5 mm below the wearer's pupils with a prescription of −4.00 DS OU, both lenses would have 2^Δ of BU prism, which cancels, leaving no imbalance. (In Section VI we will discuss partial correction of this situation by use of pantoscopic tilt.) As another example, if the wearer's monocular PDs are 28/32 for a +6.00 DS OU prescription, but the optical centers were inset equal amounts, the right lens would have 1.2^Δ BO and the left lens would have 1.2^Δ BI, which cancels. A third example would be a person with vision in only one eye; if the glasses are made with the OC in the center of the lens even though the eye with vision is not centered in the lens, the wearer will look through prism that does not affect fusion.

EXCESSIVE OR UNWANTED BASE-DOWN PRISM

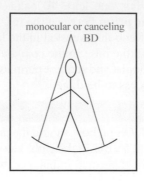

- The floor or other horizontal expanse seems concave. The wearer feels as if the floor is the bottom of a bowl.
- People and vertical objects seem taller.
- The floor seems to slant uphill.

EXCESSIVE OR UNWANTED BASE-UP PRISM

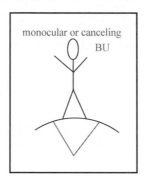

- The floor or other horizontal expanse seems convex. The wearer feels as if the floor is a pitcher's mound.
- People and vertical objects seem shorter.
- The floor seems to slant downhill.

EXCESSIVE BASE-OUT OR BASE-IN PRISM

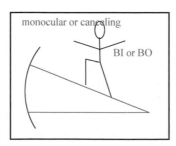

- The wearer sees a horizontal expanse as sloped. The side with the base appears higher than the side with the apex.
- The wearer sees a wall, doorframe, or other vertical expanses as curving in or out.

IMAGE JUMP

New bifocal wearers sometimes complain that the object they look down at moves, or jumps, as the eye rotates down into the bifocal segment. Experienced bifocal wearers who change bifocal style may also have this complaint. This is called *image jump* and is a function of the position of the segment optical center and the add power of the segment.

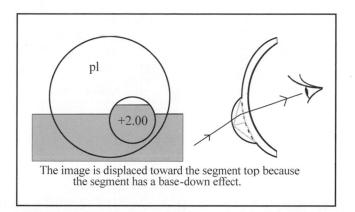

The image is displaced toward the segment top because the segment has a base-down effect.

EXAMPLE:

4-16. A round 22 segment can be thought of as a 22-mm-wide, plus-powered lens attached to the front of the distance lens. Since the segment is round, the OC of the segment is in the center of the segment, which is 11 mm from all the round edges of the segment. Therefore the OC is one half of 22 mm, or 11 mm down from the top of the segment.

The approximate prismatic effect for an Add of +2.00D can be found by use of Prentice's Law.

$$P = \frac{d \times D}{10} = \frac{11 \times 2.00}{10}$$

$$= 2.2^{\Delta} \text{ BD}$$

There is a 2.2^{Δ} image jump resulting from the direction of gaze traveling into the top of the bifocal segment. Note that this is independent of the power of the distance prescription. The amount of prism experienced through the distance portion does not undergo a noticeable sudden increase or decrease over the short distance from just above the segment top to just inside the segment.

As a rule of thumb, the OC of a segment is about:

- 11 mm from the top of a round 22 (one-half the diameter of any round segment style)
- 2.5 to 6 mm from the top of most flat-top (FT) or straight-top (ST) lenses (assume 5 mm for ST 25-28-35 if not given a segment height)
- 19 mm from the top of an Ultex A or AX lens
- 0 mm from the top of an Executive, FT-40 (or more), or a progressive lens

The position of the segment OC in an ST, FT, or D-type segment (all of these terms refer to the same style of segment) can be determined in two ways. The first is to refer to the manufacturer's literature or the lens guide published by FRAMES.[3] The second is to measure the width (diameter) of the segment and the height of the segment. The OC is at the center of the circle, which is one-half the width of the segment and is therefore one-half the diameter up from the bottom of the segment. Therefore the segment OC is:

segment center position = height of the segment – 1/2 the width of the segment

---

[3]*LENSES Product Guide,* published by FRAMES Data Inc., <u>www.FRAMESdata.com</u>, Jobson Publishing L.L.C.

4-17. An FT-28 segment measures 28 mm across (width) and 17.5 mm high. The segment OC is: 17.5 – ¹/₂(28) = 17.5 –14 = **3.5 mm from the top of the segment.**

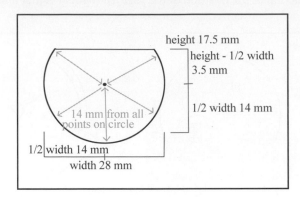

4-18. The Rx for the lens in Example 4-17 is: OD +1.00 sph, ADD +2.50. What is the image jump? The image jump is found with Prentice's Law. The distance from the top of the segment to the segment OC, 3.5 mm, is used for d, and the power of the segment, +2.50, for D. The power of the distance is not needed for this problem. So the image jump = (3.5)(2.50)/10 = 0.875$^\Delta$ BD or **0.9$^\Delta$ BD.**

23. What image jump is present for the Rx
    OD –1.00 DS   ADD +2.50 OU
    OS –1.50 DS
    made with FT-28 lenses? The segment measures 19 mm from top to bottom.

24. What image jump is present for the Rx
    OD –1.00 DS   ADD +2.50 OU
    OS –1.50 DS
    made with Executive lenses?

25. What image jump is present on the Rx
    OD –1.00 DS   ADD +2.25
    OS –1.50 DS   ADD +3.00
    made with round 22 lenses? What is the image jump if the lens is made with a round 28?

ANISOMETROPIA

Anisometropia is defined as the condition in which the eyes have different refractive errors. Anisometropia requires only that there be a difference in amount of refraction, not necessarily a difference in type of ametropia. The *a-* or *an-* prefix on a word generally means "not," and the *iso-* prefix generally means "equal." Thus *isometropia* is a condition in which the eyes have the same refractive error or no error at all.

Antimetropia is a special case of anisometropia: it is the condition in which the prescriptions have different signs. Following are some examples:

	1.	**2.**	**3.**	**4.**
OD	–3.00D	–1.00D	+1.00D	+2.25D
OS	–5.00D	+1.00D	+5.00D	+2.25D
	anisometropia	anisometropia, antimetropia	anisometropia	isometropia

Textbooks generally do not specify how much difference is needed to say that a person is anisometropic. If the person is experiencing a problem caused by a difference in magnification or prismatic effect, the person is anisometropic, or has anisometropia.

Differences in magnification result in a lack of fusion. Lenses designed to minimize this problem are called iseikonic lenses. These lenses are discussed under Spectacle Magnification in Section VI.

Differences in prismatic effect, like differences in magnification, result in a lack of fusion.

———— VERTICAL IMBALANCE ————

The wearer experiences a prismatic effect whenever looking through a point other than the optical center of the lenses. This is particularly true when the wearer is forced to look through the bifocal segment of the lens in order to read. The amount of prismatic effect depends on the prescription and how far from the optical center the wearer is looking. Vertical imbalance will be present if the two lenses have different prescriptions. If the imbalance is great enough, the person may experience *diplopia* (double vision) or may suppress one eye.

The wearer can avoid the vertical imbalance when wearing single vision lenses by adjusting the position of the head to always look through the optical center. A person wearing bifocals cannot avoid the imbalance, as this person must look through the bifocal in order to read. We have several ways to offset this imbalance.

We can dispense *two pairs of single vision glasses,* one for distance and one for reading.

We can use *two different segment styles,* giving different amounts of segment-induced prism at the reading level. This is discussed on pp. 114 to 115.

We can use special *prism-controlled segments,* which are discussed in dispensing texts such as Brooks and Borish: *Systems for Ophthalmic Dispensing.*

We can provide *reading glasses to be used over contact lenses* for distance vision, or we can fit *bifocal contact lenses,* which will not have the off-center imbalance problem.

In low amounts of imbalance we can slightly *lower the OC and raise the segment top,* splitting the imbalance between distance and reading.

We can use *bicentric grinding,* also known as *slab-off* or *reverse slab-off.* The name bicentric grinding comes from the fact that two distance optical centers are theoretically created on the same lens without changing the distance prescription.

CALCULATING VERTICAL IMBALANCE

When bifocals are made with segments having identical style, shape, size, and power, any vertical imbalance will be due to the distance prescription only. To determine how much imbalance is present, it is necessary to know what the approximate power on the 90th meridian is and how far from the distance optical center the wearer will be looking.

EXAMPLES:

4-19. Calculate the vertical imbalance present at a reading position 10 mm below the distance optical center for the following Rx:

OD –1.00D   ADD +2.00D OU
OS –4.00D

RIGHT LENS	LEFT LENS
d = 10 mm	d = 10 mm
D = –1.00D	D = –4.00D

$$P = \frac{d \times D}{10} \qquad\qquad P = \frac{d \times D}{10}$$

$$P = \frac{10 \times 1.00}{10} \qquad\qquad P = \frac{10 \times 4.00}{10}$$

P = 1$^\Delta$ BD   **P = 4$^\Delta$ BD**

The vertical imbalance is the combination of the prism in the two lenses. In this case the prisms are canceling and the vertical imbalance is **3$^\Delta$ BD** in the left lens.

CALCULATING VERTICAL IMBALANCE IN THE READING AREA (WHEN THE ADD AMOUNTS ARE THE *SAME*)

1. Determine the power from the distance Rx on the 90th meridian in each lens. (This is found by use of the oblique meridian formula.)
2. Use the reading depth below the distance OC to calculate the prism present at the reading level in each lens. Determine the base direction for each.
3. Combine the two prism amounts, based on whether they are canceling or compounding. Alternatively:
   a. If the powers found in number 1 are the same sign, the prism amounts will be canceling, so you take the difference of the prism amounts. Assign the base direction to the lens with the larger amount of prism.
   b. If the powers found in number 1 are different signs, the prism amounts will be compounding, so you will add the prism amounts together.

4-20. What is the vertical imbalance for a reading level of 9 mm below distance OC for the following Rx:

OD –7.50 –2.00 ×110   ADD +1.75
OS –5.50 –1.50 ×080   ADD +1.75

The Adds are the same, so we can use this method.

1. The powers on the 90th are –7.73 and –5.55.
2. The prism amount 9 mm below the distance OC is 7.0^Δ BD and 5.0^Δ BD.
3. BD and BD are canceling, so the imbalance is $7.0 - 5.0 = \mathbf{2.0^\Delta}$ **BD OD**.

Note: In a discussion of image jump and thickness of the lens, progressive addition lenses (PALs) are considered to have the segment OC at the top of the segment. However, since the wearer has to look much farther down in the lens (from the distance OC), and since the distance OC may not be in a predictable place if prism thinning is ground in, the methods shown in this book are not useful for calculating vertical imbalance for PALs. Imbalance for PALs should be determined by use of the lensmeter and the reading circle position indicated by the PAL manufacturer.

EXERCISES: (Round answer to one-tenth prism diopter.)

26. What is the vertical imbalance at a reading level of 8 mm below distance OC for the Rx:
    OD +1.25 –1.25 ×090   ADD +3.75
    OS pl –0.75 ×045   ADD +3.75

27. What is the vertical imbalance for the Rx:
    OD +12.50 –2.00 ×180   ADD +2.00 OU
    OS +11.00 –0.50 ×025
    The reading level is 6 mm below the distance OC.

28. The glasses wearer looks 3 mm below the top of the Franklin-style glasses to read. The segment top is set 4 mm below the distance OC. What is the vertical imbalance at the reading level for the Rx:
    OD –3.00 +0.50 ×090   ADD +2.25 OU
    OS –3.00 +2.50 ×175
    Hint: The segment top is set 4 mm below the distance OC, and the person is reading 3 mm below the segment top. How far below the distance OC is the person reading?

BICENTRIC GRINDING OR SLAB-OFF

Bicentric grinding or *slab-off* is the process used to change the amount of prism in the reading portion of the lens without affecting the prism in the distance portion of the lens. Slab-off results in added base-up prism in the reading area. It is ground on the lens that has the weakest plus or strongest minus power on the 90th meridian. On glass lenses slab-off is ground or molded on the convex (plus) surface of the lens. On plastic lenses slab-off is ground on the concave (minus) surface of the lens.

Reverse slab-off is molded on the convex (plus) side of plastic lenses and is the exact opposite of regular slab-off. Reverse slab-off results in added base-down prism in the reading area, and it is molded on the lens with the strongest plus or weakest minus power on the 90th meridian.

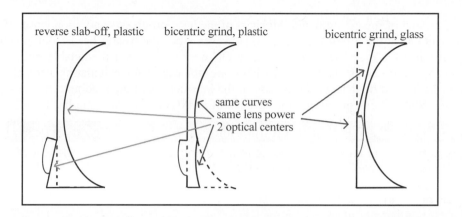

SLAB-OFF AND REVERSE SLAB-OFF

	SLAB-OFF	REVERSE SLAB-OFF
Two minus lenses	Highest minus	Lowest minus
Two plus lenses	Lowest plus	Highest plus
One plus, one minus	The minus lens	The plus lens

Usually slab-off (bicentric grind) is ordered only if the imbalance results in 1.5^Δ or more. The *LENSES Product Guide* currently lists two companies with reverse slab-off of 1.0^Δ.

When calculating the amount of prism, remember that the result is an approximation. The direction of gaze is actually in as well as down, and the oblique meridian formula results in an approximation of the power. The technique shown below results in a reasonable estimate of the vertical imbalance that must be corrected for the wearer to read comfortably.

EXAMPLE:

4-21. What is the approximate vertical imbalance at a reading level of 10 mm, and what slab-off could be ordered for the following prescription?

OD −1.00 −2.00 ×090   ADD +2.50D OU
OS +1.00 −1.00 ×060

Step 1. Find the distance power on the vertical meridian for each lens.
The right lens power on the 90th meridian is −1.00D. The left lens power in the 90th meridian is about +0.75D.

Step 2. Find the prismatic effect at the reading level for each lens.
Prismatic effect when looking 10 mm below the optical center:

RIGHT LENS

$$P = \frac{10 \times 1.00}{10}$$

$P = 1^\Delta$ BD

LEFT LENS

$$P = \frac{10 \times 0.75}{10}$$

$P = 0.8^\Delta$ BU

Step 3. Determine the total imbalance between the two prescriptions.
The prism amounts are compounding, so the vertical imbalance in this pair is about **OD 1.8^Δ BD or OS 1.8^Δ BU.**

Use a **1.75^Δ slab-off on the right lens** (most minus) or a **1.75^Δ reverse slab-off on the left lens** (most plus).

Note: Reverse slab-off is molded, so it is not available in every prism amount. The closest or the next lowest prism is fine. The imbalance that we are calculating is approximate, and we do not need to neutralize the imbalance exactly. We are reducing the imbalance to a point at which the wearer has comfortable fusion when using the near portion of the glasses. In these exercises use the prism amount calculated without considering what will actually be ordered.

Note: In a discussion of image jump and thickness of the lens, progressive addition lenses (PALs) are considered to have the segment OC at the top of the segment. However, since the wearer has to look much farther down in the lens (from the distance OC), and since the distance OC may not be in a predictable place if the lens has prism thinning ground in, the methods shown in this book are not useful for calculating vertical imbalance for PALs. Imbalance for PALs should be determined by use of the lensmeter and the reading circle position indicated by the PAL manufacturer. Slab-off can be ground on the back of a PAL once the amount has been determined.

EXERCISES: (Round the prism amounts to one-tenth diopter.)

29. What is the approximate vertical imbalance at a reading level of 8 mm for the following prescription? What slab-off could be ordered, and in which lens?
    OD −2.00 −4.00 ×030   ADD +3.00D OU
    OS −1.00 −1.00 ×030

30. Calculate the approximate vertical imbalance at a reading level of 7 mm for the following prescription. What reverse slab-off could be ordered, and in which lens?
    OD +7.50 −1.50 ×015   ADD +2.50D OU
    OS +3.50 −2.00 ×165

31. What is the approximate vertical imbalance at a reading level of 10 mm for the following prescription? What reverse slab-off could be ordered, and in which lens?
    OD +1.00 −4.00 ×060   ADD +2.00D
    OS −2.00 −1.00 ×030   ADD +2.00D

32. In the vertical imbalance exercises on p. 112, what lens would receive a regular slab-off, if applicable? What lens would receive a reverse slab-off, if applicable?

CORRECTING VERTICAL IMBALANCE IN THE READING AREA USING TWO DIFFERENT SEGMENT STYLES

Sometimes we can use unlike segments to cancel the imbalance at the reading level. Look back at the drawing on p. 109, showing the image jump for a 22-mm round bifocal. The upper half of the round segment contains base-down prism. A Franklin-style bifocal, also known as an Executive-style bifocal, has the OC of the segment at the top of the segment, so the prism induced by the Franklin-style segment is BU. Since a flat-top 22, 28, or 35 usually has the segment OC 2 to 5 mm below the top of the segment, the wearer may be looking through either BU or BD induced by the segment, depending on the reading level.

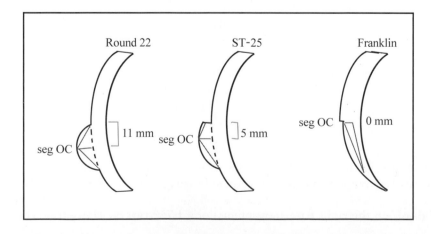

Suppose the wearer has a +2.50 Add and 1.5$^\Delta$ of imbalance at a reading level 4 mm below the top of the segment. A distance 4 mm below the top of the segment is 7 mm above the OC of the round 22, 1 mm above the OC of the FT-28, and 4 mm below the OC of the Executive. Using Prentice's Law and +2.50 Adds, to determine the induced prism in the segment, we have:

	Round 22	**FT-28**	**Executive/PAL**
Add (D)	+2.50	+2.50	+2.50
d	7 mm	1 mm	4 mm
P$^\Delta$	1.8$^\Delta$ BD	0.3$^\Delta$ BD	1.0$^\Delta$ BU

We can make use of these differing amounts of prism induced by different segment styles to minimize the vertical imbalance induced by the distance prescription. Placing a round segment over the eye with the most BU or the least BD in the distance portion and placing an FT-28 over the eye with the least BU or the most BD in the distance portion would induce a 1.5$^\Delta$ imbalance that is independent of the imbalance induced by the distance prescription.

We can use Prentice's Law to determine how much difference there should be between the segments' OCs to neutralize the distance-induced imbalance. This technique assumes that the segments will have the same Add power.

$$\text{difference} = \frac{P \times 10}{D}$$

where:
P = imbalance from the distance Rx at the reading level
D = Add power of the Rx
difference = difference between the segment OC placements

EXAMPLE:

4-22. The prescription is
−3.00 DS   ADD +1.50 OU
−1.50 DS
The reading level is 8 mm below OC, and the segments are to be set 5 mm below OC. What segments could we use to eliminate most of the imbalance at the reading level?
Step 1. First determine the imbalance at the reading level due to the distance prescription.
OD −3.00D ADD +1.50D OU
OS −1.50D

RIGHT LENS

$$P = \frac{d \times D}{10}$$

$$P = \frac{8 \times 3.00}{10}$$

P = 2.4$^\Delta$ BD

LEFT LENS

$$P = \frac{d \times D}{10}$$

$$P = \frac{8 \times 1.25}{10}$$

P = 1.2$^\Delta$ BD

The vertical imbalance at the reading level is the difference between the prism amounts for the two lenses, or **1.2$^\Delta$ BD OD**.
Step 2. Determine the difference needed between the OCs of the segments to compensate for the distance imbalance.
Using 1.2$^\Delta$ for P and +1.50D (the Add power) for D in Prentice's Law, we get:

$$\text{difference} = \frac{P \times 10}{D} = \frac{1.2 \times 10}{1.50} = 8 \text{ mm, the needed difference between segment OCs.}$$

Step 3. Decide what segments will give the needed compensating imbalance.
The difference between FT-28 OC (5 mm) and round 22 OC (11 mm) is close to the difference calculated. The round 22 will induce more BD that the FT-28 will. We want to either increase the BD effect of the left lens distance prescription or decrease the BD effect of the right lens distance prescription. Placing the FT-28 in the right lens and the round 22 in the left lens will help eliminate the imbalance at the reading level. The remaining imbalance should be small enough to cause little problem.

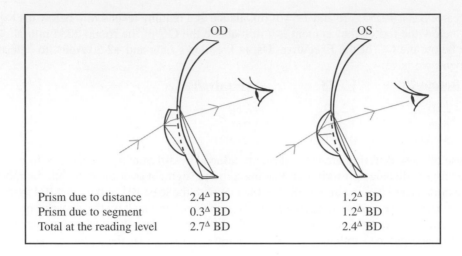

	OD	OS
Prism due to distance	2.4$^\Delta$ BD	1.2$^\Delta$ BD
Prism due to segment	0.3$^\Delta$ BD	1.2$^\Delta$ BD
Total at the reading level	2.7$^\Delta$ BD	2.4$^\Delta$ BD

Table 4-1 gives the difference in millimeters between the segments. In Step 2 of Example 4-22, we determined that we needed about 8 mm difference between the segments. Table 4-1 tells us that we can have a 6 mm difference by using an FT-28 and a round 22 in the OS, or we can use an Executive and a round 22 for 11 mm difference. The lens with the least minus power is the OS. In the pair FT-28 and round 22, the lowest OC is the round 22, so it goes on the OS. In the pair Executive and round 22, the round 22 is also the one with the lowest OC, so it goes on the OS. Of the two choices, an FT-25 in the right lens and a round 22 in the left lens would probably look better.

Table 4-1	**Segment Differences in Millimeters**				
		Segment Style			**Choosing the Lens for Each Segment**
Segment Style	**Ultex**	**Round 22**	**FT-25/28/35**	**Franklin/ST-40**	**Lensmeter Power**
Ultex	0	8	14	19	Higher power on drum
Round 22	8	0	6-9	11	
FT-25/28/35	14	6-9	0	5	Lower power on drum
Franklin/ST-40	19	11	5	0	

Rule for where to put the segments: *place the segment with the lowest OC placement on the lens with the most plus power or the least minus power in the vertical meridian.*

EXAMPLE:

4-23. The prescription reads OD +1.25 DS, OS pl, ADD +2.50 OU. The glasses have FT-28 lenses with a segment drop of 5 mm, and the reading level is 9 mm. If the wearer is experiencing problems fusing when reading, what segment change might you make?

OD +1.25D   OS pl
RIGHT LENS   LEFT LENS
d = 9 mm   d = 9 mm
D = +1.25D   D = +0D

$$P = \frac{d \times D}{10} \qquad\qquad\qquad\qquad P = \frac{d \times D}{10}$$

$$P = \frac{9 \times 1.25}{10} \qquad\qquad\qquad P = \frac{9 \times 0}{10}$$

P = 1.1$^\Delta$ BU   P = 0$^\Delta$

The imbalance at the reading level is 1.1$^\Delta$ BU in the right lens. Using Prentice's Law,

$$\text{difference} = \frac{P \times 10}{D} = \frac{1.1 \times 10}{2.5} = 4 \text{ mm, the needed difference between segment OCs.}$$

We need BD in the right lens, or BU in the left lens. Table 4-1 tells us that we can get 5 mm difference by replacing one of the FT-28 lenses with an Executive or FT-40. The FT-28 has the lower OC placement, and the lens with the most plus and least minus is the OD. So the left lens could be changed to an Executive or FT-40.

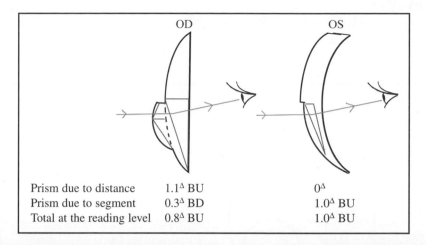

	OD	OS
Prism due to distance	1.1^Δ BU	0^Δ
Prism due to segment	0.3^Δ BD	1.0^Δ BU
Total at the reading level	0.8^Δ BU	1.0^Δ BU

EXERCISES:

33. The prescription reads
    OD −0.50 DS   ADD +2.00 OU
    OS +0.75 DS
    The reading level is 10 mm below OC, and the segments are 7 mm below OC. What segments could you use to reduce the imbalance at the reading level?

34. What is the approximate vertical imbalance at a reading level of 8 mm for the following prescription?
    If the segment top is 5 mm below the distance OC, what two segment styles could be used to reduce the imbalance at the reading level?
    OD −1.00 −1.00 ×030   ADD +2.25D OU
    OS −2.00 −4.00 ×030

———— VERTICAL IMBALANCE FOR UNLIKE ADD POWERS ————

The situation becomes a little more complex when the bifocals' Adds are of different powers or when the segments are in different positions, are different sizes, or are different styles. In this case we cannot stop with just the imbalance generated by the different distance powers. We must determine how far below the top of the segment the reading level is and how far the segment optical center is from that reading level, and add the reading imbalance to the distance imbalance.

STEPS TO DETERMINE IMBALANCE FOR UNLIKE ADDS

1. Determine the prism amount from the distance portion of each lens.
2. Determine the distance that the reading level is with respect to the OCs of the segments.
   a. Subtract: Reading level − segment drop. This is the distance from the top of the segment to the reading position.
   b. Subtract: Segment OC position − answer to a. This is the distance from the reading level to the segment OC.
3. Determine the imbalance from the segments using the Add power and the answer to number 2b.
4. Combine the prism amounts for each lens from distance and segment to give the total prism present at the reading level. (Note that, since you are combining prism in the *same* lens, BU and BD cancel, BU and BU compound, BD and BD compound.)
5. Determine the imbalance.

4-24. Given the prescription:

OD pl ADD +2.50

OS +2.00 ADD +1.50

The reading level is 9 mm below OC, and the round 22 bifocal segments are set at 5 mm below OC. What bicentric grind would be ordered?

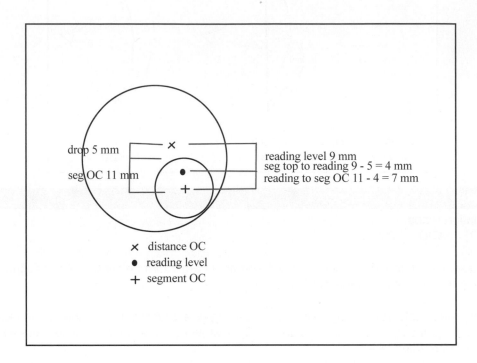

drop 5 mm

seg OC 11 mm

reading level 9 mm

seg top to reading 9 - 5 = 4 mm

reading to seg OC 11 - 4 = 7 mm

✕ distance OC

● reading level

+ segment OC

1. The prism at the reading level for the distance Rx is

 OD 0 OS 1.8$^\Delta$ BU

2. Refer back to the discussion of image jump, p. 109, for the approximate position of the segment optical center in the common bifocal styles. For this example:

 a. The drop is 5 mm and the reading level is 9 mm, so the reading level is 9 − 5 = 4 mm below the top of the segment.

 b. Segment OC is 11 mm from the top of the segment, so the reading level is 11 − 4 = 7 mm from the OC of the segment.

3. Since the wearer is looking 7 mm above the segment optical centers in these glasses, the prism resulting from the segment for the right lens is (7)(2.50)/10 = 1.75$^\Delta$ BD and for the left lens is (7)(1.50)/10 = 1.05$^\Delta$ BD.

4.

	OD	OS
Distance	0	1.8$^\Delta$ BU
Near	1.8$^\Delta$ BD	1.1$^\Delta$ BD
Total	1.8$^\Delta$ BD	0.7$^\Delta$ BU

(Note: the 1.8 BU and 1.1 BD are in the *same lens*.)

5. **Imbalance is 2.5$^\Delta$ BU OS or 2.5$^\Delta$ BD OD.** Since the left lens is the highest plus for the distance Rx, we could order either reverse slab-off of 2.5$^\Delta$ in the left lens or regular slab-off of 2.5$^\Delta$ in the right lens.

4-25. Rx: OD −1.50 −2.00 ×090 ADD +2.50

   OS −4.00 −1.00 ×045 ADD +2.00

The wearer has ST-28s. Reading level is 8 mm below OC, segment drop is 5 mm. What bicentric grind should be ordered?

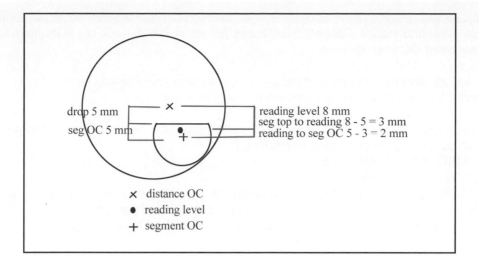

drop 5 mm
seg OC 5 mm

reading level 8 mm
seg top to reading 8 - 5 = 3 mm
reading to seg OC 5 - 3 = 2 mm

×   distance OC
●   reading level
+   segment OC

1. Determine the lens distance power on the 90th meridian, the prism amount for the distance Rx at the reading level, and the total imbalance.
   OD power on the 90th is about −1.50; prism amount is 1.2^Δ BD.
   OS power on the 90th is about −4.50; prism amount is 3.6^Δ BD.
2. Determine how far the reading level is from the segment optical center.
   a. The reading level is 8 − 5 = 3 mm below the top of the segment.
   b. The segment OC is 5 mm below the top of the segment. Therefore the reading level is 5 − 3 = 2 mm from the optical center of the segment.
3. Determine the imbalance induced by the segments.
   OD power in the segment is +2.50; prism amount is $(2)(2.50)/10 = 0.5^\Delta$ BD.
   OS power in the segment is +2.00; prism amount is $(2)(2.00)/10 = 0.4^\Delta$ BD.
4. Combine the prism for each lens.

	OD	OS
Distance	1.2^Δ BD	3.6^Δ BU
Near	0.5^Δ BD	0.4^Δ BD
Total	1.7^Δ BD	4.0^Δ BU

   (Note: you are combining prism amounts in the *same lens*.)
5. Use the combined imbalance for the amount of slab-off, and assign it to the high minus/low plus for regular slab-off or high plus/low minus for reverse slab-off.

Request approximately 2.3^Δ slab-off in the OS or 2.3^Δ reverse slab-off in the OD.

Note: The reading position is not actually on the 90th meridian. The eyes converge as they are lowered to read, so we should be calculating the prism amount about 2 mm in from the OC and 8 mm below it. Using the resultant prism calculations that we will cover next, we could find this exact answer. However, the answer we get with the method above is adequate for determining bicentric grind.

Note: The choice of segment style will change the total imbalance and could result in either less of a problem or more of a problem. For example, in Example 4-24, making the glasses from FT-40 lenses with the segment OC on the segment line will reduce the vertical imbalance at the reading level. Making the glasses in Example 4-25 with round 22s would reduce the imbalance for this pair. Prove these statements to yourself in the following exercises.

Note: Slab-off can be ground in any prism amount, but reverse slab-off is molded onto the front surface of the lens, so the choices are limited. This is not a problem because the wearer will unconsciously adjust the reading level to where vision is comfortable.

Note: For discussion of image jump or lens thickness, progressive addition lenses (PALs) are considered to have the segment OC at the top of the segment. However, since the wearer has to look much farther down in the lens (from the distance OC), and since the distance OC may not be in a predictable place if prism thinning is ground in, the methods shown in this book for calculating vertical imbalance are not useful for PALs. Imbalance for PALs should be determined with a lensmeter and the reading circle position indicated by the PAL manufacturer.

35. For Example 4-24, find the imbalance if the glasses are made with FT-40s set in the same position, where the segment OC is on the line.

36. For Example 4-25, find the imbalance if the glasses are made with Franklin lenses set in the same position. Find the imbalance if the glasses are made from round 22s.

37. What is the approximate vertical imbalance at a reading level of 8 mm for the following prescription? What slab-off could be ordered, and in which lens?
    OD −2.00 −4.00 ×060   ADD +3.50
    OS −1.00 −1.00 ×030   ADD +2.00
    a. Use an FT-28, with the segment OC 4 mm below the top of the segment, set with a below of 5 mm.
    b. Use a round 22, set with a below of 4 mm. (The accepted technique is to set the top of a round segment slightly higher than the top of a flat segment for the same wearer.)
    c. Use an ST-40, set with a below of 5 mm.
    Which of these segment styles would you recommend based just on the vertical imbalance?

38. Compute the approximate vertical imbalance at a reading level of 7 mm for the following prescription. What slab-off could be ordered, and in which lens?
    OD +7.50 −1.50 ×015   ADD +4.00
    OS +3.50 −2.00 ×165   ADD +2.50
    a. Use an FT-28, with the segment OC 4 mm below the top of the segment, set with a below of 4 mm.
    b. Use a round 22, set with a below of 3 mm.
    c. Use a Franklin-style segment, set with a below of 4 mm.
    Which of these segment styles would you recommend based just on the vertical imbalance?

RESULTANT PRISM

Prescribed prism is rarely just up, down, in, or out. Instead, the prescription may look like this:

OD pl 3$^\Delta$ BU & 5$^\Delta$ BI
OS pl 3$^\Delta$ BD & 5$^\Delta$ BI

What should you look for in the lensmeter when marking up the glasses? We call what will be seen in the lensmeter the ***resultant prism.*** (Some textbooks call resultant prism ***lab notation.***)

Or you may be neutralizing a pair of glasses and see the diagram below in the lensmeter. How would you write this in horizontal and vertical components? We call this ***resolving the prism.***

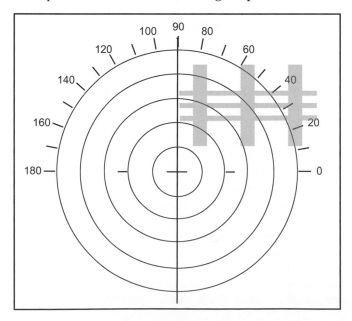

BASE DIRECTION AND PRISM AXIS

When looking at a pair of glasses from the convex side, as if you are facing the person wearing the glasses, you could imagine the lenses split into four quadrants.

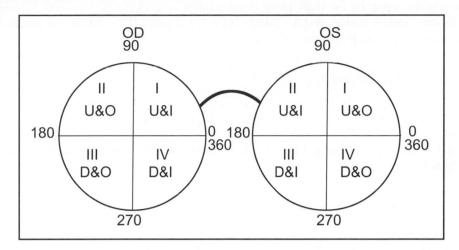

Quadrants I and II are always "UP" and quadrants III and IV are always "DOWN." II and III are on the left, and I and IV are on the right. Which two are "IN" or "OUT" depends on whether the lens is to be in front of the right eye or the left eye. (IN is toward the nose. OUT is toward the temple.)

Quadrant I has base direction UP and IN for the right lens, or UP and OUT for the left lens. The direction of the prism base is between 0 and 90 degrees.

Quadrant II has base direction UP and OUT for the right lens, or UP and IN for the left lens. The direction of the prism base is between 90 and 180 degrees.

Quadrant III has base direction DOWN and OUT for the right lens, or DOWN and IN for the left lens. The direction of the prism base is between 180 and 270 degrees.

Quadrant IV has base direction DOWN and IN for the right lens, or DOWN and OUT for the left lens. The direction of the prism base is between 270 and 360 degrees.

Prism base down and out is very different from prism base up and in, so we use 180 to 360 degrees for down. When discussing cylinder axis, we make no distinction between up and down because it is not necessary.

EXAMPLES:

4-26. The prescription is
OD pl 3^Δ BU & 5^Δ BI
OS pl 3^Δ BD & 5^Δ BI
From the diagram at right we see that the OD prism is in quadrant I and the OS prism is in quadrant III. Therefore we can expect the direction of the prism base to be between 0 and 90 degrees for the right lens and between 180 and 270 degrees for the left lens. Look first at the right lens.

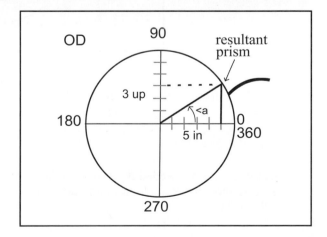

Do you see the right triangle made by the horizontal and vertical sides of the prescribed prism? The angle a in the diagram tells us where the prism is located within quadrant I and is the angle that the longest side of the triangle makes with the horizontal axis of the lens. The resultant amount of the prism is the length of the longest side of the triangle. (A right triangle is a triangle with one 90-degree angle. The longest side is called the hypotenuse and is opposite the right angle in the triangle.)

If we use P for the amount of the resultant prism, H for the amount of the horizontal prism, and V for the amount of the vertical prism, then (using Pythagoras' theorem)

$$\boxed{P^2 = H^2 + V^2}$$

The angle a shown in the diagram has

$$\boxed{\tan a = \frac{V}{H}}$$

In this example:

a. H = 5, V = 3, $P^2 = 5^2 + 3^2 = 34$, and $P = \sqrt{34} = 5.8^\Delta$, tan a = 3/5 = 0.6, and a = 31°

(Use the $\boxed{\tan^{-1}}$ key.)

b. Since 31° is between 0 and 90, which is what we wanted, the resultant prism is 5.8^Δ @ 031, or 5.8^Δ BU & I @ 031°. In the lensmeter the target will look like this:

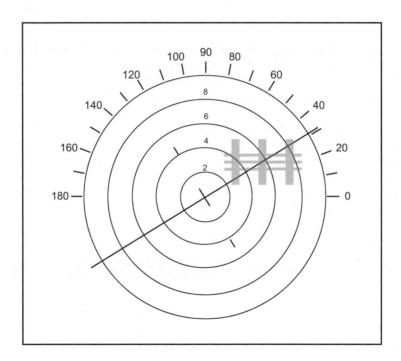

4-27. Now for the left lens: OS pl 3^Δ BD & 5^Δ BI

H = 5   tan a = 3/5 = 0.6
V = 3   a = 31°
$P^2 = 5^2 + 3^2 = 34$
P = 5.8^Δ

But this time we needed the axis to be between 180 and 270, since the prism is in quadrant III.
To find the correct angle, we add 180 degrees to the 31 from the formula. So the resultant prism is
5.8^Δ @ 211.

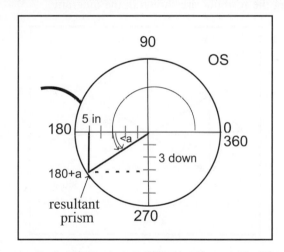

Most lensmeters only show the axis notation between 0 and 180, so we cannot read the axis directly at 211 degrees. Therefore, sometimes we show prism axis that should have been between 180 and 360 as the equivalent amount between 0 and 180 degrees. When the base direction is DOWN, subtract 180 degrees from the axis for the prism. In the example above, the answer may be written **5.8$^\Delta$ BD & I @ 031°.**

Notice that we have included the directions BD & I this time. When the prism was written 5.8$^\Delta$ @ 211°, there was no doubt where the base was: it was in the third quadrant. In the notation 5.8$^\Delta$ BD & I @ 031°, if we omit the BD & I, the base would be in the first quadrant instead of the third quadrant, and the wearer would have the prism in the worst possible wrong direction!

When we omit the base direction (BD & I, BU & O, etc.), we force the person reading the prescription to assume that we are giving the actual direction with the axis. We call this the ***360-degree notation.*** If the base were in the third or fourth quadrant, the axis would be between 180 and 360 degrees. The prism amount 1$^\Delta$ @ 028 means the prism is in the first quadrant. It cannot be in the third quadrant. The prism amount 1$^\Delta$ @ 135 is in the second quadrant; it cannot be in the fourth quadrant. Likewise, the prism amount 1$^\Delta$ @ 240 is in the third quadrant, and the prism amount 1$^\Delta$ @ 328 is in the fourth quadrant. This is 360-degree notation because we are using all of the 360 degrees in the circle.

On the other hand, if we state the base direction using BU, BD, BI, and BO, we can use the more familiar *180-degree notation,* where we do not use any degrees above 180. For the right lens:

- The prism 1^Δ @ 028 becomes 1^Δ BU & I @ 028.
- 1^Δ @ 135 becomes 1^Δ BU & O @ 135.
- 1^Δ @ 240 becomes 1^Δ BD & O @ 060 (because 240 − 180 = 060).
- 1^Δ @ 328 becomes 1^Δ BD & I @ 148 (because 328 − 180 = 148).

The upper half of the lens is always between 0 and 180 degrees, so the two notations have the same axes in quadrant I and II. In the lower half of the lens the axes for the two notations differ by exactly 180 degrees.

Remember, the base direction for prism is not like the cylinder notation, where what happens in the top of the lens also happens in the bottom of the lens. We are talking about prism base direction, where a base at 90 degrees is very different from a base at 270 degrees.

EXAMPLES:

4-28. 1^Δ BD & O @ 045 = 1^Δ @ 225 (*Note:* This is OD. Why?)

4-29. 3.5^Δ BD & I @ 120 = 3.5^Δ @ 300 (*Note:* Which lens?)

4-30. OD 4.25^Δ @ 275 = 4.25^Δ BD & I @ 095

4-31. OS 2^Δ @ 193 = 2^Δ BD & I @ 013

4-32. 1.5^Δ BU & O @ 040 = 1.5^Δ @ 040 (Why are the angles the same? Which lens is this?)

Rules for the angle, after using the formula, are shown in the diagram:

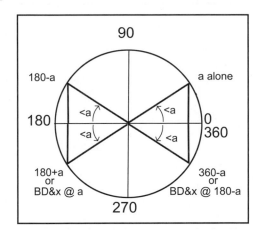

Quadrant I	$\angle a$
Quadrant II	$180 - \angle a$
Quadrant III	$180 + \angle a$, or $\angle a$ and the base direction
Quadrant IV	$360 - \angle a$, or $180 - \angle a$ and the base direction

EXAMPLES:

4-33. What are the prism amount and base direction for OD +1.50D 1.5^Δ BU & 2.5^Δ BO?
V = 1.5
H = 2.5
$P^2 = H^2 + V^2 = 6.25 + 2.25 = 8.5; P = 2.9^\Delta$
tan a = V/H = 1.5/2.5 = 0.6; a = 31°
OD BU & O is in the second quadrant, so the base direction is 180 − 31 = 149.
ANSWER: **2.9^Δ BU & O @ 149** or **2.9^Δ @ 149**

4-34. Rx: OS –4.25D 3$^\Delta$ BD & 1$^\Delta$ BO. What are the resultant prism amount and base direction?

V = 3

H = 1

P^2 = H^2 + V^2 = 1 + 9 = 10; P = 3.2$^\Delta$

tan a = V/H = 3/1 = 3; a = 72°

OS BD & O is in the fourth quadrant, so the base direction is 360 – 72 = 288.

ANSWER: **3.2$^\Delta$ @ 288** or **3.2$^\Delta$ BD & O @ 108**

EXERCISES: (Round to one-tenth prism diopter unless the prism amount is an exact quarter. Round base direction to whole angles.)

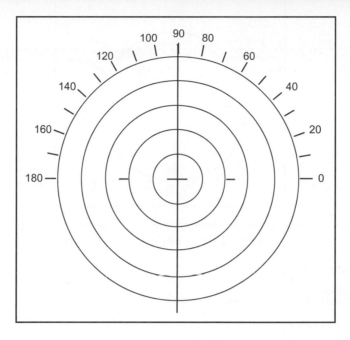

39. What are the prism amount and base direction for the prescription OD +1.00D 2.25$^\Delta$ BU & 2.25$^\Delta$ BI? Where would the resultant prism be located in the lensmeter target?

40. Rx: OS –0.50 –0.50 ×090 1.0$^\Delta$ BI & 2.0$^\Delta$ BU. What are the amount and base direction of the resultant prism? Where would the resultant prism be located in the lensmeter target?

41. If the prism prescribed is 4$^\Delta$ BD & 3$^\Delta$ BI for the right lens, what are the amount and base direction of the resultant prism? Where would the resultant prism be located in the lensmeter target?

42. If the prism prescribed is 2$^\Delta$ BD & 3$^\Delta$ BI for the left lens, what are the amount and base direction of the resultant prism? Where would the resultant prism be located in the lensmeter target?

─────────────── **RESOLVING PRISM** ───────────────

The formulas for resolving a prism into vertical and horizontal parts are

$$V = (P)(\sin a)$$
$$H = (P)(\cos a)$$

where:

P = amount of the resultant prism

V = vertical component

H = horizontal component

Note: Some textbooks call prism written in vertical and horizontal parts ***prescriber's notation.***

4-35. The prism found in the lensmeter for a pair of glasses is 2.0$^\Delta$ @ 045, and the lens is a right lens. Resolve this prism into its component parts.

On the diagram the long side P of the triangle is 2.0 and the angle ∠a that the prism makes with the axis is 45 degrees. The angle 45° is quadrant I, which is U and I for the right lens.

V = (P)(sin a) = (2.0)(sin 45) = (2)(0.707) = 1.4$^\Delta$ BU, since V is vertical

H = (P)(cos a) = (2.0)(cos 45) = (2)(0.707) = 1.4$^\Delta$ BI, since H is horizontal

The prism resolves to **1.4$^\Delta$ BI & 1.4$^\Delta$ BU.**

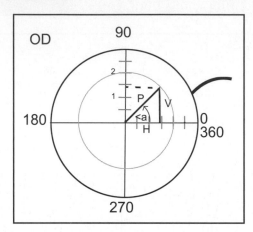

Example 4-35, Vertical Component

Type A Calculator:

2 ▣x 45 ▣sin ▣= The calculator should say 1.414...

Type B Calculator:

▣x ▣sin 45 ▣= The calculator should say 1.414...

Example 4-35, Horizontal Component

Type A Calculator:

2 ▣x 45 ▣cos ▣= The calculator should say 1.414...

Type B Calculator:

2 ▣x ▣cos 45 ▣= The calculator should say 1.414...

4-36. Resolve 4$^\Delta$ BU & I @ 105° into its component parts. Which lens is it for?

P = 4 (In these formulas, ignore the sign of the sine and cosine functions.)

V = (P)(sin a) = (4)(sin 105) = (4)(0.966) = 3.9$^\Delta$ BU

H = (P)(cos a) = (4)(cos 105) = (4)(0.259) = 1.0$^\Delta$ BI

The answer is **3.9$^\Delta$ BU & 1.0$^\Delta$ BI.** The angle 105 degrees is in quadrant II; BU & I is in quadrant II only for the left lens.

4-37. Resolve OD 3.5$^\Delta$ @ 300° into its component parts. (In these formulas, ignore the sign of the sine and cosine functions.)

P = 3.5

The angle 300° is in quadrant IV, which is BD & I for the right lens.
V = (P)(sin a) = (3.5)(sin 300) = (3.5)(0.866) = 3.0△ BD
H = (P)(cos a) = (3.5)(cos 300) = (3.5)(0.5) = 1.8△ BI
The answer is **3.0△ BD & 1.8△ BI.**

EXERCISES: (Round to one-tenth prism diopter unless the prism amount is an exact quarter. Round base direction to whole angles.)

43. Resolve OD 2.25△ @ 255° into its component parts.

44. Resolve OS 4.25△ BD & I @ 45° into its component parts.

45. What are the component parts of the prism shown in this diagram? This is a left lens. (The target is one third of the way between the two circles.)

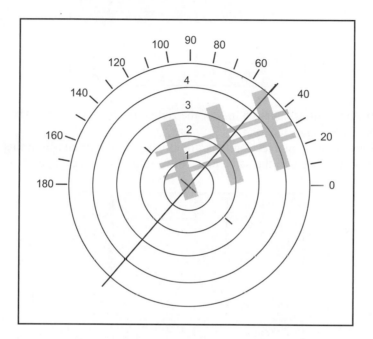

NON-FORMULA TECHNIQUES FOR FINDING RESOLVING AND RESULTANT PRISM

A non-formula charting method can be used to find resolving and resultant prism. Once you understand this method, you can use a version of it on multiple-choice examinations to verify which of the choices is the most likely to be correct. A full-color version of the chart appears on the inside back cover of this book. This chart may be photocopied onto a transparency or may be copied with a color copier and then laminated so that you can write on it with water-soluble markers.

RESULTANT PRISM

Find the horizontal prism amount on the horizontal axis.
Find the vertical prism on the vertical axis.
Using the square straight lines (blue on the chart), locate the intersection where these two meet.
Using the circular lines (red on the chart), determine what the amount of the prism is.
Using the bicycle spokes (black on the chart), determine what the axis is.
See the inside back cover for a color version of the chart.

Refer to the inside back cover for a color version of the chart.

    4-38. OD pl 3$^\Delta$ BU & 5$^\Delta$ BI

           OS pl 3$^\Delta$ BD & 5$^\Delta$ BI

This is the same problem we did in Example 4-26. We need to resolve the prism for each lens.

OD BU & I is in the first quadrant.

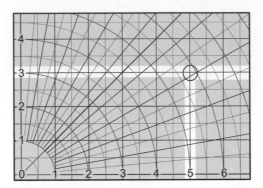

1. Using the straight (blue) lines, locate 5 in. For the right lens this will be 5 to the right, or quadrant I.
2. Using the straight (blue) lines, locate 3 up.
3. Follow the two lines to their intersection. You are looking for the intersection that is circled on the diagram above. You would get to the same place if, in step 2, you had gone up 3 on the 5 in line.

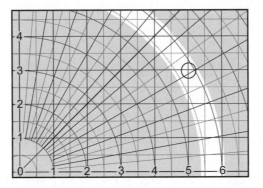

4. Look at the circular (red) lines nearest the intersection of the straight blue lines. This intersection is between the 5.5 ring and the 6.0 ring. It is a little more than halfway between them, so it is a little more than 5.75$^\Delta$. I would estimate 5.8$^\Delta$.

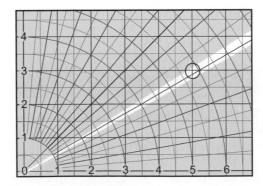

5. Look at the bicycle spokes (black). The intersection is between the 30 and the 35 degree spokes, closer to the 30. If you line up a ruler or straight edge with the 0 center and the crossing of blue lines, you will see

that the straight edge lines up with the first tick mark above the 30-degree mark at the outside edge of the circles. Each of those tick marks is one degree. So we have a degree mark of 31.
The answer is **5.8$^\Delta$ BU & I @ 31°**, or **5.8$^\Delta$ @ 31°**.

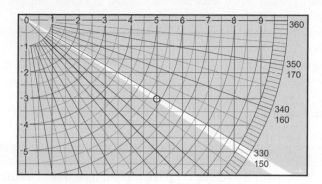

OS BD & I is in the fourth quadrant.
1. Using the straight (blue) lines on the diagram above, locate 5 in.
2. Still using the straight (blue) lines, find the 3 down line.
3. Locate the intersections of the two prism amounts. This should be in the fourth quadrant.
4. Look at the circular (red) lines nearest the intersection. They should again be the 5.5 and 6.0 rings. The prism amount is 5.8$^\Delta$.
5. Look at the bicycle spokes. This one is between the 325 and 330 spokes. If you use a straight edge between the 0 mark and the intersection and go all the way to the edge, you will note that it is at the 329, which is also the 149.
The answer is **5.8$^\Delta$ BD & I @ 149°**, or **5.8$^\Delta$ @ 329°**.

Note: There is no conversion of the angle using this chart. You use the angle that you read around the outer circle. The angle conversion that is shown in the corners is to help you remember what to do with the angle that is found using the formula.

RESOLVING PRISM

Find the prism amount on the (red) circular lines.
Find the (black) spoke that gives the meridian of the prism.
Locate the intersection where these two meet.
Using the straight lines (blue), determine the amount of the horizontal and vertical prism.
See the inside back cover for the color version of the chart.

EXAMPLE (Resolving prism):

4-39. The prism found in the lensmeter for a pair of glasses is 2.0$^\Delta$ @ 125, and the lens is a right lens. Resolve this prism into its component parts.

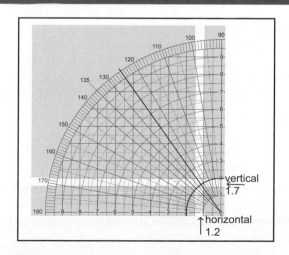

1. This is in quadrant II. Find the 2.0 prism ring (red).
2. Find the 125 bicycle spoke (black).
3. Locate the intersection of these two lines.
4. Using the horizontal lines (blue), this is between the 1.0 and 1.5 lines, but not quite halfway, so estimate as 1.2$^\Delta$. For a right lens this is OUT.
5. Using the vertical lines (blue), this is between the 1.5 and 2.0 lines, but again not quite halfway, so estimate as 1.7$^\Delta$. This is UP.

The answer from the chart is **1.2$^\Delta$ BO and 1.7$^\Delta$ BU.** Using the formulas, verify that the actual answer is 1.1 BO and 1.7 BU.

Note: The chart will not give you exact answers. If your prism amount is within 0.1$^\Delta$ and the axis is within 1°, you are doing it correctly.

EXERCISES:

46. Use the chart on the resultant prism exercises on p. 121. Compare the answers you get with the ones that you got with the formulas.

47. Use the chart on the resolving prism exercises on p. 127. Compare the answers you get with the ones that you got with the formulas.

———— MULTIPLE-CHOICE EXAMINATIONS ————

When taking multiple-choice examinations, you can use a similar charting method to find potential right choices (or eliminate definitely wrong choices). Start with the basic circle, divide it into quadrants, and then divide each quadrant into halves. You have an eight-piece pie.

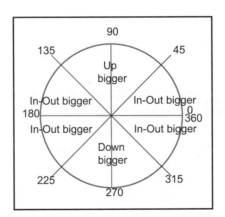

Mark the quadrants as 0-90, 90-180, 180-270, 270-360. Note the one-eighth meridians: 45, 135, 225, 315.

Now, identify in which one eighth of the pie the prism is. In the pieces that are next to the horizontal axis the horizontal amount will be greater than the vertical. In the pieces next to the vertical axis the vertical amount will be greater than the horizontal. Right on the one-eighth meridians the horizontal and vertical are equal.

Look at Example 4-39: the prism found in the lensmeter for a pair of glasses is 2.0$^\Delta$ @ 125, and the lens is a right lens. Resolve this prism into its component parts.

If this had been a multiple-choice question, the choices might be:

a. 1.1$^\Delta$ BO and 1.6$^\Delta$ BU
b. 1.6$^\Delta$ BO and 1.1$^\Delta$ BU
c. 1.1$^\Delta$ BI and 1.6$^\Delta$ BU
d. 1.6$^\Delta$ BI and 1.1$^\Delta$ BU

If you identify that the meridian of 125 is in the II quadrant and for a right lens this is BU & O, you eliminate choices c and d. If you note that meridian 125 is above the one-eighth meridian, so it is in the upper part of quadrant II, you know that the vertical amount must be greater than the horizontal amount, eliminating choice b.

Try Example 4-33: what are the prism amount and base direction for OD 1.5△ BU & 2.5△ BO? The choices might be:

a. 2.9△ BU & O @ 31
b. 2.9△ BU & O @ 149
c. 2.9△ BU & O @ 59
d. 2.9△ BU & O @ 122

Right lens UP and OUT is in quadrant II, so choices a and c are eliminated. OUT is bigger than UP, so the answer must be between 135 and 180, eliminating choice d.

Note: This technique will not give an accurate enough answer by itself for practical purposes, but it will help you check that your answer from either the chart or the formulas is reasonable.

Note: This helps only on multiple-choice examinations, and it will not necessarily eliminate all wrong choices.

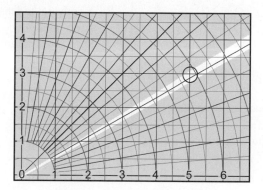

A color version of the above chart appears on the inside back cover.

The questions with an asterisk (*) in front of the question number are advanced questions. They are not likely to be on the ABO exam but might be on the ABOM exam or the COT exam.

The questions are not presented in the order of the subjects in the section. Some of these questions may require you to think about what you have read in the section, and some may depend on material covered in previous sections.

1. The image seen through a prism is
   a. displaced down.
   b. displaced up.
   c. displaced toward the apex of the prism.
   d. displaced toward the base of the prism.

2. For the Rx:
   OD −2.50   ADD +1.75 OU
   OS pl
   a. if needed, reverse slab-off would be ordered for the left lens.
   b. if needed, reverse slab-off would be ordered for the right lens.
   c. there is no need of slab-off because of the pl in the left Rx.
   d. if needed, reverse slab-off would be ordered for the right lens and regular slab-off would be ordered for the left lens.

3. The result of 3^Δ BU in the right lens and 3^Δ BD in the left lens is
   a. vertical disassociation of the eyes.
   b. no vertical disassociation but some distortion for the wearer.
   c. antimetropia.
   d. horizontal surfaces will seem sloped to the wearer.

4. The angle of deviation of a ray passing through a prism is measured from the ray
   a. to the path that the ray would have taken if the prism were not there.
   b. to the normal to the surface.
   c. to the surface.
   d. to the axis of the prism.

5. The prism diopter measures
   a. the ability of a lens to converge light rays.
   b. the amount that white light is dispersed when traveling through a prism.
   c. the amount that the eye rotates from the primary position when looking through a lens with dioptric power.
   d. the amount that an image is displaced at a given distance from a prism.

6. Antimetropia means
   a. one eye myopic and one eye hyperopic.
   b. one eye emmetropic and one eye ametropic.
   c. not the same refractive error.
   d. equal refractive errors.

7. A unit of measurement that equates to a 1:100 ratio is the
   a. prism diopter.
   b. refracting degree.
   c. Hertz.
   d. nm.

8. A converging lens shows
   a. no motion.
   b. scissors motion.
   c. against motion.
   d. with motion.

9. The Rx is OD $−3.00^\Delta$ 2 BI. To create the prism using a stock lens, the OC must be decentered an extra
   a. 15 mm out.
   b. 15 mm in.
   c. 6.7 mm out.
   d. 6.7 mm in.

10. An object is viewed through a 6^Δ prism. The image is displaced down 9 cm. The object is _____ from the prism.
    a. 54 cm
    b. 5.4 m
    c. 1.5 cm
    d. 1.5 m

11. How much will a 3.5^Δ prism displace the image of an object that is 25 cm away?
    a. 21 mm
    b. 14 mm
    c. 9 mm
    d. 7 mm

12. There is never prism present
    a. at the prism reference point of the lens.
    b. at the optical center of the lens.
    c. at the major reference point of the lens.
    d. at the geometric center on the lens.

13. A diverging lens shows
    a. against motion.
    b. with motion.
    c. no motion.
    d. scissors motion.

14. At a point 5 mm above the OC of a +2.00D lens there will be
    a. 1.0^Δ BD.   c. 2.5^Δ BD.
    b. 1.0^Δ BU.   d. 2.5^Δ BU.

15. The OC is inset 3 mm too much on a −6.50D lens. The induced prism is
    a. 2.0^Δ BO.
    b. 2.0^Δ BI.
    c. 2.25^Δ BO.
    d. 2.25^Δ BI.
16. The Rx is OD −12.00 OS −11.50. The wearer's PDs are noted on the job ticket as 59 mm. The glasses, when complete, have a distance between MRP of 61. These glasses meet ANSI standards for MRP placement.
    a. True
    b. False
17. The glasses are positioned so that the optical centers are above the wearer's pupils. If the prescription is +2.50 OU, what prism is the person experiencing?
    a. None
    c. BU
    b. BO
    d. BD
18. Slab-off prism ground on glass lenses creates
    a. BD prism in the distance area.
    b. BD prism in the reading area.
    c. BU prism in the distance area.
    d. BU prism in the reading area.
19. The amount that a prism displaces an image is dependent on
    a. the distance from the prism to the object.
    b. the distance from the observer to the prism.
    c. the distance from the image to the object.
    d. the distance from the observer to the image.
20. An object that is 50 cm from a prism appears to be displaced by 2 cm. The power of the prism is
    a. 25^Δ.
    b. 14^Δ.
    c. 8^Δ.
    d. 4^Δ.
21. When looking 8 mm below the OC of a +4.50 D lens, the wearer will experience
    a. 3.6^Δ BO.
    b. 3.6^Δ BI.
    c. 3.6^Δ BD.
    d. 3.6^Δ BU.
22. To create 5^Δ BU prism in a +6.50 lens, the OC must be decentered
    a. 13 mm up.
    b. 13 mm down.
    c. 8 mm up.
    d. 8 mm down.
23. When passing through a prism, a beam of light will be broken into its component colors. List the colors to which white light will be dispersed, from the least refracted color to the most refracted color.
    a. red, orange, yellow, green, blue, violet
    b. yellow, green, blue, violet, red, orange
    c. green, yellow, orange, red, violet, blue
    d. violet, blue, green, yellow, orange, red

24. The combination of 3^Δ BU in the right lens and 4^Δ BU in the left lens is
    a. compounding.
    b. canceling.
    c. neither compounding nor canceling.
    d. both compounding and canceling.
25. A diverging lens can be thought of as a series of progressively stronger prisms with
    a. the bases toward the center.
    b. the apices toward the center
    c. the bases toward the right.
    d. the bases oriented with the earth's magnetic poles.
26. The result of 3^Δ BI in the right lens and 3^Δ BI in the left lens is
    a. vertical disassociation of the eyes.
    b. no horizontal disassociation but some distortion for the wearer.
    c. 6^Δ of divergence of the eyes.
    d. 6^Δ of convergence of the eyes.
27. Reverse slab-off is
    a. molded on the back of plastic lenses.
    b. ground on the front of plastic lenses.
    c. molded on the front of plastic lenses.
    d. ground on the back of plastic lenses.
28. The result of 2^Δ BU in the right lens and 2^Δ BU in the left lens is
    a. vertical disassociation only of the eyes.
    b. no vertical disassociation but some distortion for the wearer.
    c. image jump.
    d. a pair of glasses that do not meet ANSI standards.
29. The Rx is OD +5.00 OS +3.50. The wearer's PDs are noted on the job ticket as 62 mm. The glasses, when complete, have a distance between MRP of 65. The induced unwanted prism is
    a. 0.2^Δ BO.
    b. 0.2^Δ BI.
    c. 1.3^Δ BO.
    d. 1.3^Δ BI.
30. The Rx is OD −12.50 OS −11.00. The wearer's PDs are noted on the job ticket as 59 mm. The glasses, when complete, have a distance between MRP of 61. The induced unwanted prism is
    a. 0.2^Δ BI.
    b. 0.2^Δ BO.
    c. 2.4^Δ BI.
    d. 2.4^Δ BO.
31. At 5 mm below the OC of the Rx −6.00 −2.50 ×030, the approximate prism amount will be
    a. 3^Δ BU.
    b. 3^Δ BD.
    c. 4^Δ BD.
    d. 5^Δ BU.

32. The Rx is:
    OD +4.00 −3.00 ×165
    OS +4.00 −1.50 ×010
    In the completed glasses the OC height for the right lens is 2 mm above the OC height for the left lens. The induced unwanted prism is
    a. 0.75^{Δ}.   c. 0.27^{Δ}.
    b. 0.51^{Δ}.   d. 0.24^{Δ}.

33. A person with anisometropia, when forced to look down through bifocal lenses, *may* experience
    a. presbyopia.
    b. esotropia.
    c. iseikonia.
    d. asthenopia.

34. The unit used by the eye care industry to compare the ability of different materials to disperse light into its component colors when the light is passed through a prism is the
    a. angle of dispersion.
    b. Abbé value.
    c. index of refraction.
    d. index of dispersion.

35. The Rx is:
    OD +4.00 −3.00 ×165
    OS +4.00 −1.50 ×010
    In the completed glasses the OC height for the right lens is 2 mm above the OC height for the left lens. The glasses meet ANSI standards for vertical OC placement.
    a. True   b. False

36. The Rx is OD +5.00 OS +3.50. The wearer's PDs are noted on the job ticket as 62 mm. The glasses, when complete, have a distance between MRP of 65. These glasses meet ANSI standards for MRP placement.
    a. True
    b. False

37. The Rx is OD pl 4^{Δ} BI OS pl 5^{Δ} BU. The comments contain the statement, "Split the prism." The glasses could be ordered:
    a. OD pl 2^{Δ} BI 2.5^{Δ} BD
       OS pl 2^{Δ} BI 2.5^{Δ} BU
    b. OD pl 2^{Δ} BI 2.5^{Δ} BU
       OS pl 2^{Δ} BI 2.5^{Δ} BU
    c. OD pl 2^{Δ} BI 2.5^{Δ} BD
       OS pl 2^{Δ} BO 2.5^{Δ} BU
    d. OD pl 2^{Δ} BI 2.5^{Δ} BU
       OS pl 2^{Δ} BO 2.5^{Δ} BU

38. A lens has the Rx +4.00 sph, ADD +2.50. The lens is made from CR-39 with a round 22 segment, a drop of 3 mm, and an inset of 2 mm. The image jump for this lens is
    a. 0.12^{Δ} BU.   c. 2.0^{Δ} BU.
    b. 0.75^{Δ} BD.   d. 2.75^{Δ} BD.

39. The image jump for an Executive lens made from crown glass with a distance Rx of −2.00 −1.00 ×090 and an Add of +1.75 is
    a. 3.0^{Δ} BD.   c. 0.
    b. 2.0^{Δ} BD.   d. 1.75^{Δ} BU.

40. Anisometropia means
    a. one eye emmetropic and one eye ametropic.
    b. one eye myopic and one eye hyperopic.
    c. equal refractive errors.
    d. not the same refractive error.

41. The most accurate measurement of prism power is the
    a. prism diopter.
    b. centrad.
    c. apical angle.
    d. degree of dispersion.

42. When looking through a prism, the eye will rotate
    a. toward the outside of the prism.
    b. toward the center of the prism.
    c. toward the base of the prism.
    d. toward the apex of the prism.

43. The Rx is:
    +4.00 sph   ADD +2.50
    +2.00 −1.00 ×180   ADD +2.50
    The vertical imbalance at a reading level of 8 mm below OC for this Rx is
    a. 1.6^{Δ} BD OD.
    b. 1.6^{Δ} BU OD.
    c. 2.4^{Δ} BD OD.
    d. 2.4^{Δ} BU OD.

44. The Rx is
    OD +1.50 sph   ADD +2.50 OU
    OS −0.50 sph
    If vertical imbalance correction is needed, reverse slab-off would be ordered for
    a. OS.
    b. OD.
    c. both lenses.
    d. the thinner lens.

45. The angle at the apex of a prism is sometimes called the
    a. dispersing angle.
    b. deviating angle.
    c. refracting angle.
    d. reflecting angle.

46. The Rx is
    −0.75 −3.25 ×035   ADD +2.50
    +0.75 −1.00 ×150   ADD +2.50
    The vertical imbalance at a reading level of 9 mm below OC for this Rx is
    a. 3.3^{Δ} BU OD.
    b. 2.6^{Δ} BD OD.
    c. 1.4^{Δ} BU OD.
    d. 0.

47. The result of 2^Δ BI in the right lens and 2^Δ BO in the left lens is
    a. vertical disassociation of the eyes.
    b. no horizontal disassociation but some distortion for the wearer.
    c. 4^Δ of divergence of the eyes.
    d. 4^Δ of convergence of the eyes.

48. A ray traveling through a -3.00 lens 5 mm to the right of the OC will be displaced
    a. 1.5^Δ to the right.
    b. 1.5^Δ to the left.
    c. 0.6^Δ to the right.
    d. 0.6^Δ to the left.

*49. 5^Δ BU & I @ 125 is the same as
    a. 5^Δ @ 305.
    b. 5^Δ @ 215.
    c. 5^Δ @ 205.
    d. 5^Δ @ 125.

*50. A prism deviated a light beam by $10°$. The prism is made from glass with an index of refraction of 1.70. What is the power of the prism?
    a. 24^Δ c. 12^Δ
    b. 18^Δ d. 7^Δ

*51. 5^Δ BU & I @ 125 is the same as
    a. 4.1^Δ BU and 2.9^Δ BI.
    b. 2.9^Δ BU and 4.1^Δ BI.
    c. 3.4^Δ BU and 1.6^Δ BI.
    d. 1.6^Δ BU and 3.4^Δ BI.

*52. A prism will be made from a flint glass having an index of refraction of 1.80. The prism will have an angle of deviation of $15°$. What apical angle will the prism have?
    a. $27.0°$
    b. $18.75°$
    c. $12.0°$
    d. $8.33°$

*53. The prescription is
    OD -2.50 sph   ADD $+1.75$ OU
    OS -0.50 sph
    The wearer has a reading problem that you trace to vertical imbalance in the reading area. The glasses are just for occasional use, and the wearer does not want to try slab-off until he is sure that it will fix the problem. If you decide to try two different segment styles to correct the imbalance, which of the following could you choose? (Assume a reading depth of 10 mm below distance OC.)
    a. OD FT-40; OS round 22
    b. OD round 22; OS FT-40
    c. OD FT-40; OS FT-25
    d. OD FT-25; OS FT-40

*54. OD 2^Δ BU and 4.5^Δ BI is the same as
    a. 4.9^Δ BU & I @ 114.
    b. 4.9^Δ BU & I @ 156.
    c. 4.9^Δ BU & I @ 066.
    d. 4.9^Δ BU & I @ 024.

*55. A beam of light is directed toward a prism made from an unknown material. The apical angle of the prism is $30°$. If the path of the beam of light is deviated by $17.6°$, what is the index of refraction of the material?
    a. 1.808
    b. 1.705
    c. 1.660
    d. 1.587

*56. OS 5^Δ BD and 3^Δ BI is the same as
    a. 5.8^Δ @ 59.
    b. 5.8^Δ @ 211.
    c. 5.8^Δ @ 239.
    d. 5.8^Δ @ 301.

*57. A prism made from 1.66 plastic has an apical angle of $10.0°$. What is the angle of deviation of a ray passing through the prism?
    a. $6.0°$
    b. $16.6°$
    c. $15.15°$
    d. $6.6°$

*58. 3.5^Δ BD & O @ 023 is the same as
    a. 3.5^Δ @ 203.
    b. 3.5^Δ @ 113.
    c. 3.5^Δ @ 293.
    d. 3.5^Δ @ 023.

SECTION V – SURFACING AND FINISHING

LENS AND FRAME MEASUREMENTS

When surfacing and cutting a lens to fit a frame, we must determine where the optical center of the lens will be. We may need to know the amount of *decentration per lens* and the *minimum blank size*. To calculate either of these values, we first need a consistent way of measuring the lens and frame opening. Two measurement systems are currently in use.

BOXING SYSTEM

In the boxing system a rectangle is drawn around each lens, allowing us to find the ***geometric center*** (GC) of the lens and frame opening. The geometric center is halfway from the top to the bottom of the lens and halfway from the right side to the left side of the lens. The horizontal size of the rectangle is called the ***eye size,*** or ***A measurement,*** and the vertical size of the rectangle is called the ***depth,*** or ***B measurement.***

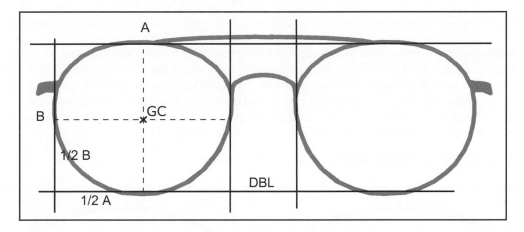

The ***distance between lenses*** (DBL) is the minimum measurement between the lenses after they have been mounted in the frame. The DBL is not necessarily the length of the bridge of the frame.

On a rimless frame or a frame with thin metal wires the DBL can be measured directly from the lenses or from the frame. It is the smallest distance between lenses.

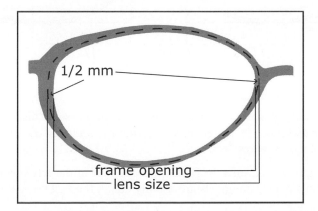

On a thick frame the edge of the lens is (or eventually will be) inside the thickness of the frame. In this case we assume that the lens bevel will be 0.5 mm inside the frame. The desired A and B measurements are taken from the inside of the eyewire, and 1 mm (0.5 mm per side) is *added* to the measurement. The DBL is measured from the inside of one eyewire to the inside of the other eyewire, and then 1 mm (0.5 mm per side) is *subtracted* from the measurement.

Manufacturers who mark their frame sizes using the boxing system may place a small box between the A and DBL: "52 □ 18" means a frame with an A measurement of 52 and a DBL of 18, using the boxing system.

DATUM SYSTEM

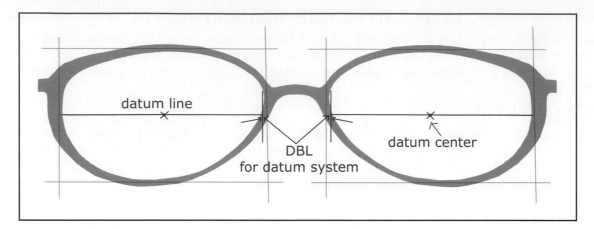

Many manufacturers use the datum system instead of the boxing system to show the measurements of the frame. In the datum system, we draw a horizontal line halfway between the top and bottom of the lens. The width of the lens at this point is the **datum measurement** or **D measurement.** The distance between the lenses at this point is the DBL. The datum system frequently gives a smaller eye size and a larger DBL than does the boxing system.

Although the measurements stamped on the frame by the manufacturer should be noted in the wearer's records, for laboratory calculations the boxing system should be used to measure the frame.

FRAME CENTER DISTANCE

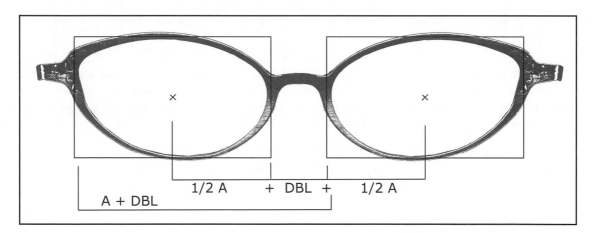

The distance between the geometric centers of the lenses in a pair of glasses ("distance between centers," or DBC) is also called the **frame center distance** (FCD), **geometric center distance** (GCD), or **frame PD** (FPD).

The DBC may be measured in two ways:

1. DBC = one half of the right lens A, plus the DBL, plus one half of the left lens A.
2. Since the right and left lens A measurements are usually equal, the FCD = A + DBL.

DECENTRATION

The distance between the wearer's pupils is called the **pupillary distance** (PD). (For a discussion of how to measure the wearer's PD, refer to a good dispensing book such as Brooks and Borish: *System for Ophthalmic Dispensing*.)

If no prism is prescribed, the completed glasses should have the optical centers of the lenses the same distance apart as the centers of the wearer's pupils. If prism is prescribed, the points on each lens where the prism amounts are exactly correct should be the same distance apart as the centers of the wearer's pupils.

The **prism reference point** (PRP) is the point on the lens where the prescribed prism is found. This point is also called the **major reference point** (MRP). The terms PRP and MRP are used interchangeably. The ANSI Z80.1-1999 standards use PRP, so PRP is used in this book. If no prism is prescribed, the optical center (OC) is the PRP.

If the wearer's PD is a binocular measurement, compare the wearer's PD and the DBC. If the DBC is equal to the wearer's PD, the PRP will be centered horizontally in the eyewire (or the frame's lens opening). If the DBC and the wearer's PD are not equal, we take one half of the difference between the wearer's PD and the DBC and offset the PRP by this amount in each lens. This process is called **decentering the lens,** because we are moving the optical center away from the geometric center of the lens.

$$\text{decentration} = 1/2 \ (DBC - PD)$$

where PD is binocular (from right pupil center to left pupil center).

When the wearer has wide-set eyes or when the frame is small with respect to the face, the decentration may be negative instead of positive. This means that the decentration will be out rather than in.

- With a zero (0) decentration the DBC and the wearer's PD are equal. In the completed glasses the PRP (or OC) will be at the frame GC.
- With a positive decentration, where the DBC is bigger than the wearer's PD, the PRP is moved from the GC toward the bridge, or in.
- With a negative decentration, where the wearer's PD is bigger than the DBC, the PRP is moved from the GC toward the temple, or out.

You may be given **monocular PDs** rather than binocular PDs. Monocular PDs are the distance from the center of the wearer's nose to the center of the pupil of each eye. Monocular PDs are typically required if the wearer's eyes are not symmetric or if you are preparing progressive addition lenses, high-power lenses, or aspheric lenses. When monocular PDs are provided, divide the DBC in half and subtract each of the two monocular PDs.

$$OD \text{ decentration} = 1/2 \ DBC - PD_{OD},$$
$$\text{where } PD_{OD} \text{ is monocular.}$$
$$OS \text{ decentration} = 1/2 \ DBC - PD_{OS},$$
$$\text{where } PD_{OS} \text{ is monocular.}$$

The **pattern differencr,** or **lens difference,** is A – B. The pattern difference is an indication of how similar the A and B measurements are. For example, the lens difference will be 0 for a round or square frame opening where A = B.

EXAMPLE:

5-1. The frame in the diagram below is a nylon suspension style. This means that the lens has a groove in it with a thin cord holding each lens to the metal frame. Determine:
a. The A, B, DBL, PFD, and lens difference using the boxing system.
b. The D and DBL using the datum system.
c. The decentration needed if the wearer's PD is 58 mm.
d. The decentration needed if the wearer's monocular PD is 28/30.

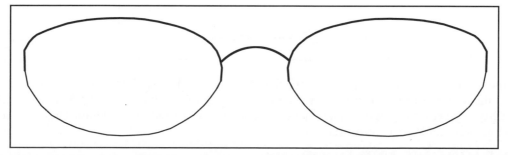

There is no bevel on the lens, so you do not need to make a 0.5-mm adjustment for the lens size. Begin by drawing rectangles around each lens, and measure one half of the A and one half of the B to locate the geometric center. Measure both lenses. They will not always be the same.

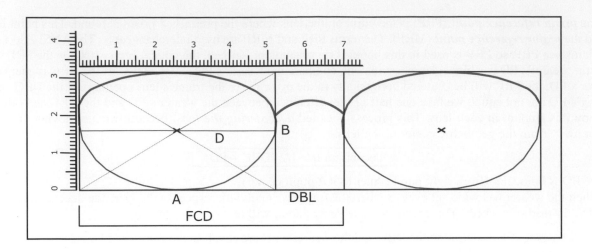

    a. A = 52 mm
        B = 32 mm
        DBL = 18 mm
        DBC = 70 mm
        Lens difference = 20 mm
    b. D = 51 mm
        DBL = 18 mm
    c. DBC – PD = 70 – 58 = 12. One half of 12 is 6 mm decentration in OU.
    d. One half of 70 is 35. OD decentration is 35 – 28 = 7 mm in.
                       OS decentration is 35 – 30 = 5 mm in.

EFFECTIVE DIAMETER

The *effective diameter* (ED) of a lens is defined as two times the longest radius of the lens. Once the geometric center of the lens has been identified, find the point on the eyewire that is the farthest from the center, measure the distance, and multiply by two. The longest measurement may be to any of the corners of the frame. The ED is *not* the longest measurement on the frame from eyewire to eyewire.

EXAMPLE:

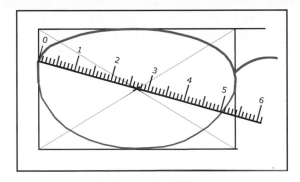

    5-2.   On the frame eyewire opening in Example 5-1 the longest radius is 27 mm, so the ED is 54 mm. Note that the longest distance from eyewire to eyewire is 52 mm (in this frame the A measurement) and the distance from eyewire to eyewire on the meridian with the longest radius is 50 mm. These would both be incorrect answers for the ED measurement.

SEGMENT HEIGHT AND DROP

On a bifocal lens we need to know where the center of the top of the segment will be with respect to the geometric center of the lens. The center of the top of the segment is sometimes called the *bifocal reference point.*

The *segment height* is the distance from the top of the bifocal segment to the lowest point of the edge of the lens. The point on the lens edge that is directly below the segment is not always the lowest point, as can be seen from the diagram. The *segment drop* or *below* is segment height – 1/2 B.

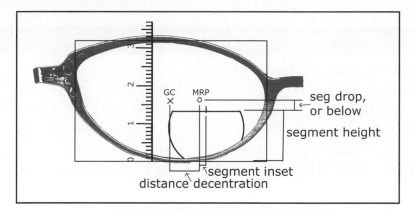

SEGMENT DROP or BELOW:

drop = segment height – 1/2 B

A negative segment drop means that the segment height is below the 1/2 B line. A positive segment drop means the segment top is above the 1/2 B line.

Note: In common usage the segment drop is referred to as a positive number when it is below 1/2 B. When the segment top is above 1/2 B, it is referred to as the *segment above* or *segment raise*.

Note: The PRP is typically placed on the 1/2 B line. If a PRP height is specified that is not 1/2 B, when the lens is prepared for surfacing, the drop will be calculated from the PRP height. In this situation when the lens is prepared for edging the 1/2 B line is used.

EXAMPLE:

5-3. In the diagram, B = 32, seg height = 13, and drop = 13 – 32/2 = 13 – 16 = –3 mm.

Note: For progressive addition lenses (PALs) the segment height is to the fitting cross and is usually *above* rather than *below*.

Note: When measuring the desired segment height for a plastic frame, add 0.5 mm to the segment height for the lower bevel of the lens.

SEGMENT INSET AND TOTAL INSET

The wearer's PD may be measured for both distance and near vision. This measurement may be either binocular or monocular. The difference between the distance and reading PDs will be the amount that the eyes converge for close work at the position where the glasses will sit.

The *segment inset* is the difference between the distance and near PD, per eye. The *total inset* or *total decentration* is the DBC – near PD, per lens.

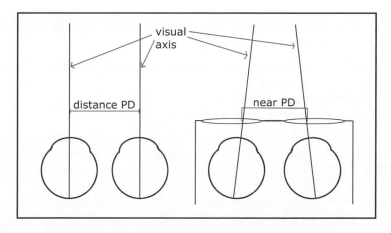

For measurements taken binocularly, so that you know only the total distance between the pupil centers for distance and close work, the segment inset is 1/2 (distance PD – near PD). For monocular measurements (each eye is measured separately) the segment inset is monocular distance PD – monocular near PD.

INSET

BINOCULAR MEASUREMENTS

Segment inset $= \frac{1}{2}(PD_{distance} - PD_{near})$

Total inset $\quad= \frac{1}{2}(DBC - PD_{near})$

$\qquad\qquad$ or

$\qquad\qquad= $ decentration + segment inset

MONOCULAR MEASUREMENTS

Segment inset $= PD_{distance} - PD_{near}$

Total inset $\quad= \frac{1}{2}(DBC - PD_{near})$

$\qquad\qquad$ or

$\qquad\qquad= $ decentration + segment inset

EXAMPLES:

5-4. In the diagram for Example 5-1 the DBC = 70 mm. If the wearer's PD measurements are recorded as 58/55, what are the distance decentration, segment inset, and total inset?

These measurements are binocular.

Distance decentration = 1/2 (DBC – PD) = 1/2 (70 – 58) = 1/2 (12) = **6.0 mm.**

Segment inset = 1/2 (distance PD – near PD) = 1/2 (58 – 55) = 1/2 (3) = **1.5 mm.**

Total inset = 1/2 (FCD – near PD) = 1/2 (70 – 55) = 1/2 (15) = **7.5 mm.**

Note: The total inset is equal to the distance decentration + the segment inset. Decentration + segment inset = 6 + 1.5 = 7.5 mm, the same answer that was calculated above. Either method for finding the total inset is acceptable.

5-5. For the same diagram, if the wearer's PD measurements are recorded as distance 28/30 and near 26/28, what are the decentration, segment inset, and total inset?

In this case the measurements are monocular.

Segment inset: OD distance PD – near PD = 28 – 26 = **2 mm.**

$\qquad\qquad\qquad$ OS distance PD – near PC = 30 – 28 = **2 mm.**

Total inset: $\quad$ OD decentration (from Example 5-1) + segment inset = 7 + 2 = **9 mm.**

$\qquad\qquad\qquad$ OS decentration (from Example 5-1) + segment inset = 5 + 2 = **7 mm.**

Verify for yourself that using 1/2 DBC – near PD gives the same answers.

EXERCISES:

On each of the following diagrams determine:

a. The A, B, DBL, DBC, ED, and frame difference using the boxing system.
b. The D and DBL using the datum system.
c. The segment height and below or above.
d-g. These questions will be different for each exercise.

1. Thin metal. Do not add 0.5 mm for bevel placement. Use the top of the round segment for the segment height. Match your ruler with the one printed here. If they agree, the measurements taken with your ruler should agree with mine.

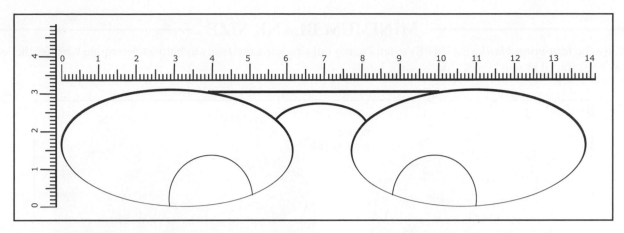

d. The distance decentration needed if the wearer's distance PD is 65 mm.
e. The distance decentration needed if the wearer's distance monocular PD is 34/31.
f. The segment inset and total inset for a PD of 65/60.
g. The segment inset and total inset for monocular PDs of distance 34/31 and near of 31/29. How would the segments have been positioned differently in this case?

2. Semi-rimless. Do not add 0.5 mm for bevel placement.

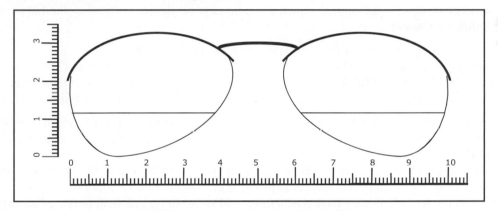

d. The distance decentration needed if the wearer's distance PD is 55 mm.
e. The distance decentration needed if the wearer's distance monocular PD is 24/27.
f. The segment inset and total inset for a PD of 57/54.
g. The segment inset and total inset for monocular PDs of distance 26/27.5 and near of 24.5/25.

3. Thick metal frame: adjust for bevel placement. Use the +, which is the fitting cross, for the segment height.

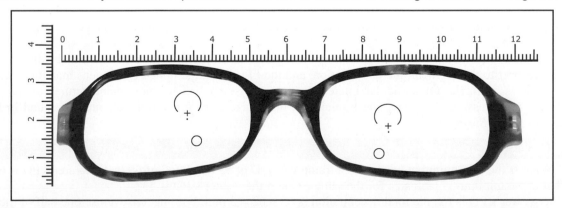

d. The wearer's distance PD, and the decentration needed to give the result shown. This should be monocular.

MINIMUM BLANK SIZE

We use the ***minimum blank size*** (MBS) when cutting out single vision lenses to help us determine whether the lens must be surfaced or can be cut from a stock lens.

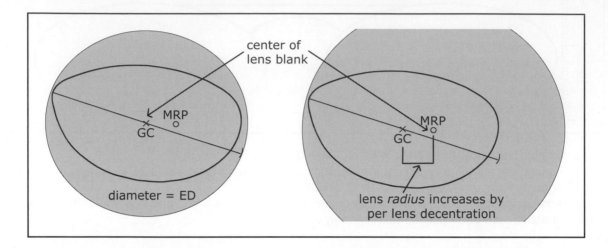

If there is no decentration of the optical center, the minimum blank size is equal to the ED of the frame. This occurs in the following situations:

- The lens is a plano power lens, or has plano power on the 180th meridian.
- No decentration is needed for the PRP from the geometric enter of the final cut lens. (The wearer's PD = DBC.)
- The lens is ground with the PRP decentered from the geometric center of the uncut lens blank. In this case the decentration has already been done, so the whole lens blank will be used for the finished, cut lens.

If the lens must be decentered from the GC of the lens blank by 1 mm, we need 1 mm in *each direction* on the lens, so we will add 2 mm to the ED. Similarly, if the decentration is 3 mm, we need 3 mm in both directions, or 6 mm plus the ED.

Since the lens moved by the amount of decentration, the *radius* of the necessary uncut lens increased by the amount of decentration and the *diameter* increased by twice the amount of decentration.

The very edge of the lens blank may have a nick or a mold seam, so for practical purposes some people add 1 to 2 mm to the amount needed for the minimum blank size. Thus

$$\boxed{\text{MBS} = \text{ED} + (2)(\text{per-lens decentration}) + 2 \text{ mm}}$$

Depending on the shape of the lens, the direction of the ED, and the condition of the edge, the lens may cut out of a smaller blank. The formula gives a "safe cutout" measurement, which is the largest size that the blank will need to be for a lens with a given decentration and ED. If the longest radius (used to calculate the ED) is toward the direction of decentration (usually toward the nasal side of the lens), this formula gives the correct minimum blank size.

Minimum blank size for a multifocal depends on the segment drop (or raise), the placement of the distance optical center with respect to the segment, the decentration, and the ED. A chart supplied by the lens manufacturer should be used if one is available. Of particular interest are the charts supplied by most manufacturers of progressive addition lens. A discussion about creating a minimum blank size chart for multifocals may be found in Brooks: *Understanding Lens Surfacing*.

EXAMPLE:

5-6. What is the minimum blank size for a frame with ED of 55 and DBC of 65 if the wearer's PD is 62? What is the minimum blank size for the same frame if the wearer's PD is 53?

If the wearer's PD is 62, the total decentration is 65 − 62 = 3 mm. For one lens we use one half of the total decentration; for minimum blank size we multiply by 2 again. So we can just use the decentration as is.

The minimum blank size is ED + twice the per-lens decentration + 2 mm = 55 + 3 + 2 = **60 mm.** The lens will cut out of a stock lens blank that has a 60-mm diameter or more.

For the person with a 53-mm PD, 65 − 53 = 12, and the minimum blank size is 55 + 12 + 2 = **69 mm.**

If the lens is ground for decentration, so that the PRP is not at the GC of the lens blank, the minimum blank size is ED + 2 mm = 55 + 2 = **57 mm** for both situations.

Note: Stock lenses (the surface curves are molded, and the optical center is at the lens blank geometric center) and unfinished lens blanks (one surface is complete, and the other surface will be created to give the Rx and PRP position desired) have a limited diameter selection determined by the manufacturer. The actual lens blank size will usually be the next larger blank from the MBS.

Note: When surfacing a high-plus lens to a 0-edge thickness, you may use the MBS to determine the final size of the uncut lens.

EXERCISES:

4. For stock lenses with the OC in the center of the lens blank, what is the minimum blank size for a wearer PD of 60, if the A = 52, B = 48, DBL = 18, and ED = 55?

5. Calculate the minimum blank size for stock lenses if the DBC is 61, A = 51, pattern difference = 2, and ED = 51, if the requested final PRP distance is 58.

6. A frame has measurements of A = 59, B = 50, DBL = 18, and ED = 63, and the requested PD is 35/37 (monocular distance). What is the minimum blank size for this pair of glasses if the lenses are ground for decentration?

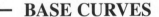

BASE CURVES

Base curve is defined in several ways.

BASE CURVE DEFINITIONS

1. *The **base curve of a lens** is the curve on the lens from which all of the other curves will be calculated.* On a spherical power single vision lens the base curve is usually the curve on the front or convex side. On a toric single vision lens the base curve is the curve on the spherical surface, which is on the front or convex side if the lens is made in minus cylinder form.
2. *The **base curve of a multifocal lens** is the curve on the surface containing the segment.* This surface will be spherical for most bifocal lenses where the segment is molded on the surface.* On a fused glass bifocal lens the surface with the segment can be given a toric surface, but it usually is not.
3. *The **base curve of a toric surface** is the flattest curve on the surface.* In a lens that has been ground in minus cylinder form, this is the flattest curve on the concave surface. In a lens that has been ground in plus cylinder form, this is the flattest curve on the convex surface.

*Some PAL designs may have cylinder molded on the surface(s) containing the segment.

Definitions one and two in the preceding box are the definitions used to choose a base curve for a prescription. Definition three will be used in the discussion of toric transposition.

BASE CURVE SELECTION

Before corrected curve series lenses were developed, base curves were chosen to keep the ocular surface as close to −6.00D as possible. For plus lenses this can be done by adding +6.00D to the spherical equivalent of the lens power. For minus lenses the rule of thumb is to add one half of the (negative) spherical equivalent to +6.00D. This rule of thumb is called ***Vogel's Rule.*** For example, if the Rx is +3.50, the base curve could be (+6.00) + (+3.50) = +9.50. But if the Rx is −3.50, the base curve is (+6.00) + (−3.50/2) = (+6.00) + (−1.75) = +4.25. (The spherical equivalent of a spherical power *is* the sphere. See the discussion of spherical equivalent in Section III.)

Vogel's Rule of base curve selection is a starting point. The lens blank chosen will be close to the result of this calculation but will rarely be exactly the result of the calculation.

> Vogel's Rule:
>
> PLUS Rx: BC = spherical equivalent + 6D
>
> MINUS Rx: BC = 1/2 (spherical equivalent) + 6D

Corrected curve design lenses were developed to minimize the lens aberrations *marginal astigmatism* (also called *oblique astigmatism*) and *curvature of field.* When you look up a lens power on a chart to determine what base curve to use, you are probably making a corrected curve lens. For any particular prescription the base curve that will minimize or eliminate marginal astigmatism is not the exact same curve that will minimize or eliminate curvature of field aberration. In addition, using the best base curve for every prescription would require stocking a very large variety of base curves. Every lens manufacturer's corrected curve series is the result of compromises between minimizing the two aberrations and controlling inventory; therefore different corrected curve lens series may recommend different (but similar) base curves for any particular prescription.

Some base curve charts require that you transpose to minus cylinder form and then look up the prescription on a table to find the recommended base curve. Others require that you determine the spherical equivalent of the prescription and then determine where it falls in a group of prescriptions, such as the following sample chart for CR-39:

SIMPLE BASE CURVE SELECTION CHART*

SPHERICAL EQUIVALENT	BASE CURVE
+7.50 to +12.50[†]	+12.25D
+4.50 to +8.75	+10.25D
+1.50 to +5.75	+8.25D
−1.75 to +1.75	+6.25D
−1.50 to −5.75	+4.25D
−4.50 to −9.25	+2.25D
−8.50 and above[†]	+0.25D

*This is not an official corrected curve chart. This chart is for illustration purposes only and is not intended for use in choosing a base curve.

[†]Aspheric curves recommended.

In a chart like this the overlapping areas allow you to choose lens blanks so that the right and left lenses are on the same base curve.

EXAMPLES:

5-7. An Rx of −5.00D would be placed on a +3.50 base curve according to Vogel's Rule. Referring to the base curve selection chart above, you would grind the Rx of −5.00D on either a +4.25D or a +2.25 base curve. The choice depends partly on the base curve of the other lens in the pair.

5-8. An Rx of +3.50 +1.00 ×090 would be placed on a +10.00D base curve according to Vogel's Rule. Referring to the base curve selection chart above, you would grind this Rx on a +8.25D base curve.

Notes:

1. Vogel's Rule gives you a place to start when taking a multiple-choice examination. Use it to find an approximate base curve, and then choose the answer that is either the closest to your approximation or the closest to +6.00: for plus power the flatter choice and for minus power the steeper choice.
2. When a base curve is specified on an order or on the Rx, ANSI standards state that the base curve supplied must be within ±0.75D of the curve requested.
3. When specifying base curve, many authorities recommend:
   a. That new lenses be placed on the same base curve as the old lens base curve *if reasonable*

b. That both lenses in a pair of glasses be on the same base curve *if reasonable* (use the base curve recommended for the strongest lens)

c. That high-plus prescriptions be placed on aspheric base curves

d. That the base curve for a plus lens be flattened for insertion in difficult frames

e. That the base curve be flattened if high prism is prescribed

4. Many wholesale laboratories stock one or two base curve series and may not be able to grind the prescription on exactly the base curve requested. Rejecting a base curve that is within ±0.75D of the curve requested may result in delays in delivery and an increased laboratory charge.

EXERCISES:

7. What base curve does Vogel's Rule call for if the Rx is –3.00 –2.00 ×180? What base curve does the selection chart on p. 146 call for?

8. What base curve does the chart indicate for a lens of power +3.00 –2.50 ×090? What does Vogel's Rule call for?

9. What base curve might be used for a –6.00 DS lens if Vogel's Rule is used? If the chart is used?

TORIC TRANSPOSITION

The purpose of *toric transposition* is to show what curves will be ground on the surfaces of the lens.

STEPS IN TORIC TRANSPOSITION

FIRST: If the written prescription is not in the correct cylinder form, transpose it. If the base curve is plus power, the Rx should be in minus cylinder form.

1. **Place the base curve on the diagram of the lens.** If the Rx is to be made in minus cylinder form, the base curve will have plus power and will be on the convex surface. If the Rx is to be made in plus cylinder form, the base curve will have minus power and will be on the concave surface.

2. **Calculate the flattest curve on the second surface of the lens.** If the Rx is in the correct cylinder form, this is the curve needed to give the spherical power of the prescription using the nominal power formula in Section III. This curve is the toric surface base curve. (See number 3 of the definitions of base curve in the box on p. 145.)

3. **Calculate the cross curve on the toric surface of the lens.** This is the curve found in step 2, plus the amount of the prescribed cylinder.

EXAMPLE:

5-9. Using a base curve of +4.25D, show the surface curves of a lens having the Rx –3.00 –1.00 ×090.

First: If the Rx had not been in minus cylinder form, we would flat transpose it.

1. The base curve of the lens is to be +4.25, on the convex side of the lens.

$$+4.25D$$
$$==================$$

2. To obtain a sphere power of –3.00D using a base curve of +4.25D, we need a toric base curve of –7.25D.
   $[D_2 = D_N – D_1 = –3.00 – (+4.25) = –7.25D]$

$$+4.25D$$
$$==================$$
$$–7.25D$$

3. For the cross curve add the amount of the cylinder to the toric base curve.
   $(–7.25) + (–1.00) = –8.25$

$$+4.25D$$
$$==================$$
$$–7.25/–8.25$$

10. Given the Rx −2.00 −1.50 ×045 and the base curve +4.25D, what are the surface curves?

11. Given the base curve −6.00 and the Rx pl + 0.50 ×180, what are the surface curves? (**Note:** The Rx is to be ground in plus cylinder form.)

12. Show the toric transposition of the Rx +5.00 +1.50 ×060, using a base curve of +10.25D.

13. What is the toric transposition for the Rx −8.50 −1.25 ×115, with a base curve of +2.00D?

REFRACTIVE POWER FORMULA

In Section II, when we discussed the surface power formula, we learned that the power of a surface depends on the radius of curvature of the surface and the index of refraction of the material of the surface. Historically, the lens clock, the surfacing laps in most ophthalmic laboratories, and most generator calibrations have been based on making or measuring curves on a material with an index of refraction of 1.530. For low-power prescriptions in crown glass, index 1.523, use of tools with index 1.530 is acceptable. We may correct for the index when using CR-39 or high-index materials. The formula used to convert the *power marked* on the tool to the *refractive power created by* the tool is

$$\frac{D_{marked}}{D_{refractive}} = \frac{0.53}{n_{refractive} - 1}$$

where:

D_{marked} = the power marked on the lap tool or the lens clock reading
$D_{refractive}$ = the actual power of the surface
$n_{refractive}$ = the index of refraction of the lens material

The tool needed (D_{marked}) to grind the curve that will have the actual power ($D_{refractive}$) is

$$D_{marked} = \frac{0.53}{n_{refractive} - 1} \times D_{refractive}$$

or, the actual power of a surface ($D_{refractive}$) that clocks at (D_{marked}) is

$$D_{refractive} = \frac{n_{refractive} - 1}{0.53} \times D_{marked}$$

EXAMPLES:

5-10. What tool would be used to grind an actual (or refractive) power of −5.00D on a lens made of CR-39?

$$D_{marked} = \frac{0.53}{n_{refractive} - 1} \times D_{refractive}$$

$$D_{marked} = \frac{0.53}{1.498 - 1} \times -5.00 = \frac{0.53}{0.498} \times -5.00 = \textbf{−5.32}$$

Corrected to the next highest 1/8D, the tool used would be **−5.37D**.

5-11. What is the actual (or refractive) surface power of a polycarbonate surface, n = 1.586, if the lens clock shows +7.25D?

$$D_{refractive} = \frac{n_{refractive} - 1}{0.53} \times D_{marked}$$

$$D_{refractive} = \frac{1.586 - 1}{0.53} \times +7.25 = \frac{0.586}{0.53} +7.25 = \textbf{+8.01}$$

Although the lens clock will read +7.25D on this surface, it actually has a power of +8.01 because it is made of polycarbonate.

Note: We do not change refractive power to one-eighth diopter steps because we are not going to make the lens using this tool, nor are we going to measure this power with a lens clock. This value is an intermediate calculation and will be used in a subsequent formula, so rounding at this point would decrease the precision of the final answer.

Note: We change marked power to one-eighth diopter steps because the marked power results in an actual tool that will be used. In some laboratories, marked powers are automatically changed to the next highest one-eighth diopter step; in the exercises below, change to the nearest one-eighth diopter.

Note: Some references call the marked power the "true" power.

EXERCISES: (Change marked power to one-eighth diopter steps. Round refractive power to two decimal places.)

14. If the lens clock reads −3.25D on a material with an index of 1.586 (polycarbonate), what is the refractive power of the curve?

15. If the lens clock reads +10.75D on a material with an index of refraction of 1.498, what is the refractive power of the surface?

16. If we want a refractive power of −7.50D on a surface made of a material with an index of 1.60, what tool would we use?

17. If we want a refractive power of −3.75 on a surface made of CR-39 (n = 1.498), what tool would be used?

18. You are to make a lens with an Rx of −8.50 −2.00 ×090 using a high-index plastic having an index of refraction of 1.66. The base curve chosen for this lens reads +1.25 on the lens clock. What tool will be used to make the back surface?
Steps:
   a. Determine the refractive power of the base curve marked +1.25 in a lens made of a material with an index of refraction of 1.66.
   b. Toric transpose for the refractive powers needed on the back of the lens.
   c. Convert each of the back powers to marked powers. The result is what the tool will be, and what the lens clock will show, when the lens is finished. Since you will choose tools with this power, change to the nearest 1/8D.
   Think about it: Using the curves found in Exercise 18, step c, calculate the power that the lens would have had if the lens were made of a material with index 1.530. Why is it difficult to estimate the power of a high-index lens just by using the readings from the lens clock?

SAGITTAL DEPTH AND LENS THICKNESS

The term *sag* refers to the *sagittal depth* of a curve or surface. If a straight edge is placed across the surface at a particular diameter, the sagittal depth is the farthest distance that the surface is from the straight edge. Notice that, for the same curve, a smaller diameter will give a smaller sagittal depth and a larger diameter will give a larger sagittal depth.

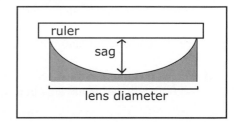

The formula for the sagittal depth of a surface is

$$sag = r - \sqrt{r^2 - \left(\frac{d}{2}\right)^2}$$

where:
d = the diameter of the surface, in mm
r = the radius of curvature of the surface, in mm

Note: The measurements may be in any unit, as long as r, d, and sag are *all the same unit.*

Note: In the diagram above, d = the distance between the two points where the ruler touches the surface. This is also called the *cord* or *cord diameter*.

Remember from Section III that r, the radius of curvature in meters, is equal to (n − 1)/D. This formula may be rewritten as

$$sag = \frac{n-1}{D} - \sqrt{\left(\frac{n-1}{D}\right)^2 - \left(\frac{d}{2}\right)^2}$$

Note: In this version of the sagittal formula the measurements must all be in meters and diopters.

EXAMPLES:

5-12. A surface made of polycarbonate has a true power of −6.00D and a diameter of 60 mm. What is the sag of the surface?

n = 1.586

r = (n − 1)/D = (1.586 − 1)/(6)

  = 0.0977 m = 97.7 mm

d = 60

$$sag = r - \sqrt{r^2 - \left(\frac{d}{2}\right)^2}$$

$$sag = 97.7 - \sqrt{97.7^2 - \left(\frac{60}{2}\right)^2}$$

$$sag = 97.7 - \sqrt{9545.29 - 900} = 97.7 - \sqrt{8645.29}$$

  = 97.7 − 93.0 = **4.7 mm**

Example 5-12

Type A Calculator:

97.7 $-$ $($ 97.7 x^2 $-$ $($ 60 $\div$ 2 $)$ x^2 $)$ $\sqrt{}$ $=$
The calculator should say 4.7199…

Type B Calculator:

97.7 $-$ x^2 $($ 97.7 x^2 $-$ $($ 60 $\div$ 2 $)$ x^2 $)$ $=$
The calculator should say 4.7199…

Note: The sign of the radius of curvature (actually the sign of the surface power) is not used in this form of the sagittal depth formula. In Section VII we deal with the sign of r. We will adjust for not using the sign of r here when combining the sagittal depths of the two surfaces of the lens.

The sag of a flat or plano surface is 0. Using the sag of the −6.00 surface made of polycarbonate, we can now find the edge thickness of a plano-concave lens with power −6.00.

5-13. If a center thickness of 1.5 mm is requested, the edge thickness of the 60-mm diameter plano-concave −6.00D polycarbonate lens in Example 4-11 will be 4.7 mm + 1.5 mm = **6.2 mm**.

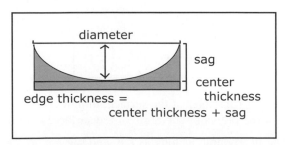

       Optical Formulas Tutorial

The formula for the edge thickness of a minus lens is

$$\text{edge thickness}_{\text{minus lens}} = \text{SAG}_{\text{back}} - \text{SAG}_{\text{front}} + \text{center thickness}$$

5-14. If a –6.00D polycarbonate lens is made with a base curve of +3.00D, a back curve of –9.00D, a diameter of 60 mm, and a center thickness of 1.5 mm, what is the edge thickness? (These powers are actual refractive power, not marked values.)

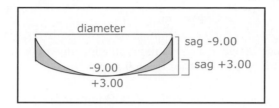

$$r = (n - 1)/D$$

$$r_{\text{front}} = (1.586 - 1)/3 = 0.1953 \text{ m} = 195 \text{ mm}$$

$$\mathbf{sag_{front}} = 195 - \sqrt{195^2 - \frac{60^2}{2}} = \mathbf{2.3215...mm}$$

$$r_{\text{back}} = (1.586 - 1)/9 = 0.0651 \text{ m} = 65 \text{ mm}$$

$$\mathbf{sag_{back}} = 65 - \sqrt{65^2 - \frac{60^2}{2}} = \mathbf{7.3371...mm}$$

The difference between the two sags is 5.0 mm, which is thicker than the plano-convex form of the lens. Adding the requested center thickness of 1.5 mm results in an **edge thickness of 6.5 mm**.

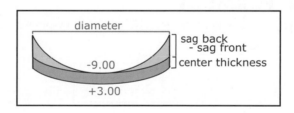

The center thickness of a plus lens is

$$\text{center thickness}_{\text{plus lens}} = \text{SAG}_{\text{front}} - \text{SAG}_{\text{back}} + \text{edge thickness}$$

5-15. What is the center thickness of a +6.00D lens made from Trivex,[1] n = 1.53, if the edge thickness is 1.00 mm, the lens diameter is 60 mm, and the base curve is = +10.00D?

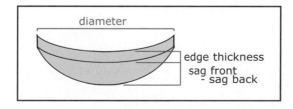

---

[1]Trivex is a trademark of PPG. Technical information is from http://corporate.ppg.com/PPG/opticalprod/en/monomers/products/Properties.htm.

$$r = (n - 1)/D$$

$$r_{front} = (1.53 - 1)/10 = 0.053 \text{ m} = 53 \text{ mm}$$

$$\mathbf{sag_{front}} = 53 - \sqrt{53^2 - \frac{60^2}{2}} = \mathbf{9.30789...mm}$$

$$D_{back} = +6.00 - (+10.00) = -4.00 \text{ D}$$

$$r_{back} = (1.53 - 1)/4 = 0.1325 \text{ m}$$

$$\mathbf{sag_{back}} = 132.5 - \sqrt{132.5^2 - \frac{60^2}{2}} = \mathbf{3.4409...mm}$$

center thickness = difference between sags + minimum edge thickness
$$= (9.3 - 3.4) + 1.0 = 5.9 + 1.0 = \mathbf{6.9 \text{ mm}}$$

5-16.   What is the approximate edge thickness of a –6.00D high-index plastic lens, n = 1.66, if the center thickness is 2.0 mm, the base curve has a refractive power of +2.00D, and the lens diameter is 50 mm?

$$r = (n - 1)/D$$

$$r_{front} = (1.66 - 1)/2 = 0.33 \text{ m} = 330 \text{ mm}$$

$$\mathbf{sag_{front}} = 330 - \sqrt{330^2 - \frac{50^2}{2}} = \mathbf{0.9483...mm}$$

$$D_{back} = -6.00 - (+2.00) = -8.00 \text{ D}$$

$$r_{back} = (1.66 - 1)/8 = 0.0825 \text{ m} = 82.5 \text{ mm}$$

$$\mathbf{sag_{back}} = 82.5 - \sqrt{82.5^2 - \frac{50^2}{2}} = \mathbf{3.8790...mm}$$

edge thickness = difference between sags + minimum center thickness
$$= (3.89 - 0.95) + 2.0 = 2.93 + 2.0 = \mathbf{4.9 \text{ mm}}$$

APPROXIMATE SAG FORMULA

The following *approximate* sag of a lens is in general use and for low-power lenses gives an acceptable approximation for the lens thickness.

$$\boxed{sag = \frac{(d/2)^2 D}{2000(n - 1)}}$$

where:
d = diameter of the lens (or surface) in mm
D = lens power (or surface power)
n = index of refraction for the material from which the lens (or surface) is made

EXAMPLES:

5-17.   What is the approximate center thickness of a +6.00D Trivex lens, n = 1.53, if the minimum edge thickness is 1.0 mm and the lens diameter is 60 mm?

CENTER THICKNESS = SAG + EDGE THICKNESS

$$sag = \frac{(d/2)^2 D}{2000(n - 1)}$$

$$sag = \frac{(30)^2 6.00}{2000(0.52)} = \frac{400}{1060} = 5.1 \text{ mm}$$

CENTER THICKNESS = 5.1 mm + 1.0 mm = 6.1 mm
In Example 5-15 the exact formula gave us 6.9 mm for this center thickness when the lens is made with a +10.00 base curve.

5-18. What is the approximate edge thickness of a –6.00D polycarbonate lens, n = 1.586, if the center thickness is 1.5 mm and the lens diameter is 60 mm?

EDGE THICKNESS = SAG + CENTER THICKNESS

$$sag = \frac{(d/2)^2 D}{2000(n-1)}$$

$$sag = \frac{(30)^2 6.00}{2000(0.586)} = 4.6 \text{ mm}$$

EDGE THICKNESS = 4.6 mm + 1.5 mm = 6.1 mm

In Example 5-13 the exact formula gave us 6.2 mm for this edge thickness in a flat form lens, and Example 5-14 gave an edge thickness of 6.5 mm for the same lens made on a +3.00 base curve.

Note: The approximate sag formula does not show the difference in thickness that results from the choice of base curve.

Note: The approximate sag formula can be used on either the lens power or the lens surfaces. The exact sag formula usually is used on lens surfaces, and the sags of the two surfaces must be combined (taking the form of the surfaces into account) to give a lens thickness. If used on the lens power, the exact sag formula results in a thickness for a lens with one plano surface.

EXERCISES: (Round radius of curvature to millimeters and sag to tenths of a millimeter.)

19. What is the approximate center thickness of a +2.50D lens with n = 1.498 if the edge thickness is to be 2 mm at a diameter of 56 mm? Use the approximation formula.

20. Redo the calculations from Question 19.
    a. Choose a base curve from the box on p. 146.
    b. Use the refractive power formula to convert to true power; then find the refractive back curve.
    c. Use these two refractive power curves to find the actual sags of the curves.
    d. Find the center thickness of the +2.50D lens using the accurate sagittal formula.

——————————— PRISM THICKNESS ———————————

The base thickness, t, of a prismatic lens with no power may be found by use of the formula

$$t = \frac{dP}{100(n-1)}$$

where:

P = prism power

t = thickness in millimeters

d = diameter of the lens in millimeters

This formula assumes that the apex of the prism is 0 mm or knife-edge.

The amount of prism may be found if the base thickness of the prism and index of the material are known, using the following form of the same formula. Either the apex thickness is 0, or t represents the difference between the apex thickness and the base thickness.

$$P = \frac{t(100[n-1])}{d}$$

EXAMPLE:

5-19. You are given a prescription of pl, 5^Δ BO OU. The wearer chooses a frame of 50 ☐ 18. The finished lens will have a minimum edge thickness of 2 mm. For a lens made of a 1.50 index plastic, what will the maximum edge thickness be?

Because this Rx has no power, we do not need to be concerned with decentration. Since the prism is base out, which is horizontal, the diameter of the lens needed is the A size of the frame, 50 mm. The base thickness is

$$t = \frac{dP}{100(n-1)} = \frac{(50)(5)}{(100)(0.5)} = \frac{250}{50} = 5 \text{ mm}$$

Adding a minimum edge thickness of 2.0 mm to the 5 mm will give a thickness of **7.0 mm** on the outside edge of each lens.

Note: The thickness of the base is equal to the prism power for a lens of diameter 50 mm and a material of index 1.50. The general rule of thumb for prism thickness is:

> For a 50-mm-diameter lens made of material of n = 1.50, the difference between thickness of the base and the thickness of the apex of the prism in mm will equal the amount of the prism power in diopters.

Based on the rule of thumb, if the material has a high index, the prism base thickness will be less than the amount of the prism. (Why?) If the lens is larger than 50 mm in diameter, the prism base thickness will be more than the amount of the prism. (Why?) If the lens is smaller than 50 mm, the prism base thickness will be less than the amount of the prism. (Why?)

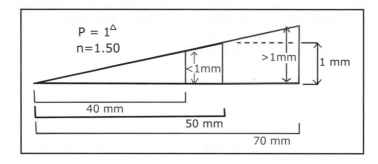

Maximum edge thickness for a prismatic lens with plano power is the sum of the prism base thickness plus the minimum edge thickness for the ED of the lens.

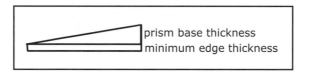

Maximum edge thickness for a prismatic lens with spherical plus power is also the sum of the prism base thickness plus the minimum edge thickness for the minimum blank size of the lens. Center thickness for a prismatic lens with plus power is the sum of the sag of the lens, the minimum edge thickness, and one half of the prism base thickness.

> For a spherical power plus lens:
>
> thickest edge = prism base thickness + minimum edge thickness
>
> center thickness = sag + minimum edge thickness + 1/2 prism base thickness

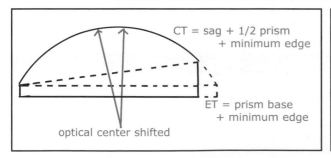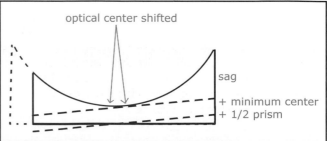

For spherical minus power prismatic lenses, adding the edge thickness, the minimum center thickness, and the prism base gives more thickness than necessary, since it results in an optical center thickness that is thicker than necessary. Using one half of the prism base thickness amount (or finding the thickness of the prism portion at one-half the ED) will give an amount that may be added to the sum of the Rx sag and minimum center thickness to approximate the thickest edge amount.

For a spherical power minus lens:

thickest edge = 1/2 prism base thickness + minimum center thickness + sag

---

Note: The calculated edge or center thickness is a maximum. Actual thickness will depend on the frame shape, the direction of the prism base, and the axis of the Rx cylinder if present.

EXAMPLES:

5-20. What are the approximate maximum edge and center thickness for the Rx +4.00 DS 2$^\Delta$ BU for a polycarbonate (n = 1.586) lens with a minimum blank size of 48, a sag of 2.1 mm, and a minimum thickness of 1.5 mm?

Step 1. Determine the prism base thickness.

$$t = \frac{dP}{100(n-1)} = \frac{(48)(2)}{(100)(0.586)} = \frac{96}{58.6} = 1.6 \text{ mm}$$

Step 2. Determine the thickest edge.
Thickest edge = minimum thickness + prism base thickness = 1.5 + 1.6 = **3.1 mm**
Step 3. Determine the center thickness.
Center thickness = minimum thickness + sag + 1/2 prism base = 1.5 + 2.1 + 1/2(1.6) = **4.4 mm**
Note: The thickness is a maximum and an approximation. Since the prism is BU, some of the thickest edge will be cut off.

5-21. What is the approximate maximum edge thickness for Rx −3.00 DS 2$^\Delta$ BI for a CR-39 lens with a minimum blank size of 54 mm, a lens sag of 2.4 mm, and a minimum center thickness of 2.2 mm? Redo the problem, using a plastic with an index of refraction of 1.66 and a lens sag of 1.9 mm.
Using CR-39:
Step 1. Determine the prism base thickness.

$$t = \frac{dP}{100(n-1)} = \frac{(54)(2)}{(100)(0.498)} = \frac{108}{49.8} = 2.2 \text{ mm}$$

Step 2. Determine the thickest edge.
Thickest edge using CR-39 = minimum thickness + sag + 1/2 prism base thickness
$$= 2.2 + 2.4 + (2.2/2) = 5.7 \text{ mm}$$
Using plastic with n = 1.66:
Step 1. Determine the prism base thickness.

$$t = \frac{dP}{100(n-1)} = \frac{(54)(2)}{(100)(0.66)} = \frac{108}{66} = 1.6 \text{ mm}$$

Step 2. Determine the thickest edge.
Thickest edge using high index = 2.2 + 1.9 + (1.6/2) = **4.9 mm**
Again, note that after the lens is edged to fit the frame, some of this thickness will have been removed.

EXERCISES: (Round to tenths of a millimeter.)

21. What are the approximate maximum edge and center thickness for the Rx +5.50 DS, 3$^\Delta$ BO, for a polycarbonate (n = 1.586) lens with a minimum blank size of 44 mm, a lens sag of 2.4 mm, and a minimum thickness of 1.5 mm?

22. What are the center thickness and maximum edge thickness for the same lens as in Exercise 21 when the material is CR-39 (n = 1.498) with a lens sag of 2.9 mm and minimum edge of 2.0 mm?

The questions with an asterisk (*) in front of the question number are advanced questions. They are not likely to be on the ABO exam but might be on the ABOM exam or the COT exam.

The questions are not presented in the order of the subjects in the section. Some of these questions may require you to think about what you have read in the section, and some may depend on material covered in previous sections.

1. The Rx is −5.00 −2.00 ×165. If Vogel's Rule of base curve selection is used as a starting point, the base curve selected would be
   a. +6.25.
   b. +4.25.
   c. +2.25.
   d. +0.75

2. The PRP is
   a. another name for the optical center.
   b. the prism reference point, which is where the prism amount is what is prescribed.
   c. The pupil reference position, which should always be in front of the patient's pupil.
   d. The patient reference point, which is also called the optical center.

3. The cross curve is
   a. the steepest curve on a toric surface.
   b. the steepest curve on a lens.
   c. the curve used to calculate the base curve of the lens.
   d. the flattest curve on a toric surface.

4. The A measurement is
   a. the maximum horizontal opening in the frame.
   b. the horizontal lens measurement at the midpoint of the lens.
   c. the largest measurement on the lens, from bevel to bevel.
   d. the maximum horizontal measurement on the lens.

5. When the Geneva lens clock is used on a lens made from crown glass, the front surface has a power of +7.25. What is the refractive power of the surface?
   a. +7.40
   b. +7.25
   c. +7.15
   d. +7.00

6. The ED is
   a. the diagonal measurement of the lens.
   b. twice the maximum radius of the lens.
   c. the longest measurement on the lens regardless of orientation.
   d. the larger of the A and B measurements.

7. A frame has the following measurements:
   A = 55
   B = 46
   DBL = 19
   ED = 57
   The wearer's distance PD is 64. The lenses will be taken from stock where the OC at the geometric center of the uncut lens is blank. There is no prescribed prism. The smallest blank size that the lenses can be cut from, including a 2-mm margin for edging, is
   a. 69 mm.   c. 59 mm.
   b. 67 mm.   d. 57 mm.

8. A frame difference of 1 indicates that
   a. the lens shape is close to round or square.
   b. the lens shape is definitely rectangular or oval.
   c. the frame has a large ED.
   d. the frame has a small bridge size.

9. The frame is marked 48 □ 19. The wearer's PD is 59 mm, and the vertical opening in the frame measures 39 mm. The frame difference is
   a. 4 mm.   c. 29 mm.
   b. 9 mm.   d. 50 mm.

10. The MRP is
    a. at the geometric center of the lens opening.
    b. the same thing as the PRP.
    c. where the markings for the patient reference are found.
    d. the point that is used to calculate all other reference points on the uncut lens.

11. The frame is marked 51 □ 20. The wearer's PD is 62 mm, and the vertical opening in the frame measures 42 mm. The job order is marked "height 19." The segment drop for this pair of glasses is
    a. 9 mm.
    b. 4 mm.
    c. −4 mm.
    d. −2 mm.

12. The frame is marked 48 □ 19. The wearer's PD is 59 mm, and the vertical opening in the frame measures 40 mm. The job ticket is marked "seg height 23 mm." The segment top position for this pair of glasses is
    a. −3 mm.
    b. 3 mm.
    c. 1.5 mm.
    d. −1.5 mm.

13. What is the toric transposition for the Rx +3.00 +0.50 ×025, with a base curve of –6.00?
    a. +6.00//–2.50/–3.00
    b. +6.00//–3.00/–3.50
    c. +9.50/+10.00//–6.00
    d. +9.00/+9.50//–6.00

14. The Rx is +1.50 –0.75 ×120. The spherical equivalent of the Rx is
    a. +1.12.
    b. +1.00.
    c. +0.75.
    d. +0.50.

15. A frame has the following measurements:
    A = 55
    B = 46
    DBL = 19
    ED = 57
    The wearer PDs are:
    distance: 33/35
    near: 31/32
    The distance decentration for the OS is
    a. 5 mm.   c. 3 mm.
    b. 4 mm.   d. 2 mm.

16. In the boxing system the DBL is the
    a. minimum distance between lenses.
    b. average distance between the lenses.
    c. distance between the lenses at the 1/2 B position.
    d. wearer's PD minus the DBC.

17. A frame has the following measurements:
    A = 55
    B = 46
    DBL = 19
    D = 57
    The wearer PDs are:
    distance: 33/35
    near: 31/33
    Decentration for SV reading glasses is
    a. 6/4.   c. 3/2.
    b. 4/6.   d. 2/3.

18. The rule of thumb for prism edge thickness is
    a. for a material index of 1.50 and a lens diameter of 50 mm there will be 1 mm edge thickness for every 1 diopter of prism power.
    b. for a material index of 1.586 and a lens diameter of 60 mm there will be 1 mm edge thickness for every 1 diopter of prism power.
    c. for a material index of 1.50 and a lens diameter of 50 mm there will be 2 mm edge thickness for every 1 diopter of prism power.
    d. for a material index of 1.586 and a lens diameter of 60 mm there will be 2 mm edge thickness for every 1 diopter of prism power.

19. A frame has the following measurements:
    A = 55
    B = 46
    DBL = 19
    ED = 57
    The wearer's distance PD is 64. The lenses will be ground for decentration. The smallest blank size from which the lenses can be cut, including a 2-mm margin for edging, is
    a. 69 mm.
    b. 67 mm.
    c. 59 mm.
    d. 57 mm.

20. The sagittal depth of a surface
    a. is the depth of the surface using the distance of the fixed pins on the Geneva lens measure.
    b. is the greatest depth that the surface has at the diameter of 72 mm.
    c. depends on the diameter of the lens.
    d. is independent of the diameter of the lens.

21. The base curve of a lens is
    a. the flattest curve on the lens.
    b. always the curve on the front (or spherical) surface.
    c. the curve from which all other curves on the lens are calculated.
    d. the curve on the concave surface of the lens.

22. The frame is marked 51 □ 20. The wearer's PD is 62 mm, and the vertical opening in the frame measures 42 mm. The per-lens decentration for this pair of glasses is
    a. 21 mm.
    b. 9 mm.
    c. 6.5 mm.
    d. 4.5 mm.

23. The Rx +2.50 –1.75 ×110 will be made from crown glass on a +7.25 base curve. The back surface curves will be
    a. –10.75/–9.00.
    b. – 9.00/–10.75.
    c. –4.75/–6.50.
    d. –5.50/–6.50.

24. The base curve of a toric surface is
    a. the steepest curve on the lens.
    b. the curve from which all other curves on the lens are calculated.
    c. the flattest curve on the surface.
    d. the steepest curve on the surface.

25. The frame is marked 48 □ 19. The wearer's PD is 59 mm, and the vertical opening in the frame measures 39 mm. The DBC is
    a. 53.5 mm.   c. 59 mm.
    b. 57.5 mm.   d. 67 mm.

26. The base curve of a multifocal lens is
    a. the curve on the surface where the segment is.
    b. the steepest curve on the surface where the segment is.
    c. the flattest curve on the surface.
    d. the steepest curve on the surface.

27. The datum or D measurement
    a. is equal to the A measurement.
    b. is greater than or equal to the A measurement.
    c. is less than or equal to the A measurement.
    d. is never equal to the A measurement.

28. A frame has the following measurements:
    A = 55
    B = 46
    DBL = 19
    ED = 57
    The wearer PDs are:
    distance: 33/35
    near: 31/32
    The segment inset for the OD is
    a. 5 mm.
    b. 4 mm.
    c. 3 mm.
    d. 2 mm.

29. The Rx is +2.00 –0.75 ×110. The following are the BC selections for a given lens manufacturer. The BC that you will select is
    a. +10.25.
    b. +9.25.
    c. +7.25.
    d. +5.25.

30. The BC of a lens does not affect the total thickness of the lens.
    a. True   b. False

31. The Rx is:
    OD –5.00 sph
    OS –6.00 sph
    Comments: BC +2.75
    The BC supplied by the lab is a +2.25.
    a. The glasses meet ANSI standards for BC selection.
    b. The glasses do not meet ANSI standards for BC selection.
    c. The glasses cannot be ground on this BC.
    d. ANSI does not set standards for base curve selection.

32. The frame is marked 51 □ 20. The wearer's PD is 30/32 mm, and the vertical opening in the frame measures 42 mm. The decentration for the left lens is
    a. 6.5 mm.
    b. 5.5 mm.
    c. 4.5 mm.
    d. 3.5 mm.

33. The Rx is +1.50 –1.00 ×120. If Vogel's Rule for base curve selection is used, the base curve will be
    a. +8.50.
    b. +7.00.
    c. +6.50.
    d. +6.00.

34. A lens blank has a finished front surface with a marked power of +7.01 D. The lens is made from polycarbonate. The refracting power of the surface is
    a. +7.95.
    b. +7.75.
    c. +7.41.
    d. +7.01

*35. A minus power lens has a front surface sag of 1.5 mm and a back surface sag of 2.3 mm. If the minimum thickness on the lens is 2.0, what is the edge thickness of the lens?
    a. 2.0 mm
    b. 2.8 mm
    c. 3.5 mm
    d. 5.8 mm

*36. The ocular surface of a 1.60 index plastic lens is to have a refracting power of –6.00/–6.75. What tool will be used to create this surface if the tools are marked on the standard index?
    a. 6.75/7.50
    b. 6.37/7.00
    c. 6.00/6.75
    d. 5.37/6.00

*37. The minimum and maximum edge thicknesses for a 45-mm prism made from 1.66 plastic are 1.5 mm and 5.8 mm. What is the power of the prism?
    a. 8.5^Δ
    b. 6.7^Δ
    c. 6.3^Δ
    d. 5.0^Δ

*38. The sagittal depth of a +6.50 surface on a 72-mm crown glass lens blank is
    a. 28 mm.
    b. 12.9 mm.
    c. 8.5 mm.
    d. 5.4 mm.

*39. A plus lens made from 1.50 plastic has a refractive front surface power of +10.00, a refractive back surface power of –5.00, a diameter of 60 mm, and a minimum edge thickness of 1.5 mm. What is the center thickness of the lens?
    a. 6.9 mm
    b. 6.0 mm
    c. 5.4 mm
    d. 4.8 mm

*40. A lens is to be made from a 1.66 high-index plastic. The power is to be +5.00 −2.50 ×156. The base curve on the lens blank has a marked power of +8.05. The lap chosen to fine and polish the toric surface will be
a. 4.12/6.62.
b. 4.12/6.12.
c. 3.12/5.12.
d. 3.12/5.62.

*41. The base thickness of a crown glass 60 mm 3.5$^\Delta$ lens with no power and 0 apical thickness is
a. 4.6 mm.
b. 4.0 mm.
c. 2.0 mm.
d. 1.4 mm

*42. A minus power lens has a front surface sag of 1.5 mm and a back surface sag of 2.3 mm. If the minimum thickness on the lens is 2.0, what is the center thickness of the lens?
a. 2.0 mm
b. 2.8 mm
c. 3.5 mm
d. 5.8 mm

SECTION VI – ADVANCED LENS FORMULAS

MARTIN'S FORMULA FOR LENS TILT

The position of a lens in front of the eye changes the effect of the lens on the optical system that is a combination of lens and eye. One example, discussed in Section III, is vertex distance change. Pantoscopic tilt and face form also change the effective power of the lens with respect to the eye. Changing the tilt of the lens induces the lens aberration *marginal astigmatism*, also called *oblique astigmatism*.

Pantoscopic tilt changes the effective sphere power of the lens and induces cylinder power on the 180 meridian. For a plus sphere lens, plus cylinder is induced. For a minus sphere lens, minus cylinder is induced. Face form changes the sphere power of the lens and induces cylinder power on the 90 meridian. For small amounts of tilt, the formula for the new effective power of the lens is:

$$S' = S\left[1 + \frac{(\sin \alpha)^2}{2n}\right]$$
$$C' = S'(\tan \alpha)^2$$

where:
S' = new spherical power
S = original sphere power
α = degrees of tilt
n = index of refraction of the lens material
C' = induced cylinder on the axis of rotation

EXAMPLES:

6-1. A +10.00D lens made of CR-39 (n = 1.498) is tilted 15°. What is the effective power of this lens on the combined eye/lens system?

$S' = S[1 + (\sin \alpha)^2/2n]$
$= (+10.00)(1 + [\sin 15]^2/2[1.498])$
$= (+10.00)(1 + 0.06699/2.996)$
$= (+10.00)(1.02235)$
$= \mathbf{+10.22D}$

$C' = S' (\tan \alpha)^2$
$= (+10.22)(\tan 15)^2$
$= (+10.22)(0.0718)$
$= \mathbf{+0.73 \times 180}$

Effective Rx +10.22 +0.73 × 180

The answers are not changed to 1/8D because this effective power will not be ordered from a laboratory or recorded in the wearer's records.

This formula assumes that the optical center (OC) of the lens is directly in front of the wearer's pupil. Changing the position of the OC can change the effect of pantoscopic tilt on the prescription. The general rule is:

Lower the optical center 1 mm for every 2 degrees of pantoscopic tilt

Note: You may have seen the new sphere formula in the form $S' = S[1+(\sin \alpha)^2/3]$. This formula works for CR-39 and for crown glass and is a close and usually acceptable approximation for high-index materials.

6-2. What is the effective power of the lens on the eye if the following glasses are fitted with the OC in front of the pupil and with 10 degrees of pantoscopic tilt? The glasses are made of polycarbonate, n = 1.586.
Rx: OD –8.50 DS
     OS –9.25 DS
OD: $S' = S[1+(\sin \alpha)^2/2n]$
      $= (–8.50)(1 + (\sin 10)^2 /2(1.586)$

$$= (-8.50)(1 + (0.030)/(3.172)$$
$$= (-8.50)(1.0095)$$
$$S' = -8.58D$$
$$C' = S'(\tan \alpha)^2$$
$$= (-8.58)(\tan 10)^2$$
$$= (-8.58)(0.031)$$
$$C' = -0.27D$$

Example 6-2, OD S′

Type A Calculator

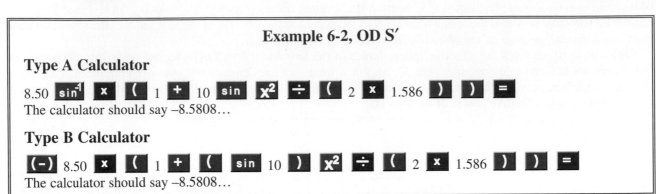

The calculator should say −8.5808...

Type B Calculator

The calculator should say −8.5808...

Example 6-2, OD C′

Type A Calculator

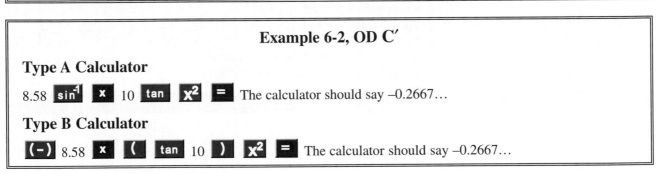

8.58 $\boxed{\text{sin}^{-1}}$ $\boxed{\times}$ 10 $\boxed{\text{tan}}$ $\boxed{x^2}$ $\boxed{=}$ The calculator should say −0.2667...

Type B Calculator

$\boxed{(-)}$ 8.58 $\boxed{\times}$ $\boxed{(}$ $\boxed{\text{tan}}$ 10 $\boxed{)}$ $\boxed{x^2}$ $\boxed{=}$ The calculator should say −0.2667...

OS $S' = S[1+(\sin \alpha)^2]$
$$= (-9.25)(1 + (\sin 10)^2/2(1.586)$$
$$= (-9.25)(1 + (0.030)/(3.172)$$
$$= (-9.25)(1.0095)$$
$$S' = -9.34D$$
$$C' = S'(\tan \alpha)^2$$
$$= (-9.34)(\tan 10)^2$$
$$= (-9.34)(0.031)$$
$$C' = -0.29D$$

Effective Rx: OD −8.58 −0.27 ×180
OS −9.34 −0.29 ×180

6-3. What is the effective power for the following Rx if the glasses have 15 degrees of face form and the PRP distance is made normally? The glasses are made of 1.66 plastic.
Rx: +7.00 −2.00 ×180 OU
The prescription already has some cylinder in it. Since the tilt will induce cylinder on the 90 meridian, first transpose the problem to the 90 meridian and then use the sphere power in the exercise.
Transposed Rx: +5.00 +2.00 ×090
$S' = S[1+(\sin \alpha)^2/2n]$
$$= (+5.00)(1 + (\sin 15)^2/2(1.66)$$
$$= (+5.00)(1 + (0.067)/(3.32)$$
$$= (+5.00)(1.020)$$
$$S' = +5.10D$$

$$C' = S'(\tan \alpha)^2$$
$$= (+5.10)(\tan 15)^2$$
$$= (+5.10)(0.072)$$

C' = +0.37 ×090

C' is added to the old cylinder power, since they are at the same axis. The new cylinder power is +2.00 +0.37 = **+2.37D**

The effective lens power is +5.10 +2.37 ×090 or +7.47 −2.37 ×180.

Note: Compensating the Rx for tilt, increasing the PRP distance 1 mm for every 2 degrees of face form, and using retroscopic tilt to correct for an OC that is above the pupil *are NOT recommended procedures.*

What if the prescription has cylinder with an axis other than 90 or 180? The result of the cylinder and axis calculations will be obliquely crossed cylinders and involves the use of both Martin's formula and Thompson's formula, on pp. 161 and 170. Calculation of the sphere power, however, is beyond the scope of this book. Note that if the cylinder is small with respect to the sphere power, an approximation may be calculated using just the sphere of the prescription. An alternative method of determining the answer would be to place the lens at the desired angle in the lensmeter.

Note: The amount of face form that should be present in a pair of glasses depends on the amount of decentration of the PRP from the geometric center of the frame lens opening. If there is no decentration, there should be no face form. If there is a small amount of decentration, there should be a small amount of face form. If there is "a lot" of decentration, there should be "a lot" of face form.

In the following exercises, notice that low pantoscopic tilt or a small amount of face form introduces very little error.

EXERCISES: (Round answers to hundredths of a diopter.)

1. If a −6.00D polycarbonate (n = 1.586) sphere is given 20 degrees of pantoscopic tilt, what are the effective sphere power and the amount of cylinder induced at the OC?

2. If a +10.00D sphere made of n = 1.66 plastic is given 5 degrees of pantoscopic tilt, what is the effective lens power at the OC?

3. Given a +4.50 polycarbonate (n = 1.586) lens with 20 degrees of positive face form because the wearer insists it gives him side protection when riding his bike, what is the effective lens power?

SPECTACLE MAGNIFICATION

Plus lenses are often considered to be magnifiers. A hyperope wears a plus lens because this lens adds just enough power to the eye system to bring the focal plane to the retina, not because it magnifies the image. A presbyope wears extra plus power (or less minus power) because that is what is needed to bring the image of a close object to a focus on the retina. *Magnification* induced by the glasses lens or the contact lens *is a side effect* of the lens power.

The amount of magnification that any particular lens will add to the eye system depends on a variety of factors, including:

- Thickness of the lens
- Material used to make the lens
- Distance the lens is from the eye
- Curvature of the front surface of the lens

These factors all have to work together to give the correct focal length. For any particular prescription, many different combinations of the factors will give the correct focal length. A particular combination, however, may give a different amount of magnification from another combination.

When the wearer has good corrected vision in each eye but requires a different prescription in each lens, the difference in magnification between the two lenses *may* result in visual problems. A person who has different prescriptions has *anisometropia*. If the difference in magnification or image size caused by the different prescriptions causes visual problems, usually the breaking of fusion, the wearer has *aniseikonia*. Specially designed lenses that attempt to correct the magnification or image size difference without changing the focal lengths of the lenses are called *iseikonic lenses.*

Some types of anisometropia, when corrected with glasses, do not induce aniseikonia. In this case, fitting the person with contact lenses may induce image size differences. If glasses do induce aniseikonia, the fitting of contact lenses may correct the image size differences.

Spectacle magnification (SM) is a number that shows how much a particular lens will magnify the image on the retina. An SM of 1 means the image on the retina is the same size it would be if the eye focused correctly with no glasses or contact lens added. An SM of 0.95 would be a 5% reduction in retinal image size; an SM of 1.05 would be a 5% increase in retinal image size.

The formula for spectacle magnification is:

$$SM = \left[\frac{1}{1 - \frac{t}{n}D_1} \right] \left(\frac{1}{1 - hD} \right)$$

(shape factor) (power factor)

where:

t = thickness of the lens in meters
n = index of refraction of the lens material
D_1 = base curve (BC) or front surface power of the lens
D = actual power of the lens
h = vertex distance + 3 mm, converted to meters

The first of these fractions is called the *shape factor* because it is determined by the BC selection and the thickness of the lens. Changes in BC, lens material, and thickness affect the shape factor. The second of the fractions is called the *power factor* because it is determined by the power of the lens. Changes in vertex distance affect the power factor. The h in the power factor actually represents the distance from the back of the lens to the center of the pupil inside the eye, not to the apex of the cornea, which is the definition of the vertex distance. We cannot measure the distance to the center of the pupil. The average distance from the corneal apex to the pupil center is 3 mm, so we add 3 mm to the vertex distance.

The percentage of spectacle magnification, or %SM, is found by subtracting 1 from the SM and then multiplying by 100:

$$\%SM = (SM - 1)100$$

An SM of 1.05 gives %SM = (1.05 − 1)100 = (0.05)100 = +5%, or 5% magnification. An SM of +0.95 gives %SM = (0.95 − 1)100 = (−0.05)100 = −5%, or 5% minification.

While doing the exercises, notice that all minus lenses have an SM between 0 and 1, which means that they will minify the image, and all plus lenses have an SM greater than 1, which means that they will magnify the image.

Once a wearer's problems are determined to be caused by different SM in the right and left lenses, it is necessary to estimate how much change will occur in each lens if changes are made to the shape or the vertex distance. The formulas to approximate the changes in SM are:

$$\Delta\%SM = \Delta D_1 t/15$$
$$\Delta\%SM = D_1 \Delta t/15$$
$$\Delta\%SM = \Delta hD/10$$

where:
$\Delta\%SM$ = change in the percent of magnification
ΔD_1 = change in front BC only
Δt = change in thickness only *in mm*
t = thickness *in mm*
Δh = change in vertex distance only *in mm*

Note: The symbol Δ used here symbolizes "change in." It is not a variable, nor does it refer to prism.

Note: When using these formulas, change only one factor at a time. If you try a 1D BC change, use the thickness in the original problem. If you then try a 2 mm thickness change, use the front curve from the original problem.

The change formulas are approximate. Changing one factor changes the others. For example, a change in BC may change the thickness and the vertex distance. On high prescriptions a change in vertex distance may require compensation of the lens power (see pp. 81-84). The approximation magnification changes may be made to determine what types of change will be most likely to help the wearer; the full formula could be used with all of the proposed changes to come up with a final answer.

Note: When changing factors that will affect magnification, do not aim to eliminate the differences in magnification completely.

EXAMPLE:

6-4.   What is the spectacle magnification for each of the lenses in the prescription below, and what is the difference in magnification percent for the two lenses?

The Rx is: +1.50

+4.50

The glasses fit at 12 mm. The lenses are made of CR-39, n = 1.498, BCs +6.25 and +9.25.

Use of calipers on the completed lenses shows thicknesses of 3 mm and 5 mm.

USING THE CALCULATOR

Do each fraction separately and then multiply the results.

Use five decimal places for the intermediate results, since we are using the final result to four significant digits.

Make sure you use parentheses ( ) around the denominator in each fraction when punching it into the calculator.

OD:

$$SM = \frac{1}{1 - \left(\frac{t}{n}\right)D_1} \times \frac{1}{1 - hD}$$

$$SM = \frac{1}{1 - \left(\frac{0.003}{1.498}\right)(+6.25)} \times \frac{1}{1 - (0.015)(+1.50)}$$

$$SM = \frac{1}{1 - 0.0125167} \times \frac{1}{1 - 0.0225}$$

SM = (1.01268)(1.02302) = **1.036**

%SM = (SM − 1)100 = (1.036 − 1)100 = **3.6%**

OS:

$$SM = \frac{1}{1 - \left(\frac{t}{n}\right)D_1} \times \frac{1}{1 - hD}$$

$$SM = \frac{1}{1 - \left(\frac{0.005}{1.498}\right)(+9.25)} \times \frac{1}{1 - (0.015)(+4.50)}$$

$$SM = \frac{1}{1 - 0.0308745} \times \frac{1}{1 - 0.0675}$$

SM = (1. 03186)(1. 07239) = **1.107**

%SM = (SM − 1)100 = (1.107 − 1)100 = **10.7%**

The right lens has 3.6% magnification, and the left lens has 10.7% magnification. The wearer has a magnification difference of 10.7 − 3.6 = **7.1%**.

If the wearer has good vision in each eye when corrected, this person might have a problem with fusion. What can be done to decrease the 7.1% magnification difference?[1]

---

[1]If the anisometropia is *axial*, meaning that the two eye globes are different lengths, the glasses wearer may not have aniseikonia and no negative effect will result from the difference in magnification of the two lenses. If the anisometropia is *refractive*, meaning that the eyes are the same length but the amount of curvature in the two corneas is different, the glasses will induce the aniseikonia. For axial aniseikonia, contact lenses may induce aniseikonia that glasses do not. For refractive aniseikonia, glasses may induce aniseikonia that contact lenses do not.

1. **BC changes:** Putting both lenses on a +8.25 BC increases D_1 from +6.25 to +8.25 for the right lens, a change of +2D, and decreases D_1 from +9.25 to +8.25 for the left lens, a change of –1D.
   OD ΔD_1 = +2, $\Delta SM\% = \Delta D_1 t/15 = (+2)(3)/15 = $ **+0.4% increase;** with this change OD magnification would be 3.6 + 0.4 = 4.0%.
   OS ΔD_1 = –1, $\Delta SM\% = \Delta D_1 t/15 = (-1)(5)/15 = $ **–0.3% decrease;** with this change OS magnification would be 10.7 – 0.3 = 10.4%.
   Together, they decrease the difference from 7.1% to about **6.4%.**
   Note: This may increase lens aberrations, creating other potential problems for the wearer.

2. **Thickness changes:** Make the OD 5 mm thick; decrease the OS to 3 mm. The right lens changes from 3 mm to 5 mm, a change of +2 mm. The left lens changes from 5 mm to 3 mm, a change of –2 mm.
   OD Δt = +2, $\Delta SM\% = D_1 \Delta t/15 = (+6.25)(+2)/15 = $ **+0.8% increase;** with this change OD magnification would be 3.6 + 0.8 = 4.4%.
   OS Δt = –2, $\Delta SM\% = D_1 \Delta t/15 = (+9.25)(-2)/15 = $ **–1.2% decrease;** with this change OS magnification would be 10.7 – 1.2 = 9.5%.
   Together, they decrease the difference from 7.1% to about 5.1%.
   Note: On the OS, this change may not be safe without refitting to a smaller frame (which, if it were possible, should have been done before the whole exercise was started!).

3. **Vertex distance changes:** Move the bevel on one lens, or give the glasses co-planar misalignment, resulting in an OD vertex distance (VD) of 13 mm and OS VD of 11 mm. The right lens changes from 12 mm to 13 mm, a change of +1 mm. The left lens changes from 12 mm to 11 mm, a change of –1 mm.
   OD Δh = +1, $\Delta SM\% = \Delta hD/10 = (+1)(+1.50)/10 = $ **+0.2% increase;** with this change OD magnification would be 3.6 + 0.2 = 3.8%.
   OS Δh = –1, $\Delta SM\% = \Delta hD/10 = (-1)(+4.50)/10 = $ **–0.5% decrease;** with this change OD magnification would be 10.7 – 0.5 = 10.2%.
   Together, they decrease the difference from 7.1% to about 6.4%.
   Note: Bevel placement changes are more practical on minus lenses than on plus lenses.
   If each of these changes were made to the prescription, the difference would seem to decrease from 7.1% to about 3.7%. Why?
   OD: 3.6 + 0.4 + 0.8 + 0.2 = 5.0%
   OS 10.7 – 0.3 – 1.2 – 0.5 = 8.7%
   8.7 – 5.0 = **3.7% difference between lenses.**
   Reworking the original question but using the new parameters: BCs of +8.25, t = 5 mm and 3 mm, and VDs of 13 mm and 11 mm:
   OD:

$$SM = \frac{1}{1 - \left(\dfrac{t}{n}\right)D_1} \times \frac{1}{1 - hD}$$

$$SM = \frac{1}{1 - \left(\dfrac{0.005}{1.498}\right)(+8.25)} \times \frac{1}{1 - (0.016)(+1.50)}$$

$$SM = \frac{1}{1 - 0.0275367} \times \frac{1}{1 - 0.024}$$

SM = (1.02832)(1.02459) = **1.054**
%SM = (SM – 1)100 = (1.054 – 1)100 = **5.4%**
OS:

$$SM = \frac{1}{1 - \left(\dfrac{t}{n}\right)D_1} \times \frac{1}{1 - hD}$$

$$SM = \frac{1}{1 - \left(\dfrac{0.003}{1.498}\right)(+8.25)} \times \frac{1}{1 - (0.014)(+4.50)}$$

$$SM = \frac{1}{1 - 0.0165220} \times \frac{1}{1 - 0.063}$$

SM = (1.01680)(1.06724) = **1.085**

%SM = (SM − 1)100 = (1.085 − 1)100 = **8.5%**

The right lens now has 5.4% magnification, and the left lens has 8.5% magnification, giving a difference of **3.1%** for the two lenses.

Note:
- Aspheric design for at least one of the lenses may reduce the difference in SM to tolerable limits without use of an iseikonic design. *Aspheric design lenses should be the first choice for solving anisometropic Rx problems.*
- Some of the changes discussed here may not be reasonable. Iseikonic lens designers rarely change all three factors.
- Choosing a smaller, rounder frame that fits closer to the face may make a substantial change without the special designs. In Example 6-4 use the original specifications, but with a VD of 8 mm and thicknesses of 2.5 mm and 4 mm, respectively, to prove this change to yourself.

If the wearer could not fuse before, but decreasing the magnification difference allows binocular vision, the cosmetics of these glasses may be perfectly acceptable to the wearer. If the wearer suppresses one eye, or for some other reason does not notice a difference in binocular vision, however, the cosmetics of the iseikonic lenses may be totally unacceptable.

Not all anisometropia results in image size problems, so this process should not be attempted unless there is an indication that the glasses are inducing aniseikonia.

When SM is calculated for spherocylindrical lenses, the magnification must be calculated on each of the major meridians separately. For example, an Rx of −1.00 −4.00 ×180 will have a very different magnification on the 180 meridian than on the 90 meridian. The SM should be calculated for the major meridian powers, in this case, for −1.00D and for −5.00D.

For all lenses, remember the rules in the box below.

RULES FOR SPECTACLE MAGNIFICATION

	PLUS LENS	**MINUS LENS**
Increase BC	More magnification	Less minification
Increase t	More magnification	Less minification
Increase VD	More magnification	More minification

Refractive anisometropia is better corrected with contact lenses and may necessitate iseikonic design lenses when corrected with glasses. Axial anisometropia is better corrected with glasses where the inherent differences in spectacle magnification will correct differences in image size on the retina that results from the eye globes being different sizes. Not everyone with anisometropia gets aniseikonia from their glasses, so iseikonic lenses are considered only if the wearer is having problems associated with magnification changes.

Several tools other than the formulas are available for the design of iseikonic lenses, and several factors should be considered before becoming involved in designing iseikonic lenses. A complete discussion of this problem and potential solutions may be found in Fannin and Grosvenor: *Clinical Optics*, ed. 2, pp 300-325.

EXERCISES: (Round all magnification percents to one decimal place.)

4. The Rx is OD −14.50 OS −10.00. Center thickness is 1.5 mm OU, material is polycarbonate (n = 1.586), fitting vertex distance 9 mm, BC +1.50 OU. What is the SM for each lens, and what is the difference between the lenses? What could be done to decrease the difference? Try:
   a. Increasing the center thickness of the OD by 1 mm
   b. Moving the bevel placement on the OS to increase the VD by 2 mm and on the OD to decrease the VD by 1 mm
   c. Increasing the BC one diopter for OD, decreasing one diopter for OS
   Which changes make the most difference? Are they practical? (Not coming up with the answers in Appendix 7? Remember to add 3 mm to the VD but not to the change in VD, and watch the signs in the denominators.)

5. What is the SM for contact lenses (VD = 0) for the prescription OD +1.50, OS +4.50? For contact lenses we use only the power factor because the shape factor is essentially 1. (Why?) Notice that this is the same prescription used for Example 6-4. Compare the difference in magnification between glasses and contact lenses.

ANGULAR MAGNIFICATION[2]

The size of an image on the retina depends on the size of the object and the distance of the object from the eye. To measure the size of the image on the retina, we use the angle from the visual axis to the top of the object. In the diagram below we will assume that the object, the large E, is 25 cm (about 10 inches) from the eye.

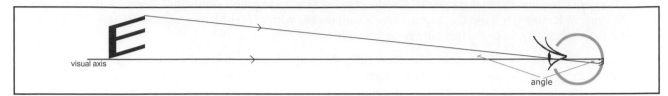

Suppose we do something that allows the object to be brought closer to the eye than 25 cm while still allowing the eye to focus the image on the retina. The ratio of the new angle made by the object and the visual axis to the original angle is called ***angular magnification***. In this case we made the image on the retina larger by bringing the object closer. If we bring the object E to 12.5 cm, the angle will be about twice the original angle, the image on the retina will be about twice the size of the original image, and the angular magnification that results from the change in position is 2.

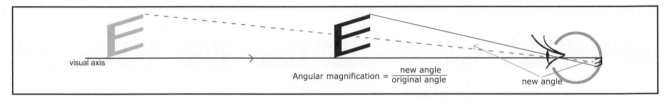

Simple hand-held magnifiers use a plus lens to change this angle. If the magnifier is held so that the object is at the focal point of the lens, the rays diverging from the object will emerge from the lens as if the object were at infinity, allowing the eye to look at the image without accommodation. The angle made by image rays to the optical axis gives an angular magnification of about 1/4D when the angle is compared with the angle if the object was at 25 cm. This is the *nominal magnification* of the lens. Thus a 2 DS lens would have a nominal magnification of 1/2 because the object would be at 50 cm and its size would be compared with the size of the object at 25 cm. This formula requires two factors:

- The object is at the focal point of the lens, resulting in the emerging rays that are parallel to one another. Thus the emmetropic eye will see the image in focus without accommodation.

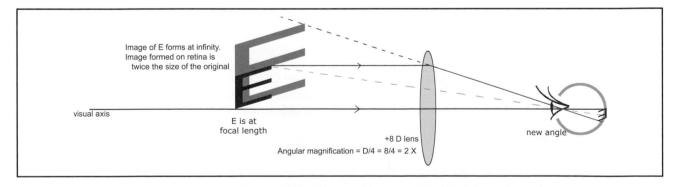

- The comparison is with the angle that is made by the object when it is 25 cm from the eye.

---

[2]Information in this section derived from April 29, 2005, e-mail communication with Darryl Meister.

Since the rays are emerging parallel with one another, the distance between the eye and the lens does not matter.

Note: Usually when the division by 4 occurs, a comparison is being made with an object at 25 cm.

Used in this manner, a lens of +4.00 DS power placed immediately in front of the eye would allow the emmetropic eye to see the object placed at 25 cm at its correct size without the use of accommodation. With the eye at any other distance from the lens, the image will appear to be the size it would be if the object were 25 cm *from the observer,* resulting in the in-focus image with the perception of magnification.

In the diagram below, the lens with +8 DS power has a focal length of 12.5 cm. Regardless of the position of the eye, an object that is placed at a distance of 12.5 cm from the +8 DS lens will result in an image for the eye that is twice the size the object would be at 25 cm from the lens. Because the object is at the focal point, the rays emerge parallel, and the eye (without accommodating) sees an in-focus image that appears to be 12.5 cm from the eye.

If the object is placed closer to the lens than the focal length, the image on which the eye will focus will form between infinity and the object. The image will also be bigger than the object. If the object is positioned so that the image formed by the lens is at 25 cm from the eye, the angular magnification will be about 1/4D + 1. This is the *conventional magnification* or *maximum angular magnification.* The formula 1/4D + 1 assumes that:

- The object will be inside the focal length of the magnifying lens.
- The image will form at 25 cm from the lens.
- The eye will be as close as possible to the lens.

Note that in this instance the position of the eye with respect to the magnifying lens is important, and that to see the image clearly, the eye will have to accommodate.

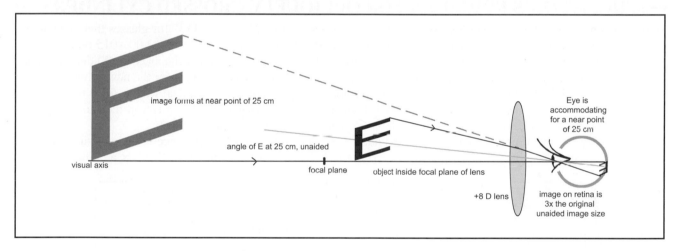

When a hand-held magnifier is used, the actual magnification will be up to 1/4 D + 1, depending on the eye-to-image and lens-to-object distances.

ANGULAR MAGNIFICATION

- Nominal magnification = 1/4D. Object is at focal plane of lens; result is compared to size of object when 25 cm from eye.
- Conventional or maximum angular magnification = 1/4D + 1. Object is inside focal length of lens; eye is as close to the lens as possible or practical.

There is a practical limit to how strong a simple magnifier can be. Lens aberrations make the image either distorted or fuzzy on the edges. Strong plus lenses used this way have a limited field of view. Use of aspheric curves for the lens or of a series of specially designed lenses can extend both of these limits.

Manufacturers of magnifiers may state the angular magnification using either 1/4D (nominal magnification) or 1/4D + 1 (conventional or maximum magnification). To compare two magnifying lenses, we must know which formula is being used.

6. Take a +2.00D lens and hold it about 16 inches away from you and a few inches above a piece of lined paper. Notice the difference in size of the spaces between the lines where you are looking through the lens and where you are looking directly at the paper. By moving the magnifier to various distances from the paper and from your face, you will discover that the best you can do is have the lines 1.5 times as far apart with the lens as they are without it. Based on the maximum angular magnification formula, what magnification are you seeing?

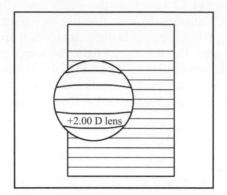

— THOMPSON'S FORMULA FOR OBLIQUELY CROSSED CYLINDERS —

What happens if an aphake has an Rx that says "over-refracted OD +1.25 –1.25 ×113" for glasses that have an Rx of +12.50 –2.25 ×085? What if over-refraction of a new contact lens wearer gives –1.25 –2.00 ×015 on a lens that is –5.00 –1.00 ×180? If the two prescriptions being combined are at the same axis or the axes are 90 degrees apart, transpose if necessary to put both prescriptions in the same axis, add the sphere powers for the new sphere, and add the cylinder powers for the new cylinder. If the axes are not 90 degrees apart, the practical way to solve this problem is to dot a lens with the over-refraction Rx on axis, place it and the glasses in the lensmeter at the same time, and neutralize the result. This book is a formulas reference, however, so we will use formulas.

First, transpose the prescriptions to plus cylinder. (Transposing is not strictly necessary but will make the calculations easier.) Label the Rx with the *lower value axis* $S_1 \, C_1 \times a_1$, and the other $S_2 \, C_2 \times a_2$. The angle γ is $a_2 - a_1$.

$$C^2 = C_1^2 + C_2^2 + 2C_1C_2 \cos 2\gamma \text{ gives the amount of the new cylinder power}$$

$$S = S_1 + S_2 + \frac{C_1 + C_2 - C}{2} \text{ gives the amount of the new sphere power}$$

$$\tan 2\theta = \frac{C_2 \sin 2\gamma}{C_1 + C_2 \cos 2\gamma} \text{ gives } \theta, \text{ the amount to be added to } a_1 \text{ to give the new axis}$$

If the result is a negative axis, remember that what is on the lower half of the lens is the same as what is 180 degrees away on the upper half. Just add 180 to the negative answer to find the new prescription axis. Or, if the resulting axis is over 180, subtract 180 from it.

6-5. The current Rx in the glasses is OS +10.50 +2.00 ×015.
The over-refraction is –0.50 +0.75 ×045.
What lens power should be ordered?
Step 1. Put the prescriptions in plus cylinder form.
Label the Rx with the lower value axis as $S_1 \, C_1 \times a_1$ and the other as $S_2 \, C_2 \times a_2$.
The prescriptions are in + cylinder form and are in the correct order. So:

$S_1 = +10.50$	$S_2 = -0.50$
$C_1 = +2.00$	$C_2 = +0.75$
$a_1 = 015$	$a_2 = 045$

Step 2. The angle γ is $a_2 - a_1 = 45 - 15 = 30$; $2\gamma = 60$

Step 3. Calculate the new cylinder power.

$C^2 = C_1^2 + C_2^2 + 2C_1C_2 \cos 2\gamma$

$\quad = (2.00)^2 + (0.75)^2 + 2(2.00)(0.75)(\cos 60)$

$\quad = 4 + 0.5625 + (3)(0.5) = 6.0625$

$C = \sqrt{6.0625} = \textbf{+2.46, the new cylinder power}$

Step 4. Calculate the new sphere power.

$S = S_1 + S_2 + \dfrac{C_1 + C_2 - C}{2}$

$\quad = +10.50 - 0.50 + \dfrac{2 + 0.75 - 2.46}{2}$

$\quad = +10.00 + 0.145$

$\textbf{S = +10.15, the new sphere power}$

Step 5. Calculate the new axis.

$\tan 2\theta = \dfrac{C_2 \sin 2\gamma}{C_1 + C_2 \cos 2\gamma}$

$\tan 2\theta = \dfrac{(0.75)\sin 60}{(2) + (0.75)\cos 60} = \dfrac{0.6495}{2.375} = 0.27347$

So, $2\theta = 15.29$, and $\theta = 7.6$, which rounds to 8 degrees. The 8-degree change is added to a_1, so $15 + 8 = \textbf{23, the new axis}$.

The combined Rx is now $+10.15\ +2.46\ \times023$. This answer, changed to the nearest eighth so that it may be ordered or surfaced, is $\textbf{+10.12 +2.50} \times\textbf{023}$.

This set of formulas is shown in a variety of forms in different textbooks. The problems may also be solved graphically by use of vector analysis. Possible sources are Fannin and Grosvenor: *Clinical Optics,* ed. 2, pp 43-48; Epting and Morgret: *Ophthalmic Mechanics and Dispensing,* pp 106-110; and Jalie: *The Principles of Ophthalmic Lenses,* ed. 4, pp 287-296. The formulas shown here seem to be the easiest combination of several different versions.

6-6. The Rx is $+12.50\ -3.50\ \times180$. Over-refraction is $+1.75\ -1.00\ \times135$. What should be ordered?

Step 1. Transpose and rearrange: $+0.75\ +1.00\ \times045$

$\qquad\qquad\qquad\qquad\qquad +9.00\ +3.50\ \times090$

$S_1 = +0.75 \qquad\quad S_2 = +9.00$

$C_1 = +1.00 \qquad\quad C_2 = +3.50$

$a_1 = 045 \qquad\qquad a_2 = 090$

Step 2. $\gamma = 45$, $2\gamma = 90$

Step 3. $C^2 = C_1^2 + C_2^2 + 2C_1C_2 \cos 2\gamma$

$\qquad\quad = (1.00)^2 + (3.50)^2 + 2(1.00)(3.50)(\cos 90)$

$\qquad\quad = 1 + 12.25 + (2)(3.5)(0) = 13.25$

$\qquad\ C = \sqrt{13.25} = \textbf{+3.64, the new cylinder power}$

Step 4. $S = S_1 + S_2 + \dfrac{C_1 + C_2 - C}{2}$

$\qquad\ S = +0.75 + 9.00 + \dfrac{1 + 3.50 - 3.64}{2}$

$\qquad\qquad = +9.75 + 0.43$

$\qquad\ \textbf{S = +10.18, the new sphere power}$

Step 5. $\tan 2\theta = \dfrac{C_2 \sin 2\gamma}{C_1 + C_2 \cos 2\gamma}$

$\qquad\quad \tan 2\theta = \dfrac{(3.5)\sin 90}{(1) + (3.5)\cos 90} = \dfrac{3.5}{1} = 3.5$

So, $2\theta = 74$, and $\theta = 37$ degrees. The 37-degree change is added to a_1.

So, $45 + 37 = \textbf{82, the new axis}$.

The new Rx is +10.18 +3.64 ×082, or +13.82 −3.64 ×172. Changed to eighths so that it may be ordered or surfaced, it is **+13.87 −3.62 ×172.**

Note: It is a good practice to call the refractionist so that the final lens Rx can be recorded in the wearer's records.

EXERCISES:

7. Combine −6.50 −2.00 ×054 with −1.50 −0.75 ×010. (Remember: Start by transposing to plus cylinder form. Finish by rounding to 1/8 diopter steps.)

8. A glasses wearer hands you an Rx that reads: "Over-refraction of +0.25 +1.75 ×123 on current right lens." Neutralizing the current right lens, you find an Rx of +10.50 −1.25 ×088. What lens will you order? Note: Round to 1/8 diopter steps when you are finished. (Then call the refractionist so that the final lens Rx can be recorded in the wearer's records.)

FRESNEL'S EQUATION FOR REFLECTION

When a light ray travels from one transparent material to another material, one of three things happens: it is refracted, which was discussed in Section II; it is absorbed, which will be discussed on pp. 175-179; or it is reflected. The amount of incident light reflected from the interface between two transparent materials depends on the refractive indexes of the two materials.

The approximate percentage of incident light that is reflected from a transparent surface is equal to

$$100 \frac{(n_r - n_i)^2}{(n_r + n_i)^2}$$

where:

n_i = index of refraction of the material from which the light is traveling
n_r = index of refraction of the material the light is entering

Since the difference in the numerator is squared, the percent of incident light reflected from the surface is the same regardless of which is the incident material, so the order in which n_i and n_r are listed is not important.

The version of this equation that we use when the lens is in air is

$$100 \frac{(n - 1)^2}{(n + 1)^2}$$

where n = the index of refraction of the lens material

If I_0 is the intensity of light falling on a lens, the amount of light entering the lens will be I_1, which is I_0 − the amount reflected. Thus:

$$I_1 = I_0 - I_0 \times \frac{(n - 1)^2}{(n + 1)^2}$$

I_1 is the intensity of light that travels through the non-absorptive lens to the back surface of the lens. I_2, then, will be what is not reflected from the back surface of the lens and therefore exits the lens through the back surface.

$$I_2 = I_1 - I_1 \times \frac{(n - 1)^2}{(n + 1)^2}$$

EXAMPLE:

6-7. What percentage of the incident light is transmitted through a white (or clear) lens made of crown glass? I_0 will be 100% of the incident light.
n = 1.523.

$$\frac{(n - 1)^2}{(n + 1)^2} = \frac{(0.523)^2}{(2.523)^2} = \frac{0.2735}{6.3655} = 0.043$$

100(0.043) = 4.3% of the incident light reflects from the front surface of the lens.

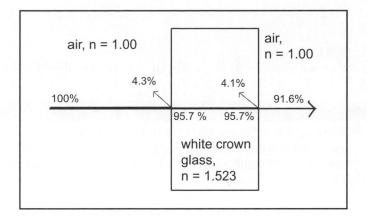

Or, given that 0.043 of the light reflects from the surface,

$I_0 = 100\%$

$I_1 = I_0 - I_0(\text{reflection})$

$\quad = I_0 - I_0(0.043)$

$\quad = 100 - (100)(0.043)$

$\quad = 95.7\%$

$\mathbf{I_2} = I_1 - I_1(\text{reflection})$

$\quad = I_1 - I_1(0.043)$

$\quad = 95.7 - 95.7(0.043)$

$\quad = 95.7 - 4.1$

$\quad = \mathbf{91.6\%}$

In words, what the formula tells us is that 100% – 4.3% = 95.7% of the incident light travels into the lens. Since the lens is white, or clear, all of this light reaches the back surface of the lens. Of the light reaching the back of the lens, 4.3% is reflected back into the lens. So (0.043)(95.7%) = 4.1% of the light reflects from the back surface, and 95.7% – 4.1% = 91.6% of the incident light actually travels through the lens.

Now take the same lens and immerse it in water. Of the light traveling through the water, the amount that reflects from the first surface is

$$\frac{(n_1 - n_2)^2}{(n_1 + n_2)^2} = \frac{(1.523 - 1.33)^2}{(1.523 + 1.33)^2} = \frac{(0.193)^2}{(2.853)^2} = 0.0046, \text{ or } 0.5\%$$

Since 0.5% of the incident light reflects from the front surface, 99.5% of the light enters the lens; (0.005)(99.5%) = 0.5% more of the original light reflects back into the lens, leaving 99% of the incident light to travel through the lens back into the water. Why do you suppose a clear lens is harder to see in water than in air? If you don't believe this, drop a clear, uncoated lens into a fish tank.

Notice in the drawing above that the light reflecting from the back surface of the glass reaches the front surface, and some of it reflects back inside the glass instead of reentering air on the front of the glass. Increasingly smaller amounts will reflect back and forth, some of it exiting the lens through the back surface. So the actual total of the light transmitted through the lens is a little larger than the amount we get from this series of calculations. An approximation for the total amount of light transmitted through the lens material is found with this equation[3]:

$$\boxed{\text{Transmission} = \frac{2n}{1 + n^2}}$$

Using the crown glass lens in Example 6-7 the total transmission equation gives:

$$\text{Transmission} = \frac{2n}{1 + n^2}$$

$$= \frac{(2)(1.523)}{1 + (1.523)^2}$$

---

[3]From Bruneni J: Ask the labs, *Eye Care Business,* April 1998, p 40.

$$= \frac{3.046}{3.3195}$$

$$= 0.9176\ldots = \mathbf{91.8\%}$$

The total transmission for crown glass of 91.8% is slightly larger than the 91.6% that the surface reflection formula gave, as expected.

EXERCISES:

9. What percentage of incident light is reflected from the front surface of a clear CR-39 lens? What percentage of the original incident light reflects back into the lens from the back surface? What percentage of the incident light is transmitted through the lens? Based on the transmission formula, what is the total transmission through this lens?

10. What percentage of incident light is reflected from the front and back surfaces of a polycarbonate lens? What percentage of the incident light is transmitted completely through the polycarbonate lens?

11. Perform the calculations again for a high-index lens material with index of refraction of 1.66. Do you see the trend? Why do reflections bother high-index wearers more than CR-39 wearers, regardless of prescription?

ANTI-REFLECTIVE COATINGS

Several conditions should be met for an anti-reflective (AR) coating to work at its best. One condition is that the amount of light reflected from the coating should be equal to the amount of light reflected from the lens. Another condition is that the wave of light reflected from the coating should cancel the wave of light reflected from the lens. (These conditions assume that the amplitudes of the incident and reflected waves are equal.)

If the *index of refraction of the coating material is equal to the square root of the index of refraction of the lens material*, the exact same amount of light will be reflected from the surface of the coating and from the interface between the coating and the lens material. Since the coating must have several other attributes, such as being insoluble in water, the best coating materials do not meet this criterion exactly.

> When the coating index = the square root of lens material index, the reflections from the coating surface and the lens surface have equal intensity.

Two waves traveling exactly out of phase with each other cancel each other, or show ***destructive interference.***

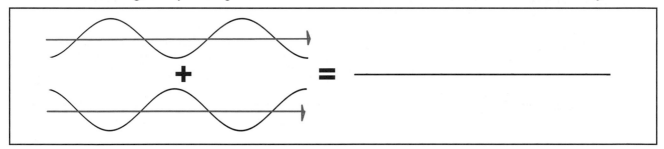

Two waves traveling in phase with each other compound each other. They show ***constructive interference.***

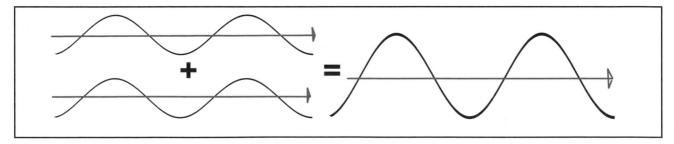

If the thickness of the lens coating is one fourth of the wavelength of the incident light, the reflections from the coating and from the lens will cancel each other, or have destructive interference. If the thickness of the lens coating is 1/2 of the wavelength of the incident light, the reflections from the coating and the lens will compound each other. They have constructive interference.

> When the optical thickness of coating = 1/4λ or 3/4λ or 5/4λ or ...., the reflections cancel, or show **destructive interference**.

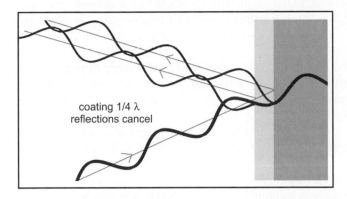
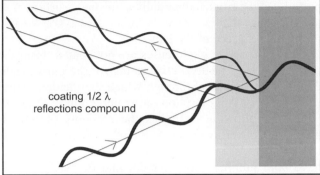

coating 1/4 λ
reflections cancel

coating 1/2 λ
reflections compound

The rule of thumb and diagrams are extremely simplistic representations of what happens. The optics sections in some college physics textbooks or advanced optical theory books go into more detail about the mechanics of the reflections. What is important to us is that the coating thickness should be an odd multiple of 1/4 of the wavelength of the incoming light. Most manufacturers use 1/4λ.

The visible spectrum ranges from about 380 nm to about 760 nm. One fourth of 760 nm is 190 nm. But 190 nm is one half of 380 nm, so the coating thickness that would cancel the high-end red waves would also compound the low-end violet waves. Similarly, for any wavelength between, the coating that would cancel one color would at least partially compound other colors. Therefore coating manufacturers apply several layers of varying thickness to cancel a majority of the reflected light waves. The colored sheen that is seen on AR coatings is what is left based on a particular manufacturer's combination of coatings and thicknesses. Each manufacturer of AR coating is careful to keep the resulting colored sheen consistent from batch to batch.

——— TRANSMISSION THROUGH ABSORPTIVE LENSES ———

Once a light ray enters the front surface of lens, it can be either absorbed by the lens material or transmitted through to the back surface of the lens.

Making absorptive lenses from CR-39 and other plastic materials requires dyeing the lenses. When the lens is immersed in a warm dye bath, pigments that will absorb some of the incident light are incorporated into the lens material in an even layer less than 0.5 mm thick. Thus the absorption of light does not depend on the thickness of the lens, only on the amount of pigment absorbed by the material. A lens that has been dyed to 15% absorption transmits 85% of the entering light. For an uncoated CR-39 lens, 4% of the incident light is reflected from the front surface, so $I_1 = 96\%$.

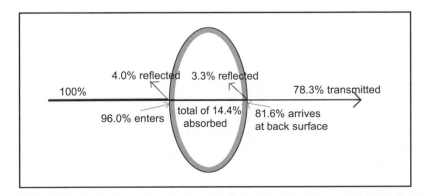

4.0% reflected   3.3% reflected

100%   78.3% transmitted

96.0% enters   total of 14.4%   81.6% arrives
                absorbed   at back surface

If 85% of the light entering the lens is transmitted, then (0.85)(96) = 81.6% of the incident light is transmitted to the back surface of the lens. Since the lens is uncoated, 4% of 81.6% will be reflected back into the lens at the back surface; that is, (0.04)(81.6) = 3.3% is reflected at the back surface, and 81.6 – 3.3 = 78.3% of the original light falling on the lens is actually transmitted through the lens. (See the discussion of Fresnel's equation for reflection, pp. 172-174.)

Sometimes white (or clear) glass lenses are given an absorptive coating. When this process is performed, the transmission as shown above works the same way. A lens' absorptive ability is indicated as one number, regardless of whether the absorption occurs at one surface or both surfaces. In the plastic lens above, the 15% absorption occurs partially at the front and partially at the back surface. A 15% absorptive coating on a glass lens would all be absorbed at the surface that is coated. In either case 100% – 15% = 85% of the light entering the lens is transmitted through to the back surface of the lens.

Most absorptive *glass* lenses are not coated. Instead the absorptive oxides are distributed evenly throughout the glass material. The absorptive rating for the glass material is indicated by a percentage per 2 mm thickness. Every 2 mm of lens material through which the incident light travels absorbs more light. The transmission rating for the material is 100 – absorption rating per 2 mm of thickness.

In the following examples the amounts of light are sometimes expressed as decimals and sometimes as percents. Convert from one to the other by multiplying or dividing by 100. Thus 0.56 → 56%; 82% → 0.82. Round the numbers to one decimal in percent form or three decimals in decimal form. When *adding* or *subtracting*, have *both* numbers in either decimal or percent form. When *multiplying*, either use both numbers in decimal form (the answer will be in decimal form) or have one in percent and one in decimal (the answer will be in percent form).

EXAMPLE:

6-8. What is the total transmission through the center of a crown glass lens with 15% absorption per 2 mm of thickness, if the center thickness of the lens is 6 mm?

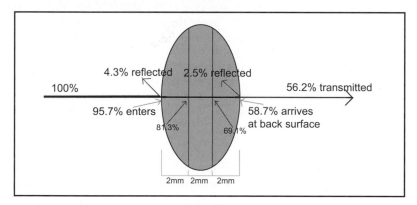

1. The reflection from the front surface is **4.3%**, or 100% – 4.3% = **95.7%** of the incident light enters the lens. (See the discussion of Fresnel's equation for reflection, pp. 172-174.)
2. The first 2 mm of the lens absorbs 15% of the light that reaches it, or it transmits 85% → 0.85 of the light reaching it. Therefore (0.85)(95.7) = **81.3%** of the incident light is transmitted through the first 2 mm of thickness of the lens.
3. In the next 2 mm of lens 15% of the 81.3% will be absorbed, or 85% → 0.85 of the 81.3% will be transmitted. Therefore (0.85)(81.3) = **69.1%** of the incident light is transmitted through the second 2 mm of thickness of the lens.
4. In the last 2 mm of the lens 15% of the 69.1% will be absorbed, or 85% → 0.85 of the 69.1% will be transmitted. Therefore (0.85)(69.1) = **58.7%** of the incident light is transmitted through to the back surface of the lens.
5. Of the light reaching the back of the lens, 4.3% is reflected back into the lens, or 95.7% → 0.957 will pass through the back surface. Therefore (0.957)(58.7) = **56.2% of the incident light is transmitted through the lens at the center**.

Notice that the 15% absorptive CR-39 lens allowed 78% of the incident light through the lens, which is about what will be transmitted through this glass lens at the 2 mm edge, but the center of the 15% absorptive glass lens allowed just over half of the incident light through.

Lambert's equation for lens transmission can be used to determine the absorption of the glass lens in fewer steps. Let q = thickness/2 (in mm). In the lens above, q = 6/2 = 3. Let T be the amount of incident light transmitted per 2 mm thickness. Then the amount of light transmitted through the lens from front surface to back surface is

$$I_2 = I_1 T^q$$

where:

I_2 = intensity of light reaching the back surface of the lens
I_1 = intensity of light entering the lens
T = transmission factor per 2 mm of lens thickness (in decimal form)
q = thickness of the lens in mm divided by 2 mm

In Example 6-8, I_1 = 95.7%, T = 100% – 15% = 85% = 0.85, and q = 6/2 mm = 3. So the amount of light transmitted to the back surface of the lens is:

I_2 = (95.7)(0.85)³ = (95.7)(0.614) = 58.8%

The 58.8% answer using this equation is what the series of calculations above gave. (The 0.01% difference is the result of rounding when we did the transmission step by step.) Use the transmission in decimal form for this equation. (You still need to calculate the reflection from the back surface.)

If your calculator has the sin/cos/tan functions, somewhere on it is a key labeled x^y, y^x, or ^. (If your calculator *also* has a key labeled x^n or y^n, do *not* use that key.) Enter the transmission amount, in the above example 0.85, press the x^y or y^x or ^ key, enter 3, and press =. The result is 58.7717.... What you are doing when you enter this sequence is telling the calculator what x is, then that you want to raise it to the y power, then what y is.

Example 6-8, Second Try, Lambert's Equation

Type A Calculator

95.7 | **×** | 0.85 | **x^y** | 3 | **=**   The calculator should say 58.7717…

Type B Calculator

95.7 | **×** | 0.85 | **^** | 3 | **=**   The calculator should say 58.7717…

What if the thickness of the lens is 4.7 mm? Now q = 4.7/2 = 2.35. How will you do this with your calculator? Enter the intensity, in this example 95.7, press the multiply key, enter the transmission amount, in this example 0.85, press the x^y or y^x or ^ key, enter 2.35, and press =. The result is 65.3200....

EXAMPLE:

6-9. An uncoated crown glass lens has an absorptive rating of 25%/2 mm of thickness. The lens is ground to an Rx of –5.00D, with a center thickness of 2.2 mm. What is the transmission through the center of the lens? If the lens edge calipers to 7.1 mm, what is the transmission through the thickest edge of the lens?

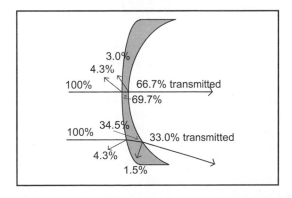

1. The reflection from the front surface at both the center and the edge will be 4.3%, so **95.7%** of the incident light will enter the lens.

2. At the center of the lens,
   thickness = 2.2 mm,
   q = 2.2/2 = 1.1, and
   T = 100 − 25 = 75% = 0.75.
   The transmission through the lens at the center is
   $I_2 = (95.7)(0.75)^{1.1}$
   $= (95.7)(0.729)$
   $= \mathbf{69.7\%}$

3. Of the 69.7% of the incident light that reached the back surface at the center of the lens, 4.3% = 0.043 is reflected back into the lens at the back surface. So (69.7)(0.043) = 3.0% of the incident light is reflected, leaving 69.7 − 3.0 = **66.7% transmission through the center of the lens.**

4. At the edge of the lens,
   thickness = 7.1,
   q = 7.1/2 = 3.55,
   T = 100 − 25 = 75% = 0.75,
   and 95.7% of the incident light enters the lens at the edge. So the transmission to the back surface of the lens is
   $I_2 = (95.7)(0.75)^{3.55}$
   $= (95.7)(0.3601)$
   $= \mathbf{34.5\%}$

5. Of the 34.5% of the incident light that reached the back surface at the edge of the lens, 4.3% = 0.043 is reflected back into the lens at the back surface. So (34.5)(0.043) = 1.5% of the incident light is reflected, leaving 34.5 − 1.5 = **33.0% transmission through the edge of the lens.**

The thick edge of a minus power absorptive glass lens will be much darker than the center of the lens. Similarly, the thick center of a plus power absorptive glass lens will be darker than the edge of the lens.

Photochromatic lenses do not lend themselves to the use of Lambert's equation. Plastic photochromatic lenses have a thin layer of photoreactive material on the front surface of the lens, and therefore they have an even distribution of absorption over the surface of the lens, regardless of lens thickness. Photochromatic glass has silver halide mixed evenly throughout the material, so it seems that it would work the way absorptive glass works. The amount of transmission or absorption, however, depends on the amount of ultraviolet (UV) light reaching the silver halide. Since the UV rays are absorbed by the change in the lens material, the transmission of UV decreases as the ray penetrates the lens. The amount of change in the lens material decreases as the ray penetrates the lens. In the full dark state the innermost 2 mm of a thick lens does not change as much and therefore does not absorb as much light as the outer 2 mm absorbed.

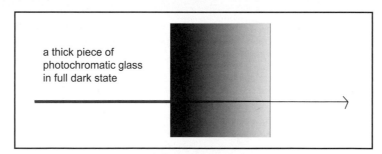

a thick piece of photochromatic glass in full dark state

As a result the variation in darkness from the thinnest point on the lens to the thickest point on the lens is not as great as the variation in darkness on a non-variable absorptive glass lens.

Look at what happens when several absorptive lenses are lined up in a row. If the total transmission through the first lens is 75% and the total transmission through the second lens is 50%, the total transmission through the two lenses will be 50% = 0.50 of 75%, or (0.5)(75) = 37.5%. Consider a person driving in a car with tinted windshields. If the windshield has a total transmission of 80% and the driver is wearing sunglasses with a total transmission of 20%, the driver is actually seeing (0.20)(80) = 16% of the incident light. What if the same driver wears lenses with a 30% to 0% gradient tint when driving at night? If the person drives looking through the top of the lenses (most of us do) where the transmission is 70%, the driver is receiving (0.80)(70) = 56% of the incident light. A transmission of 56% will not block enough of the glare from oncoming car headlights but may well keep the driver from seeing people, objects, or animals in the low-light, low-contrast conditions at the side of the road.

EXERCISES: (Round answers to one tenth of a percent.)

12. What is the total transmission through a plastic lens having an index of refraction of 1.66, tinted with a 15% cosmetic tint?

13. What is the total transmission through an AR coated glass lens having an absorptive rating of 15% per 2 mm thickness? The glass lens has a center thickness of 2.2 mm, and the thickest edge is 5.7 mm. (Since the lens is AR coated, you may ignore surface reflections.)

14. Suppose a plano photochromatic lens has an absorptive rating of 18% in its unexposed state and 56% in the car during the day. If the lens is not AR coated and the wearer is driving a car with windshields tinted to 15% absorption, what is the total transmission to the driver in bright sunlight? What is the total transmission at night? (Assume that the indexes of refraction for the photochromatic glass and for the windshield are both 1.523.) Steps:
    a. Determine the final transmission through the car windshield. Assume the window index is 1.523 and absorption is 15%. (Keep in decimal form.)
    b. Determine the final transmission through the photochromatic lens only, with 56% absorption and index 1.523. (Keep in decimal form.)
    c. Multiply the two final transmission numbers from parts a and b. Convert to a percent. This is how much of the incident light this wearer sees while driving during the day.
    d. Determine the final transmission through the photochromatic lens only, with 18% absorption and index 1.523. (Keep in decimal form.)
    e. Multiply the two final transmission numbers from parts a and d. Convert to a percent. This is how much of the incident light this wearer sees while driving at night.

POLARIZING FILTERS

Normal diffuse sunlight contains "waves" that are vibrating in every direction perpendicular to the direction of travel of the sunlight. The light beam is said to be *unpolarized* if it contains waves oscillating in random directions. The light beam is said to be *polarized* if it contains waves oscillating on or near only one plane.

The light in a light beam can be limited to oscillate on only one plane, or *polarized,* in essentially two main ways. A beam of unpolarized light can be polarized by reflection from the surface of a material that does not conduct electricity (a dielectric material). Examples of dielectric, or non-conducting, materials are water, snow, sand, glass, and pavement. Or the beam can be polarized by being passing through a material with a crystalline structure that only allows transmission of rays vibrating in a particular direction. Examples of crystals that polarize transmitted light are quartz, tourmaline, and iodine in a particular compound or matrix. Iodine impregnated in a sheet of polyvinyl alcohol is used in ophthalmic polarizing lenses.

A beam of light that is completely polarized, so that all rays are oscillating in only one direction, is called *linearly polarized* or *plane polarized.* There is also a circular polarization, which will not be discussed here. A beam of light that is not completely polarized is called *partially polarized.* Most of the light that reflects from the surface of water is partially polarized. The ray will be fully polarized if the angle of incidence of the ray satisfies *Brewster's equation:*

$$\tan \angle i = n_i / n_r$$

where:
$\angle i$ = angle of incidence of the incident light
n_i = index of the incident material
n_r = index of the reflecting material

For a pond sitting out in the sunshine of mid-morning or mid-afternoon, $n_i = 1$, $n_r = 1.33$. Brewster's formula gives: $\tan i = n/n_r = 1/1.33 = 0.7519$; therefore $\angle i = 37°$

When the sun is at an angle of 37° with the normal to the surface of the water (which means 53° up from the horizon), the light reflecting from the surface of the water is linearly polarized. At any other angle the reflected sunshine is partially polarized.

Unpolarized light passing through a polarizing crystal or film will be polarized. If polarized light passes through a second polarizing film, the final total transmission depends on the relationship between the axes of the two filters. If the second filter is oriented in the same direction as the axis of the first filter, all the light that passes through the first will pass through the second. (We are ignoring the surface reflections and the absorbing pigments present in the filter material.) If the axis of the second filter is at 90° to the first, none of the polarized light will emerge from the second filter. At any other orientation, the percent of the polarized light that is transmitted through the second filter can be found from *Malus' Law:*

$$I_2 = I_1 \cos^2 \theta$$

where:

I_1 = intensity of light emerging from the first filter
I_2 = intensity of light emerging from the second filter
θ = angle between the axis of the two filters

$\cos^2 0° = 1$, so when the filters have their axes oriented in the same direction, $I_2 = I_1$. $\cos^2 90° = 0$, so when the filters are at 90° to each other, $I_2 = 0$. In these two situations the equation verifies what you already knew. If the filters are at 30° to each other, $I_2 = I_1 \cos^2 30 = I_1 \times 0.75$, or 75% of the light traveling through the first filter will travel through the second filter. If the filters are at 45° to each other, 50% of the light transmitted through the first filter will be transmitted through the second filter.

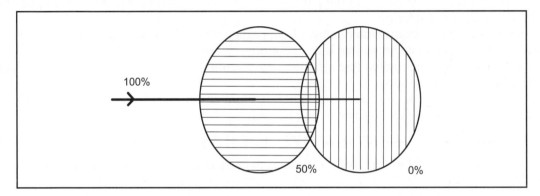

When unpolarized light passes through one linearly polarizing filter, 50% of the incident light is transmitted through the single filter regardless of the orientation of the filter. If 50% of the incident light passes through the first filter and the second filter is held with the polarizer at 45° to the first, (0.50)(50%) = 25% of the originally incident light passes through the two filters.

What happens when three polarizing filters are in a row, with the axis of the second filter 45° from the axis of the *first*, and the axis of the third filter 90° from the axis of the *first*? It seems that no light should go through, since the first and third are at 90°. But, according to Malus' Law, 50% of what travels through the first filter will travel through the second filter, and 50% of what travels through the second filter will travel through the third filter. Therefore placing a second filter between the first and third filters means that 12.5% of the light that was incident on the first filter will be transmitted through the third filter.

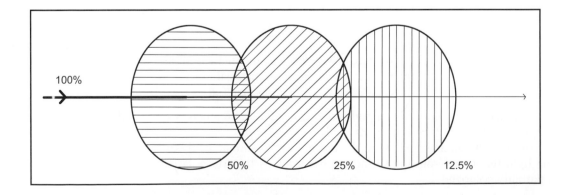

The fact that introducing a third polarizing element between two polarizers crossed at 90° will permit light to come through the third element is the basis for the polariscope, or colmascope, which is used in the ophthalmic laboratory to see stress patterns. Heat tempering a glass lens creates stress patterns in the lens that partially polarize the light. Placing a heat-treated lens between two polarizing filters allows the light to come through in the areas where the stress is created, giving the characteristic pattern. Similarly, uneven pressure on the edge of a lens of any material, which results from uneven tension in mounting the lens, creates stress that polarizes light. Thus the use of the polariscope, or colmascope, to see this induced stress is another application of Malus' Law.

EXERCISES:

15. What is Brewster's angle (in air) for crown glass, n = 1.523?

16. What percentage of incident light will emerge from a series of four polarizing filters, each at 30° to the one before?

The questions with an asterisk (*) in front of the question number are advanced questions. They are not likely to be on the ABO exam but might be on the ABOM exam or the COT exam.

The questions are not presented in the order of the subjects in the section. Some of these questions may require you to think about what you have read in the section, and some may depend on material covered in previous sections.

1. Angular magnification is equal to
   a. the angle of the object on the retina.
   b. the angle of the image on the retina.
   c. the ratio of the size of the object to the size of the image on the retina.
   d. the ratio of the size of the image to the size of the object on the retina.

2. AR coatings work on the principles of
   a. absorption and constructive interference.
   b. absorption and destructive interference.
   c. reflection and constructive interference.
   d. reflection and destructive interference.

3. The rule of thumb for the relationship between OC height and pantoscopic tilt is
   a. raise OC 2 mm for every 1 degree of pantoscopic tilt.
   b. lower OC 2 mm for every 1 degree of pantoscopic tilt.
   c. lower OC 1 mm for every 2 degrees of pantoscopic tilt.
   d. raise OC 1 mm for every 2 degrees of pantoscopic tilt.

4. The Rx
   OD +1.50 −1.50 ×110
   OS +6.50 sph
   is an example of
   a. amblyopia.
   b. antimetropia.
   c. anisometropia.
   d. all of the above.

5. Increasing the BC of a lens will _____ the spectacle magnification.
   a. increase
   b. decrease
   c. have no effect on
   d. have a negative impact on

6. When light travels from air to a clear material,
   a. all of the light is reflected.
   b. all of the light is refracted.
   c. a small amount of light is refracted and the rest is reflected.
   d. a small amount of light is reflected and the rest is refracted.

7. Increasing the thickness of a lens will
   a. increase the spectacle magnification.
   b. decrease the spectacle magnification.
   c. increase the magnification of a plus lens and decrease the magnification of a minus lens.
   d. increase the magnification of a minus lens and decrease the magnification of a plus lens.

8. What is the magnification of a +10 lens, with the object at the focal length of the hand-held magnifier?
   a. 2.0×
   b. 2.5×
   c. 3.5×
   d. 5×

9. Iseikonic design lenses
   a. correct for prismatic imbalance in anisometropic prescriptions.
   b. completely correct magnification differences between the right and left lenses.
   c. decrease magnification differences to the point where fusion is possible.
   d. decrease the difference between prismatic lenses to the point where fusion is broken.

10. The transmission through clear, uncoated crown glass is
    a. 99.5%.
    b. 92%.
    c. 89.5%.
    d. 88%.

11. The new Rx is
    OD +2.50 sph
    OS +4.75 sph
    The right lens in the old glasses is +3.50 sph. The wearer tells you that with the new glasses her vision in each eye is good but she is having trouble with depth perception. The first method to try to correct the image size differences would be
    a. tonometric lenses.
    b. slab-off.
    c. iseikonic design lenses.
    d. aspheric design lenses.

12. The reason that AR coatings make more difference on high-index materials than on standard-index materials is
    a. high-index materials have more chromatic aberrations than standard index materials.
    b. high-index materials have a slight color cast that standard index materials lack.
    c. psychological.
    d. high-index materials have more surface reflection than standard-index materials.

13. Placing a polarized lens between two polarizers that are at 90 degrees to each other will result in
    a. no transmission because two polarizers at 90 degrees to each other block all light transmission.
    b. some transmission, depending on the intensity of the light source.
    c. some transmission, depending on the orientation of the middle lens.
    d. no transmission because the iodine in the polarizers absorbs all visible radiation.

14. The maximum magnification that a +8.00 D lens can give when used as a simple hand-held magnifier is
    a. 8×.
    b. 4×.
    c. 3×.
    d. 2×.

15. Factors that can change the effective power of an Rx that was made correctly according to the prescriber script are
    a. change in vertex distance and incorrect distance between PRPs.
    b. incorrect distance between PRPs and change in BC.
    c. change in BC and vertical OC placement.
    d. incorrect vertical OC placement and change in vertex distance.

16. If a cylinder of a clear plastic material with an index of refraction of 1.52 is imbedded in a clear glass material with an index of refraction of 1.52,
    a. it will be invisible because both the materials are clear.
    b. it will be invisible because no light will be reflected or refracted at the surfaces.
    c. it will be visible because light will be reflected and refracted at the surfaces.
    d. it will be visible because one is plastic and one is glass.

17. Decreasing the vertex distance of a lens will
    a. increase the spectacle magnification.
    b. increase the magnification of a plus lens and decrease the magnification for a minus lens.
    c. increase the magnification of a minus lens and decrease the magnification for a plus lens.
    d. decrease the spectacle magnification.

18. A glasses wearer is having trouble adjusting to new glasses that use her old prescription. You check everything against her old glasses and the only thing that you can find is that the OCs are 2 mm above her pupil center. One acceptable solution is to give the glasses 4° of retroscopic tilt.
    a. True
    b. False

19. AR coatings have a slight color cast because
    a. it is not practical to completely cancel all reflections of all wavelengths in the visible spectrum.
    b. the manufacturers want to ensure that eye care professionals can tell their coatings from other companies' coatings.
    c. if all reflections were cancelled, birds might try to fly through the lens.
    d. the lenses will still show up in photographs.

20. A glasses wearer comes to you with a spectacle Rx of –6.50 OU and asks to be fitted with contact lenses. The minification that the person will experience with the contact lenses will be
    a. less than with the glasses.
    b. more than with the glasses.
    c. the same as with the glasses.
    d. either more or less, depending on the method of manufacture of the contact lenses.

21. The laboratory instrument that uses the principle of crossed polarizers is the
    a. tonometer.
    b. polaroptic.
    c. malusoptic.
    d. colmascope.

22. The amount of light that reflects from one surface of a plastic material with an index of refraction of 1.50 (when in air) is
    a. 20%.   c. 6%.
    b. 8%.   d. 4%.

*23. What is the spectacle magnification for the following lens: +7.25 sphere, BC +10.25, high-index plastic with n = 1.66, center thickness of 3.5 mm, vertex distance 9 mm?
    a. 119%
    b. 12%
    c. 10%
    d. 8.5%

*24. A pair of glasses with a 15% cosmetic pink tint has clip-on sunglass lenses with 85% absorption. The transmission through the combination of lenses is
    a. 0.
    b. 13%.
    c. 81%.
    d. 87%.

*25. An Rx of +12.50 made with an aspherical design of a 1.60 plastic has the OC positioned in front of the pupil center. The glasses have the frame manufacturer's recommended face form of 10 degrees. What is the effective power of the Rx for the wearer?
a. +12.62 +0.37 ×090
b. +12.62 −0.37 ×090
c. +12.37 +0.37 ×090
d. +12.37 −0.37 ×090

*26. What is Brewster's angle for a polycarbonate window pane?
a. 32°
b. 37°
c. 39°
d. 51°

*27. The amount of light that reflects from one surface of a high-index plastic material with an index of 1.60 is
a. 23%.
b. 8.8%.
c. 5.3%.
d. 4.5%.

*28. The ideal thickness for an AR coating that will completely cancel a yellow ray of light (λ = 550 nm) is
a. 275 nm.
b. 138 nm.
c. 106 nm.
d. 23 nm.

*29. A spectacle magnification of 0.95 means
a. 5% minification of the image.
b. 5% magnification of the image.
c. 95% minification of the image.
d. 95% magnification of the image.

*30. A polarizing lens is placed with its polarizing axis at 35° to a second polarizing lens. Taking both polarizing lenses into account and ignoring surface reflections and absorption from lens color, the amount of light that will be transmitted through the pair will be
a. 67%.
b. 34%.
c. 28%.
d. 0.

*31. The Rx is
OD −12.75 sph
OS −9.00 sph
The wearer is having problems with binocular vision that are the result of image size differences. Of the following, which would result in the best single change in the image?
a. increase in thickness for the right lens
b. increase in thickness for the left lens
c. increase in vertex distance for the left lens by a change in the bevel placement on the lens
d. increase in vertex distance for the right lens by a change in the bevel placement on the lens

*32. A pair of goggles has 25 degrees of face form. The Rx is −7.50 OU, and the Rx is made from Trivex. What effective power will the wearer experience when wearing these goggles?
a. −7.95 −1.73 ×090 OU
b. −7.95 −0.98 ×090 OU
c. −8.56 −0.98 ×090 OU
d. −8.56 −1.73 ×090 OU

*33. A contact lens wearer has one toric lens with the Rx −6.50 −1.50 ×180. On over-refraction you find that the vision is improved with −1.00 −0.50 ×25. What Rx would be your starting point in refitting this patient? (Round to the nearest 0.25D.)
a. −7.50 −2.00 ×006
b. −9.50 +1.75 ×011
c. −7.50 −2.00 ×016
d. −7.00 −1.75 ×011

*34. A glass material has an absorption rating of 15% per 2 mm of thickness. If you ignore surface reflections, what is the transmission at the center of a plus lens made from this material if the center is 5.5 mm thick?
a. 64%
b. 69%
c. 76%
d. 85%

*35. The transmission through a clear, uncoated lens with an index of refraction of 1.66 is
a. 12%.
b. 75%.
c. 88%.
d. 99.5%.

SECTION VII – IMAGE FORMATION

IMAGE SIZE AND PLACEMENT: MIRRORS

In Section II we discussed the law of reflection, which states that the angle of incidence is equal to the angle of reflection. Reflection from a plane (or flat) mirror will change the direction of a ray of light but will not change the *vergence* of two rays, meaning the relationship of the rays to each other. If the rays are traveling away from each other, they are diverging from a source. How much the rays diverge, and at any particular plane how far they are from their source, determines their vergence at that plane. If the rays are traveling toward each other, they are converging toward a point. How much the rays converge, and how far they will travel from a particular plane until they meet, determines their vergence at that plane. A flat reflecting surface will not change the vergence of the rays striking it, so an image seen in a mirror appears to be as far behind the mirror as the object is in front of the mirror.

If the surface of the reflecting material is curved, the vergence of the reflected rays will change. We can think of a spherical reflecting surface as if it were made up of a series of small, flat, reflecting surfaces. If a small light source is placed at the center of the sphere that created the curved surface, the light rays traveling from the center to the small, flat surface will be perpendicular to the surfaces and will travel right back to the little light. (After the rays reflect from the surface and arrive back at the center of the curve, the rays continue on to the left, diverging from the source.)

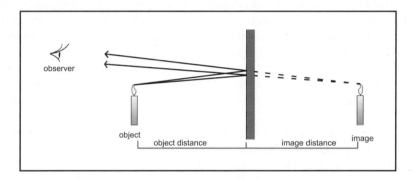

If the small light source is placed one half of the distance between the center of curvature and the surface of the spherical mirror, the rays will reflect back parallel to the line between the center and the light.

In each of the diagrams below, the light rays are diverging from the small light source and the spherical concave reflecting surface changes the vergence of the rays. In the case where the light source is at the center of curvature of the surface, the rays change from diverging to converging rays. They converge back toward the source (and then diverge again in the new direction). In the diagram where the light source is at half the length of the radius of the curve, the rays change from diverging to zero (or no) vergence.

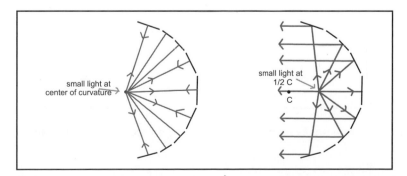

A concave reflecting surface is a converging surface, just as a convex refracting surface (or lens) is a converging surface. The point from which diverging rays are reflected parallel to each other is the focal point of the reflecting surface. Therefore the focal length of a curved mirror is equal to one half of the radius of curvature of the surface. When we discussed lenses, we agreed to call a converging lens a plus lens and to call its focal length a positive focal length. Therefore a concave mirror has a positive focal length.

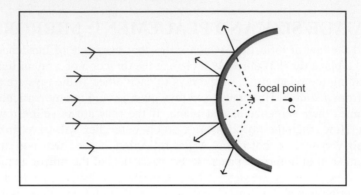

A convex reflecting surface has a negative focal length and is a diverging surface. Incident parallel rays of light diverge after reflection from the surface. Their vergence is the same as it would have been had they originated at a point, called the focal point, that is to the right of the convex mirror. Rays of light converging toward each other with the exact vergence that would result in their meeting at the focal point are reflected parallel to each other by the convex mirror.

We should define several terms. The ***center of curvature*** is the point that is equidistant from every point of the sphere that describes the curved mirror. The ***axis*** of the mirror can be any ray that passes through the center of curvature. In the following discussion we use as the axis a ray that goes through both the object and the center of curvature. The ***focal point*** is the point on the axis that is half the distance from the center of curvature to the mirror. Rays of light emerging from a small light at the focal point reflect from a converging mirror parallel to the axis. The ***vertex*** is the point where the axis touches the mirror. Spherical mirrors have only one center of curvature but an infinite number of axes, focal points, and vertices. For every axis that can be chosen there is only one focal point and only one vertex.

Look at what happens to the light rays that bounce off an object and travel toward a concave mirror. Rays of light bounce off every point on the object, and many travel toward the mirror. The rays that are reflected back from the surface of the mirror will cross at some point and continue on. The light rays will appear to an observer to be diverging from the point where they all crossed. The image appears to be at that point. When an observer looks toward the mirror, the object will appear to be where the rays crossed.

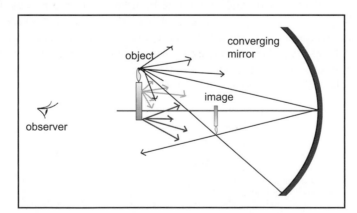

Consider several particular rays that just happen to travel in directions that allow us to predict their paths after reflection.

CURVED MIRROR PRINCIPAL RAYS

- The ray that travels parallel to the axis is reflected so that it passes through the focal point.
- The ray that travels through the focal point reflects back parallel to the axis. This statement is a definition of the focal point.
- The ray that travels through the center of curvature is reflected back on itself.
- The ray that touches the mirror at the vertex is reflected back at the exact same distance below the axis that it had been above the axis.

In the next diagram the particular rays that are drawn are a *pencil of rays* that come from the head of the object and are traveling toward the mirror. The reflected image of the head of the object that an observer sees *appears* to form where the rays cross and continue on. To an observer to the left of the mirror, the rays *appear* to originate at the point where they cross, since they are diverging from that point. The rays may originate at the object, or they may originate elsewhere and reflect from the object. In either case the brain interprets the origin or source of the rays to be at the object because that is where they last crossed.

We need an agreement on what is negative and what is positive. We already agreed that the concave mirror has a positive focal length. We will now state that the object distance, p, is positive if it is to the left of the mirror. (For single mirrors, p is always positive. If several mirrors or lenses are lined up in a series, p may not be always positive.) For mirrors, if the image is to the left of the mirror, we will consider the image distance, q, to be positive. We will also state that if the object or the image is above the axis, its height (or the distance to the axis) will be positive. In the previous diagram the *image distance q is positive* but the distance from the axis to the *top of the image* is negative. For horizontal distances the direction in which the light is traveling is positive and opposite that direction is negative. For mirror exercises, before reflection left to right is positive and after reflection right to left is positive.

Note: Some texts use l and l' for image and object distance, some use s and s', some use u and v, and some use p and q. We will use p and q in this text. We chose to use p and q rather than l and l' or s and s' because the notation using $'$ is hard to see and can cause unnecessary confusion.

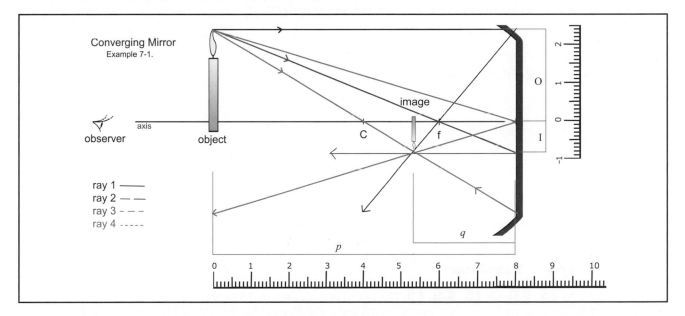

When p is used to represent the distance from the object to the mirror and q is used to represent the distance from the mirror to the point where the image forms, the image distance formula is

$$\frac{1}{f} = \frac{1}{p} + \frac{1}{q}, \text{ or } \frac{1}{q} = \frac{1}{f} - \frac{1}{p}$$

We will now define the object size, or the distance from the axis to the top of the object, to be O, and the image size, or the distance from the axis to the point where the top of the image *forms*, to be I. The ***linear magnification***, or ratio of image size to object size, will be M.

The linear magnification is

$$M = -\frac{q}{p} = \frac{I}{O}$$

where:

M = linear magnification

O = distance of the tip of the object from the axis

I = distance of the tip of the image from the axis

For practical purposes, use

$$I = (M)(O)$$

We will try a few examples. A good way to practice is with graph paper and colored pencils. As you do the drawings yourself, you will notice one potentially disturbing fact: the four rays, when correctly drawn, do not cross at exactly the same point. The rule that the focal point is at one-half the radius of curvature is actually true only if the object size O is small with respect to the focal length of the mirror. In our drawings O is not small with respect to the focal length. This disparity in the drawings is a demonstration of ***spherical aberration***. Spherical aberration means that peripheral rays have a shorter focal length than the rays that are ***paraxial***, or parallel to and close to the axis. Spherical aberration is corrected by use of parabolic curves for the mirror (or for a lens), rather than spherical curves. The focal length of any spherical mirror or lens is shorter at the periphery of the lens than at its optical center. The placement of the focal point F at 1/2 C is for the paraxial rays.

Note: In the formulas for image size and placement the values for f, *p*, and *q* may be in any unit of measure, as long as they are in the *same* unit. Similarly, I and O may be in any unit of measure, as long as they are in the same unit. They need not be in the same unit as f, *p*, and *q*. M is a ratio and has no unit.

EXAMPLES:

7-1. A concave mirror has a focal length of 20 mm. If a 24-mm object is 80 mm from the mirror, where does the image form? What are the size and orientation of the image?

f = 20 mm

p = 80 mm

O = 24 mm

Using the image distance formula,

$$\frac{1}{q} = \frac{1}{f} - \frac{1}{p}$$

$$= \frac{1}{20} - \frac{1}{80}$$

$$= 0.05 - 0.0125$$

$$= 0.0375$$

Since $1/q = 0.0375$, *q* = 1/0.0375 = **27 mm.**

Example 7-1, *q*

Type A Calculator:

20 ⊞ ⊟ 80 ⊞ ＝ ⊞ The calculator should say 26.6666…

Type B Calculator:

20 x^{-1} ⊟ 80 x^{-1} ＝ x^{-1} The calculator should say 26.6666…

Using the magnification formula,

$$M = \frac{q}{p} = -\frac{27}{80} = -0.34$$

Therefore **I** = (M)(O) = (24)(–0.34) = **–8 mm.**

You can verify both the 27-mm distance for q and the –8-mm length for I by using a centimeter ruler and the previous diagram.

If we had not already drawn the diagram to show where the image is, we would be able to tell several facts from these numbers.

1. q is positive, so the image is to the left of the mirror (the direction the ray travels after reflection).
2. M is negative, so the image is inverted or has the opposite orientation to the orientation of the object.
3. I is negative, so the image is forming inverted, below the axis.
4. |M| is less than 1, so the image is smaller than the object.[1] It is **_minified._**

7-2.   Suppose a concave converging mirror has a center of curvature of 50 mm, and an 11-mm object is placed 37 mm from the vertex of the mirror surface. Where does the image form, what is the linear magnification, and what is the image size?

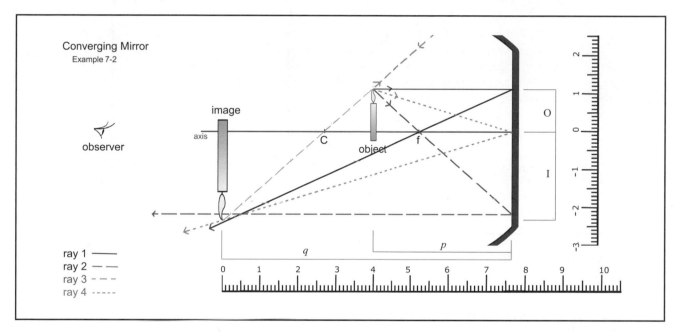

f is one half the distance of the center of curvature, so f = 50/2 = 25 mm. p = 37 mm, and O = 23 mm.

$$\frac{1}{q} = \frac{1}{f} - \frac{1}{p}$$

$$= \frac{1}{25} - \frac{1}{37} = 0.04 - 0.0270 = 0.0130$$

Since $1/q$ = 0.0130, q = 1/0.0130 = **77 mm.**

Using the magnification formula,

$$M = -\frac{q}{p} = -\frac{77}{37} = -2.1$$

Therefore **I** = (M)(O) = (11)(–2.1) = **–11 mm.**

We may now state several facts from these numbers.

---

[1] |M| means the absolute value of M, or the value of M if you ignore the sign. Therefore saying that |M| is less than 1 means that M is between –1 and +1.

1. *q* is positive, so the image is to the left of the mirror.
2. M is negative, so the image is inverted from the orientation of the object.
3. I is negative, so the image is forming inverted, below the axis.
4. |M| is greater than 1, so the image is larger than the object. It is ***magnified.***

Notice that in both Example 7-1 and Example 7-2 it was necessary to draw only rays 3 and 4. These two rays do not depend on the rule that f is one half of the radius of curvature, so they do not result in spherical aberration. We will not be so lucky when we do drawings with lenses. Draw rays 1 and 2 on the diagrams so you can see that they give image positions similar to, but not exactly the same as, the positions given by rays 3 and 4.

Now we will try a convex, diverging mirror.

EXAMPLE:

7-3. This mirror has a negative focal length. The rays are drawn from the object so that they *would have* gone through the center or through the focal point, *had the mirror not been there*, and then would have reflected according to the rules on p. 187.

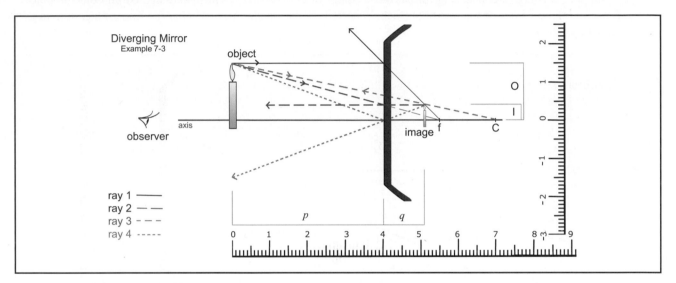

Based on this drawing, the distances are f = –15 mm, *p* = 40 mm, and O = 15 mm.

$$\frac{1}{q} = \frac{1}{f} - \frac{1}{p}$$

$$= \frac{1}{25} - \frac{1}{37} = -0.0667 - 0.02570 = -0.0917$$

Since $1/q = -0.0917$, ***q*** = 1/(–0.0917) = **–11 mm.**
Based on the magnification formula,

$$\mathbf{M} = -\frac{q}{p} = -\frac{-11}{40} = \mathbf{+0.28}$$

I = (M)(O) = (15)(0.28) = **4 mm.**

1. *q* is negative, so the image is to the right of the mirror.
2. M is positive, so the image has the same orientation to the object.
3. I is positive, so the image is forming erect, above the axis.
4. |M| is less than 1, so the image is smaller than the object. It is *minified.*

We are ready to state more rules of the road.

RULES OF IMAGE FORMATION

- If the linear magnification, M, is positive, the image has the same orientation as the object. If M is negative, the image has the opposite orientation from the object.
- If the length of the image, I, is positive, the image is above the axis. If I is negative, the image is below the axis.
- If the image distance, q, is positive, the image is to the left of the mirror. This image is *real.* It will actually form on a screen or a piece of film placed at the plane where the rays cross.
- If the image distance, q, is negative, the image is to the right of the mirror. This image is *virtual.* The rays appear to diverge from there, so it appears to be present to the observer, who is to the left of the mirror. But the rays of light do not ever actually pass through the position where the image appears to form, so it cannot be formed on a piece of film at that place.
- If the absolute value of the linear magnification, |M|,* is between 0 and 1, the image is smaller than the object, or *minified.* If |M| is greater than 1, the image is larger than the object, or *magnified.* If M is equal to 1, the image and the object are the same size. (In using this rule, use the absolute value of M; ignore the sign of M.)

*The absolute value of a number, in this case M, is expressed as |M| and means the number without the sign. Therefore, if M is from –0.99 to +0.99, |M| is less than 1 and the object is minified. For example, if M = –2.50, |M| is 2.50 and it is greater than 1, so the image is magnified. If M = –0.25, |M| = 0.25 and this is less than 1, so the image is minified.

When there is only one imaging element, such as one mirror or one lens, an erect image is always virtual. Therefore both the negative M and the negative I indicate that the image is real, and a positive M and a positive I indicate that the image is virtual. However, the object for a lens or mirror could be either real or virtual when there is more than one element, such as in a telescope or in a microscope. In a multiple-element system, a negative M simply means that the image has the opposite orientation from the object. The only time the image must be virtual is when the image distance, q, is negative.

The following exercises will be easier if you use graph paper. For some of the exercises you may find it easier to use the formulas first to see where the image should be forming; for others it may be easier to make the drawings first. Remember, the most accurate rays are those that do not use the focal point.

EXERCISES: (Round all measurements to whole millimeters.)

1. Do a series of drawings, all with a concave converging mirror having a focal length of 40 mm and an object size of 20 mm. Use the formulas to calculate q, M, and I.
   a. $p = 100$ mm
   b. $p = 80$ mm (where the center of curvature is)
   c. $p = 60$ mm
   d. $p = 40$ mm (where the focal point is)
   e. $p = 20$ mm
   What conclusions can you make from these drawings about image formation in a converging mirror?

2. Do a series of drawings, all with a convex diverging mirror having a focal length of –40 mm and an object size of 20 mm. Use the formulas to calculate q, M, and I.
   a. $p = 80$ mm
   b. $p = 40$ mm
   c. $p = 20$ mm
   What conclusions can you make from these drawings about image formation in a diverging mirror?

3. The focal length of a plano mirror is infinity. As f becomes very large, 1/f approaches 0. Use the image placement and linear magnification formulas to demonstrate the truth of the placement of the image in the flat mirror at the beginning of this section.

4. Where does the image form, and what is its orientation, if an object is between the center of curvature and the focal point of a concave mirror? Is the image real or virtual, and is the image larger or smaller than the object?

THINK ABOUT IT:

1. Most dispensaries have a magnifying mirror. Demonstrate the answers you got in problem 1, by analyzing the image of yourself in the mirror when you are at various distances from the mirror. What is the approximate focal length of your mirror? What is the length of the radius of curvature of your mirror?
2. What kind of mirror is the left-side rear view mirror mounted on most cars? Notice that the images are smaller, but also closer than the objects, yet we interpret the images to be farther away than the actual objects are. Why?

——————— IMAGE SIZE AND PLACEMENT: THIN LENSES ———————

We are going to do the same things with lenses that we did with mirrors. Lenses have a few differences from mirrors, and we will make a few assumptions:

1. Assume that the lens in infinitely thin. We will discuss what happens with thick lenses next.
2. Assume that all light waves have the same refractive index in a material, so that all colors have the same focal point for a given lens. (The fact that this assumption is not true results in chromatic aberrations, as was discussed briefly in Section II.)
3. Assume that the lens has the same material on both sides. We normally think of the lenses as being in air. They could just as well be in water, as long as the water is on both sides of the lens. We will look at what happens when materials are different on each side of the lens on pp. 202-203.
4. For mirrors, the ray through the center of curvature, which reflected back on itself, has no corresponding ray when lenses are used. So we have only three principal rays, and only one of them does not depend on the assumption that the rays are paraxial, or parallel to and "close" to the axis.
5. A positive image distance q, resulting in a real image, is on the right of the lens. A negative image distance q, resulting in a virtual image, is on the left of the lens.
6. For a mirror, any line passing through the center of curvature could be an axis. For lenses, the *axis* is the line that passes *through the centers of curvature of both surfaces*.
7. For now, the point where the axis passes through the lens will be called the ***optical center***. The optical center takes the place of the vertex for the mirrors.
8. For a plus lens the ***primary focal point*** is the point on the axis where all the rays diverging from a small source will emerge from the lens traveling parallel to the axis. For a minus lens the ***primary focal point*** is the point on the axis *toward which* rays are converging before they reach the lens; when they emerge from the lens, however, they are traveling parallel to the axis.

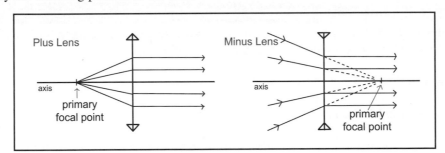

9. For a plus lens, the ***secondary focal point*** is the point on the axis where all incident rays traveling parallel to the axis cross after emerging from the lens. (For mirrors the primary and secondary focal points coincide.) For a minus lens the ***secondary focal point*** is the point on the axis from which all incident rays traveling parallel to the axis appear to be diverging after emerging from the lens.

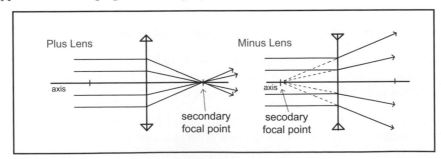

A straight line with a base-down prism at the top and a base-up prism at the bottom will represent a plus lens. (In other words, the prism bases are diagrammed toward the center of the lens.) A straight line with a base-up prism at the top and a base-down prism at the bottom will represent a minus lens. (In other words, the prism apices are diagrammed toward the center of the lens.)

The rules for ray tracing are as follows.

THIN LENS PRINCIPAL RAYS

- The ray that travels through the optical center is not deviated.
- The ray that travels through (or toward) the primary focal point emerges parallel to the axis.
- The ray that travels parallel to the axis emerges traveling toward (or from) the secondary focal point.

The formulas remain exactly the same as the mirror imaging formulas.

EXAMPLES:

7-4. A lens with focal length of +30 mm (what is its dioptric value?) has a 10-mm-tall object that is 50 mm away. What type of image is produced, how tall is it, and where is it located?

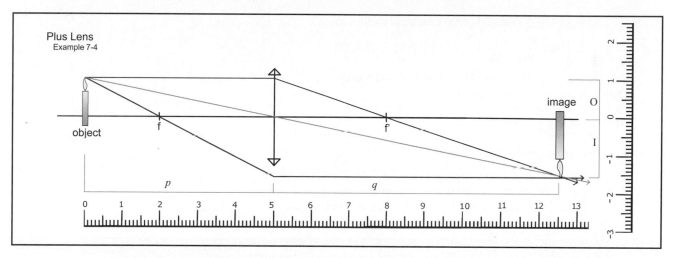

$$\frac{1}{q} = \frac{1}{f} - \frac{1}{p} = \frac{1}{30} - \frac{1}{50} = 0.0333 - 0.02 = 0.0133$$

Since $1/q = 0.01333$, $q = 1/0.01333 = $ **75 mm.**
Using the magnification formula,

$$\mathbf{M} = -\frac{q}{p} = -\frac{75}{50} = \mathbf{-1.5}$$

$$\mathbf{I} = (M)(O) = (10)(-1.5) = \mathbf{-15\ mm.}$$

1. q is positive, so the image is to the right of the lens. It is real.
2. M is negative, so the image forms with the opposite orientation to the object.
3. I is negative, so the image formed is inverted, below the axis.
4. |M| is greater than 1, so the image is larger than the object. It is magnified.
   (Dioptric power is D = 1/f = 1/0.030 = +33.33D.)

Example 7-5 involves a diverging lens. Remember, when we are drawing the rays, they are the rays that *would have gone through a particular point* had the lens not been there. The emerging rays are diverging from one another, so we draw back to see where they *would have originated* in order to be traveling in their observed direction. The point where the rays appear to begin diverging is where the image *appears* to form. Since the rays do not actually come from this point, however, the image is virtual.

7-5. A 10-mm object is 50 mm from a lens with a power of –33.33D. What is the image distance and size?

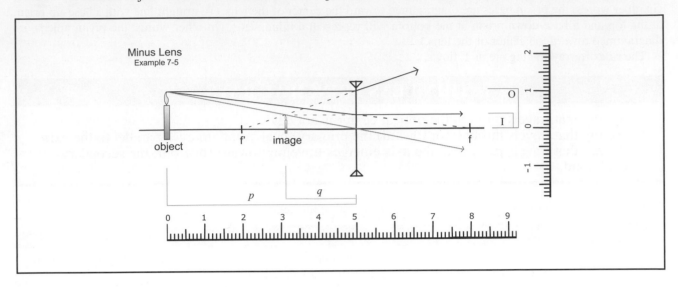

f – 1/D = 1/(–33.33) = –0.030003 meters = –30 mm.

$$\frac{1}{q} = \frac{1}{f} - \frac{1}{q} = \frac{1}{-30} - \frac{1}{50} = 0.0333 - 0.02 = -0.0533$$

Since 1/q = –0.05333, **q = 1/(–0.05333) = –19 mm.**
Using the magnification formula,

$$\mathbf{M} = -\frac{q}{p} = -\frac{-19}{50} = \mathbf{+0.38}$$

I = (M)(O) = (10)(0.38) = **4 mm**

1. q is negative, so the image is to the left of the lens. It is virtual.
2. M is positive, so the image has the same orientation to the object.
3. I is positive, so the image is forming erect, above the axis.
4. |M| is less than 1, so the image is smaller than the object. It is minified.

EXERCISES: (Round all measurements to whole millimeters.)

5. Do a series of drawings, all with a convex converging thin lens with a power of +25.00D and an object size of 20 mm. Use the formulas to calculate q, M, and I.
   a. p = 100 mm.
   b. p = 40 mm (where the primary focal point is).
   c. p = 20 mm.
   From these drawings, what can you conclude about image formation in a converging lens?

6. Do a series of drawings, all with a concave diverging lens having a power of –25.00D and an object size of 20 mm. Use the formulas to calculate q, M, and I.
   a. p = 80 mm.
   b. p = 60 mm.
   c. p = 20 mm.
   From these drawings, what can you conclude about image formation in a diverging lens?

Try it: Demonstrate the answers you got in Exercises 5 and 6. Use a spherical lens with 3 diopters or more of plus power, and another with 3 diopters or more of minus power. Hold each lens out at a normal reading distance, and notice the size and orientation of the images of objects at various distances on the other side of the lens. What is the approximate focal length of the converging lens? If you hold the converging lens close to your eye, why are all of the images formed magnified and erect?

When drawing the principal rays for image formation, we assumed that the thickness of the lens was not important. In Section III we discovered that the front and back vertex powers of a thick lens are not equal. The front vertex power is derived from the distance between the front vertex, where the optical axis enters the front surface of the lens, and the primary focal point. The back vertex power is derived from the distance between the back vertex and the secondary focal point. (See the discussion of back and front vertex power on pp. 84-86.)

We are going to deal only with single lenses having two spherical surfaces and having a particular thickness. The lenses are spherical, so each surface has a center of curvature. In an earlier section we defined the radius to be *positive* for convex surfaces and *negative* for concave surfaces, which is the way most of us think of lenses in real life. Most physics and optical theory books define positive and negative radii based on whether the center of curvature is to the left (negative) or right (positive) of the lens surface. Using this definition a lens with two positive power surfaces has a front surface radius that is positive and a back surface radius that is negative. A meniscus lens has two surfaces with positive radii. We also defined the surface power formula as $D = (n - 1)/r$. It is now $D = (n_r - n_i)/r$. When a ray enters the front surface of a lens from air, this formula reduces to $D_1 = (n - 1)/r_1$. When the ray leaves the lens traveling back into air, the formula reduces to $D_2 = (1 - n)/r_2$.

The *axis of the lens* is the imaginary ray traveling through both the centers of curvature. The *front surface* will be the surface on the left in our drawings; for meniscus lenses the plus power surface will be the front surface. The *front vertex*, V_1, will be where the axis touches the front surface and enters the lens. The *back vertex*, V_2, will be where the axis touches the back surface and exits the lens. Aside from the radius of curvature, *for lenses positive distances* are distances where the travel is measured from left to right. All vertical measurements made above the axis are *positive distances*. All thicknesses and radii of curvature are measured in *meters*. We will assume that all the rays we trace are *paraxial;* that is, they are close to the axis. The assumption that all rays are paraxial allows us to ignore the effects of spherical lens aberrations.

As we go through the concepts and formulas below, keep in mind that some formulas can be written in several forms, so you may have seen them written differently in physics books or optical theory books. In this book the formulas are in forms consistent with the way we use the concepts in our more basic formulas. We will use D for dioptric power and f for focal length because these initials are what opticians use every day.

PRINCIPAL PLANE LOCATION IN THICK LENSES

When we diagrammed thin lenses, we constructed a single principal plane and called it the plane where all the refraction occurred. Because we were assuming that the lens had only one focal length, using only one plane was acceptable. Since thick lenses have two focal lengths based on the lens vertices, as shown by the thick lens formulas, we will diagram the thick lens with two principal planes: P_1 and P_2. We find the location of the *first principal plane* by determining where the ray that enters the lens from the primary focal point would bend *just one time* to exit parallel to the axis. We find the location of the *second principal plane* by determining where the ray that enters the lens parallel to the axis would bend *just one time* to exit toward the secondary focal point.

The front focal length is the distance from f_1 to V_1. The back focal length is the distance from V_2 to f_2. They are equal only if the front and back surfaces have equal curvature. The formulas for the front and back vertex powers (see Section III) are:

$$D_B = \frac{D_1}{1 - \left(\dfrac{t}{n_L}\right)D_1} + D_2 \qquad D_F = \frac{D_2}{1 - \left(\dfrac{t}{n_L}\right)D_2} + D_1$$

where:

    t   = distance between the front and back vertices in meters

    n_L = index of refraction of the lens material

The two focal lengths (see Section III) are:

    $f_1 = n_s/D_F \ (= 1/D_F$ in air) $\qquad f_2 = n_s/D_B = (1/D_B$ in air)

where n_s is the index of the material surrounding the lens.

Note: Physics textbooks use F rather than D in these formulas. The value being quantified is actually the ***vergence*** and not the dioptric value represented by the focal length f. We will continue to use D rather than F for the vergence to keep the notation consistent with the rest of this book.

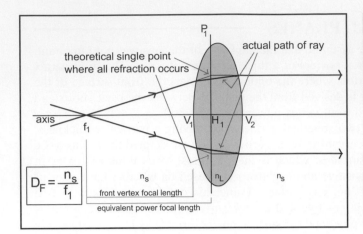

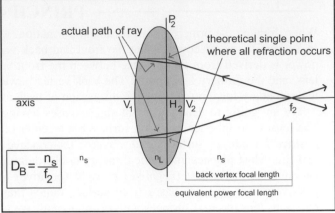

Next we need the *equivalent power formula.* The equivalent power has two uses. When several lenses are lined up in series, the equivalent power is the power needed for a single lens to provide the same power as the series of lenses. This definition is the more general concept. For a lens system with a single thick lens, the equivalent power formula provides the position of the principal planes *with respect to the first and second focal points.* The equivalent power formula for a single thick lens is:

$$D_{eq} = D_1 + D_2 - \frac{t}{n}D_1D_2$$

and $f = n_s/D_{eq}$ (= $1/D_{eq}$ when the lens is in air).

Using the above definition of f, we can now locate the principal planes with respect to the lens vertices. H_1 and H_2 are the *principal points,* the points where the principal planes cross the axis. f is the distance from f_1 to H_1, as well as the distance from H_2 to f_2. (See the next drawing.)

When we do ray tracings on thin lenses, we assume that the two principal planes coincide and that the point where that plane crosses the axis is the optical center. For a thin lens the principal points, H_1 and H_2, coincide. For a thick lens the concept of optical center is not meaningful.

Let's analyze the principal plane positions for a few lenses before we eliminate the surfaces and use the principal planes to predict where images will form.

EXAMPLES:

7-6. A thick lens in air made of a material with index of refraction of 1.50 has a front surface power of +15.00D, a back surface power of +5.00D, and a thickness of 32 mm.

D_1 = **+15.00D**
D_2 = **+5.00D**
n = **1.50**
t = 32 mm = **0.032 m**
r_1 = (n − 1)/D_1 = 0.5/15 = **+0.0333 m**
r_2 = (1 − n)/D_2 = −0.5/5 = **−0.1 m** (See Section III for the change in the formula for r.)

$$D_B = \frac{D_1}{1 - \left(\frac{t}{n}\right)D_1} + D_2 = \frac{+15}{1 - \left(\frac{0.032}{1.5}\right)(15)} + 5 = \frac{15}{0.68} + 5 = 22.06 + 5$$

D_B = **+27.06D**
f_2 = 1/D_B = 1/27.06 = 0.037 m = **37 mm**

$$D_F = \frac{D_2}{1 - \left(\frac{t}{n}\right)D_2} + D_1 = \frac{+5}{1 - \left(\frac{0.032}{1.5}\right)(5)} + 15 = \frac{5}{0.893} + 15$$

D_F = 5.60 + 15 = **+20.60D**
f_1 = 1/D_F = 1/20.60 = 0.049 m = **49 mm**
D_{eq} = D_1 + D_2 − (t/n)D_1D_2 = +15 +5 − (0.032/1.5)(15)(5)

$\mathbf{D_{eq}} = 20 - 1.6 = \mathbf{+18.40D}$
$\mathbf{f_{eq}} = 1/D_{eq} = 1/18.40 = 0.054 \text{ m} = \mathbf{54 \text{ mm}}$

Notice on the following drawing that the principal planes have shifted toward the surface with the steeper curve.

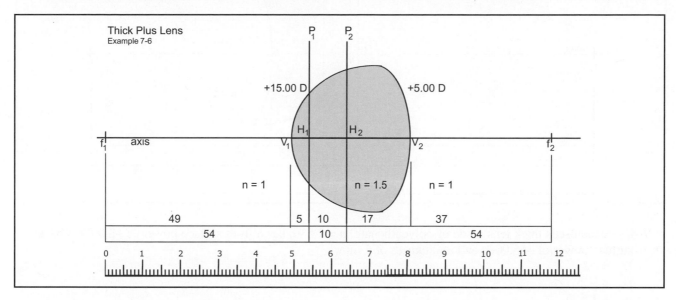

7-7. A meniscus thick lens made of flint glass, n = 1.70, has a front surface power of +20.00D, a back surface power of –5.00D, and a thickness of 19 mm.

$\mathbf{D_1} = \mathbf{+20}$
$\mathbf{D_2} = \mathbf{-5}$
$\mathbf{n} = \mathbf{1.70}$
$\mathbf{t} = 19 \text{ mm} = \mathbf{0.019 \text{ m}}$
$\mathbf{r_1} = (n - 1)/D_1 = 0.7/20 = \mathbf{+0.035 \text{ m}}$
$\mathbf{r_2} = (1 - n)/D_2 = -0.7/(-5) = \mathbf{+0.14 \text{ m}}$

$$D_B = \frac{D_1}{1 - \left(\dfrac{t}{n}\right)D_1} + D_2 = \frac{+20}{1 - \left(\dfrac{0.019}{1.7}\right)(20)} - 5 = \frac{20}{0.776} - 5$$

$\mathbf{D_B} = 25.76 - 5 = \mathbf{+20.76D}$
$\mathbf{f_2} = 1/D_B = 1/20.76 = 0.048 \text{ m} = \mathbf{48 \text{ mm}}$

$$D_F = \frac{D_2}{1 - \left(\dfrac{t}{n}\right)D_2} + D_1 = \frac{-5}{1 - \left(\dfrac{0.019}{1.7}\right)(-5)} + 20 = \frac{-5}{1.056} + 20$$

$\mathbf{D_F} = -4.74 + 20 = \mathbf{+15.26D}$
$\mathbf{f_1} = 1/D_F = 1/15.26 = 0.066 \text{ m} = \mathbf{66 \text{ mm}}$
$\mathbf{D_{eq}} = D_1 + D_2 - (t/n)D_1D_2 = +20 - 5 - (0.019/1.7)(20)(-5)$
$\mathbf{D_{eq}} = 15 + 1.12 = \mathbf{+16.12D}$
$\mathbf{f_{eq}} = 1/D_{eq} = 1/16.12 = 0.062 \text{ m} = \mathbf{62 \text{ mm}}$
Now the principal planes have shifted even farther toward the steeper curve.

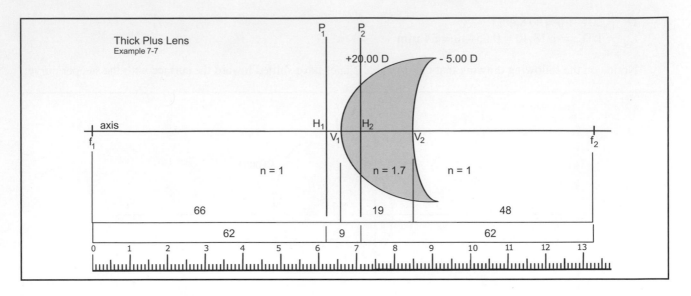

Thick Plus Lens
Example 7-7

+20.00 D   -5.00 D

axis

n = 1   n = 1.7   n = 1

66   19   48

62   9   62

7-8. A meniscus thick lens made of polycarbonate, n = 1.586, has a front surface power of +2.00D, a back surface power of −25.00D, and a thickness of 5 mm.

D_1 = +2

D_2 = −25

n = **1.586**

t = 5 mm = **0.005 m**

r_1 = $(n − 1)/D_1$ = 0.586/2 = **+0.293 m**

r_2 = $(1 − n)/D_2$ = −0.586/(−25) = **+0.023 m**

$$D_B = \frac{D_1}{1 - \left(\dfrac{t}{n}\right)D_1} + D_2 = \frac{+2}{1 - \left(\dfrac{0.005}{1.586}\right)(2)} - 25 = \frac{2}{0.994} - 25$$

D_B = 2.01 − 25 = **−22.99D**

f_2 = $1/D_B$ = 1/22.99 = −0.044 m = **−44 mm**

$$D_F = \frac{D_2}{1 - \left(\dfrac{t}{n}\right)D_2} + D_1 = \frac{-25}{1 - \left(\dfrac{0.005}{1.586}\right)(-25)} + 2 = \frac{-25}{1.079} + 2$$

D_F = −23.17 + 2 = **−21.17D**

f_1 = $1/D_F$ = 1/21.17 = 0.047 m = **−47 mm**

D_{eq} = $D_1 + D_2 − (t/n)D_1 D_2$ = +2 −25 − (0.005/1.586)(2)/(−25)

D_{eq} = −23 + 0.16 = **−22.84D**

f_{eq} = $1/D_{eq}$ = 1/22.84 = −0.044 m = **−44 mm**

The steeper side is to the back of the lens, so the principal planes moved toward the back. On some thick minus lenses, P_1 and P_2 change sides.

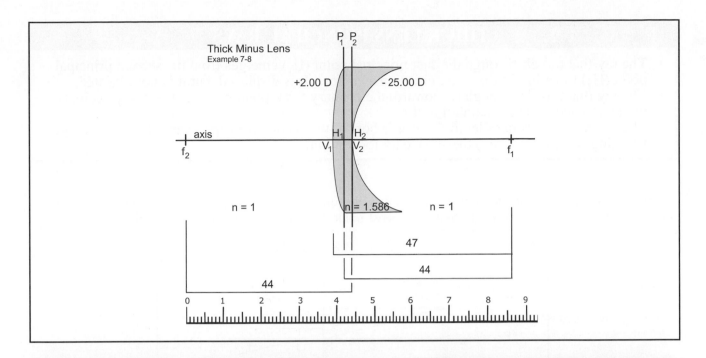

Thick Minus Lens
Example 7-8

+2.00 D   − 25.00 D

axis

P_1 P_2

f_2 H_1 H_2 f_1
          V_1 V_2

n = 1   n = 1.586   n = 1

47

44

44

0 1 2 3 4 5 6 7 8 9

EXERCISES: (Round all measurements to millimeters.)

7. Locate the principal planes for a bi-convex lens made of index 1.50 plastic, if the front surface has a surface power of +35D, the back has a surface power of +1D, and the thickness at the vertices is 35 mm.

8. Locate the principal planes for a meniscus lens made of index 1.50 plastic, if the front surface has a radius of curvature of +20 mm, the back surface has a radius of curvature of +50 mm, and the vertices are 50 mm apart.

──── IMAGE SIZE AND PLACEMENT: THICK LENSES ────

Now that we can find the position of the principal planes for any lens, we can determine where the image forms for any thick lens. The rules for ray tracing differ from those for the thin lens in only one way. All rays are drawn parallel to the axis as they travel from P_1 to P_2. Otherwise, the rules are the same.

Keep in mind as we go through the drawings that we are not showing the actual path of the ray as it traverses the lens. We are showing the exact path of the ray *before it enters* the lens and *after it exits* the lens. What happens between the vertices and the principal planes is *constructed* so that we can explain mathematically the result of the refractions that occur at the two surfaces.

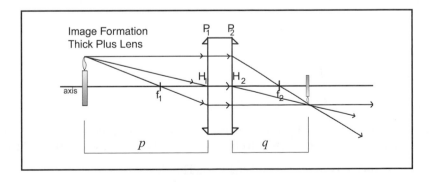

Image Formation
Thick Plus Lens

P_1 P_2

H_1 H_2

axis

f_1 f_2

p   q

- The ray that travels through the first principal point (H_1) emerges from the second principal point (H_2) traveling in the same direction as before. It is displaced, but it is not deviated.
- The ray that travels through (or toward) the primary focal point bends at the first principal plane (P_1) and emerges parallel to the axis.
- The ray that travels parallel to the axis is bent at the second principal plane (P_2) and emerges traveling toward (or from) the secondary focal point.

The diagram below is a thick minus lens, with P_1 to the left of P_2. For the occasional thick minus lens where P_1 is on the right of P_2, the rays go to P_1 first and emerge in the correct direction from P_2 even though it is on the left side of P_1.

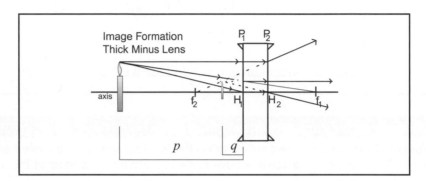

This leads us to the image formation formulas. They remain exactly the same as for the thin lens and the mirror. The object distance p is measured from the object to P_1, and the image distance q is measured from P_2 to the image. The focal length f is derived from the equivalent power D_{eq}. Look at the definition of D_{eq} again. It is the power needed to give the observed results using only a single thin lens. The equivalent power and the principal planes are fabricated. We create imaginary planes so that we can use formulas and ray tracings to predict the size and position of the image formed.

EXAMPLES:

7-9. Example 7-6 is a lens with $D_1 = +15D$, $D_2 = +5D$, and $f_{eq} = 54$ mm. If an object is placed 75 mm to the left of the front vertex, where does the image form and what is the magnification?

For this lens, f_1 is 49 mm to the left of the front vertex, and f is 54 mm. Therefore P_1 is 5 mm to the right of the front vertex, and the object distance p, which is measured to P_1, is 75 + 5 = 80 mm.

Based on the image formation formula,

$$\frac{1}{q} = \frac{1}{f} - \frac{1}{p} = \frac{1}{54} - \frac{1}{80} = 0.0185 - 0.0125 = 0.0060185\ldots$$

Since $1/q = 0.0060185$, $q = 1/0.0060185 =$ **166 mm.**

Based on the magnification formula,

$$\mathbf{M} = -\frac{q}{p} = -\frac{166}{80} = -2.0769\ldots = \mathbf{-2.1}$$

q is 166, which is the distance from P_2 to the image. f_2 is 37 mm and f is 54 mm, so P_2 is 17 mm to the left of the back vertex. Therefore the image will form 166 – 17 = **149 mm to the right of the back vertex V_2.**

1. q is positive, so the image is to the right of the lens. The image is real.
2. M is negative, so the image has the opposite orientation from the object.
3. I (not calculated) would be negative for a real, or positive, object, so the image is forming inverted, below the axis.
4. |M| is larger than 1, so the image is magnified.

Optical Formulas Tutorial

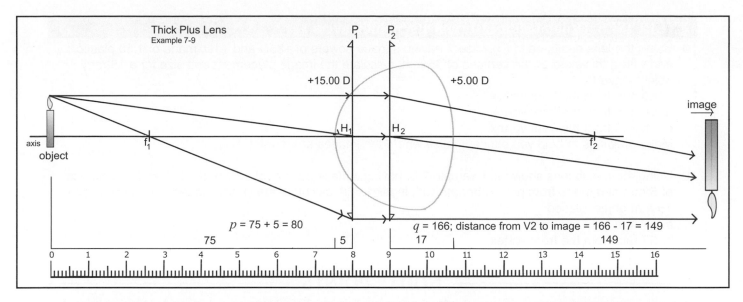

Thick Plus Lens
Example 7-9

+15.00 D   +5.00 D

image

axis

object

$p = 75 + 5 = 80$

$q = 166$; distance from V2 to image = 166 - 17 = 149

75   5   17   149

A good way to deal with each of these exercises is to get some graph paper and draw the whole system to scale. Trace the rays, and verify for yourself that the formulas give the correct answer. Remember, the rays will give you only the approximate location and size, since the drawings violate the paraxial rule for spherical lenses. The rays that are not close to the axis show spherical aberration.

7-10.   Look at the negative lens in Example 7-8. For this lens $f_{eq} = -44$ mm. Where will the image be located if an object is placed 50 mm from the front surface? What is the magnification for this image?

f_1 is –47 mm and f is –44 mm, so P_1 is 3 mm to the right of the front vertex. The object distance, p, is 50 + 3 = 53 mm from P_1.

$$\frac{1}{q} = \frac{1}{f} - \frac{1}{p} = \frac{1}{-44} - \frac{1}{53} = -0.023 - 0.019 = -0.042$$

Since $1/q = -0.042$, $q = 1/(-0.042) = \mathbf{-24\ mm}$, or the image forms 24 mm to the left of P_2, which is coincident with the back vertex V_2. Based on the magnification formula,

$$\mathbf{M} = -\frac{q}{p} = -\frac{-24}{53} = \mathbf{+0.5}$$

1. q is negative, so the image is to the left of the lens. The image is virtual.
2. M is positive, so the image is in the same orientation to the object.
3. I will be positive for a real, or positive, object, so the image will form above the axis.
4. |M| is less than 1, so the image is smaller than the object, or minified.

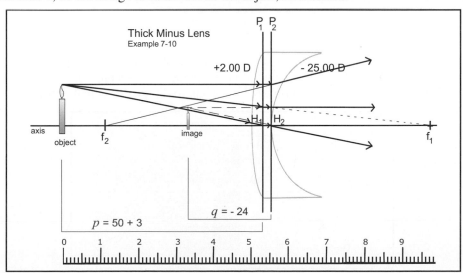

Thick Minus Lens
Example 7-10

+2.00 D   - 25.00 D

axis

object f_2 image f_1

$q = -24$

$p = 50 + 3$

9. Using the lens designed in Exercise 7 having surface powers of +35D and +1D, made of 1.50 plastic, and with a thickness at the vertices of 35 mm, calculate the image placement and size for a 15-mm object placed:
   a. 60 mm from the front vertex.
   b. 28 mm from the front vertex.
   c. 15 mm from the front vertex.
   Make drawings to help you conceptualize where the images are forming.

10. Using the minus lens shown in Example 7-8, having surface powers of +2D and −25D and a thickness of 5 mm and made from polycarbonate with index 1.586, calculate the image placement and size for a 15-mm object placed:
    a. 57 mm from the front vertex.
    b. 27 mm from the front vertex.
    Make drawings to help you conceptualize where the images are forming.

NODAL POINTS

We have one assumption left to explore. In all of our ray tracings the lenses have been surrounded by air. Immersing the lens in water or some other medium with index of refraction n_i would affect only the calculations of focal length from surface powers and of surface power from radius of curvature. Go back to Section III to review the way to adjust these calculations.

What if the lens is separating two different materials? A prescription diver's mask would have air on one side and water on the other side. The eye has air on one side and aqueous and vitreous on the other. Many lenses in optical instruments are composed of two or more different materials sandwiched together. Look at the path of a light ray when it enters the eye. There are several different refractions, separating a variety of media. Consider a lens made of a material with index of refraction of n_2, separating two other media with indices of n_1 (on the left) and n_3 (on the right). For our examples the index of refraction of the lens, n_2, is higher than either n_1 or n_3.

In the last several pages we have discussed the principal planes and briefly mentioned H_1 and H_2, where the principal planes cross the axis. H_1 and H_2 are called the ***principal points***. When $n_1 = n_3$, the principal points are the points where the incident light ray exits the lens displaced but not deviated.

When n_1 and n_3 are not equal, the points where the incident light ray exits displaced but not deviated are the ***nodal points*** N_1 and N_2. The nodal points coincide with the principal points when $n_1 = n_3$. For a plus thick lens the nodal points move away from H_1 and H_2 toward the side of the lens where the denser material is; if $n_3 > n_1$, the nodal points move to the right on the diagram. For a minus thick lens the nodal points move away from H_1 and H_2 toward the side of the lens where the rarer material is; if $n_3 > n_1$, the nodal points move to the left on the diagram. The two nodal points move equal amounts: the distance from H_1 to N_1 is equal to the distance from H_2 to N_2. The distance HN that the nodal points move from the principal points is equal to

$$HN = H_2f_2 - f_1H_1$$

where:

HN $\;=$ offset of the nodal point from the corresponding principal point
$H_2f_2 \;=$ distance from the second principal point to the second focal point
$f_1H_1 \;=$ distance from the primary focal point to the first principal point

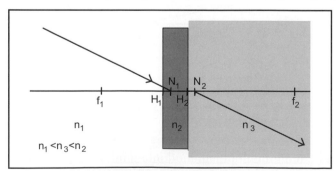

When the materials on each side of the lens have unequal indices, the focal points will no longer be the same distance from the principal points. The formula for the surface powers now becomes

$$D_S = (n_2 - n_1)/\text{radius of curvature}$$

The *cardinal points* for a lens are the focal points, the nodal points, and the principal points.

EXAMPLE:

7-11. A bi-convex lens made of a material with n = 1.5 separates air, n = 1, from water, n = 1.33, and has a center thickness of 18 mm. The radius of curvature of the surface in contact with air is 25 mm. The radius of curvature of the surface in contact with water is –25 mm. An 11-mm object is placed 50 mm from the front lens surface on the side where the air is. Find the positions of all six cardinal points and the image size, orientation, and location. Verify all results with a drawing.

n_1 = **1.0**

n_2 = **1.5**

n_3 = **1.33**

r_1 = 25 mm

    = **0.025 m**

D_1 = $(n_2 - n_1)/r_1$

    = 0.5/0.025

    = **+20D**

r_2 = –25 mm

    = **–0.025 m**

D_2 = $(n_3 - n_2)/r_2$

    = –0.17/–0.025

    = **+6.80D**

t = 18 mm

    = **0.018 m**

$$D_B = \frac{D_1}{1 - \left(\dfrac{t}{n_2}\right)D_1} + D_2 = \frac{20}{1 - \left(\dfrac{0.018}{1.5}\right)(20)} + 6.80 = \frac{20}{0.76} + 6.80$$

D_B = 26.32 + 6.80 = **+33.12D**

V_2f_2 = n_3/D_B = 1.33/33.12 = 0.040 m = **40 mm**

$$D_F = \frac{D_2}{1 - \left(\dfrac{t}{n_2}\right)D_2} + D_1 = \frac{6.8}{1 - \left(\dfrac{0.018}{1.5}\right)(6.8)} + 20 = \frac{6.8}{0.9184} + 20$$

D_F = 7.40 + 20 = **+27.40D**

f_1V_1 = n_1/D_F = 1/27.40 = 0.036 m = **36 mm**

D_{eq} = $D_1 + D_2 - (t/n_2)D_1D_2$ = 20 + 6.80 – (0.018/1.5)(20)(6.80)

D_{eq} = 26.80 – 1.63 = **25.17D**

f_1H_1 = n_1/D_{eq} = 1/25.173 = 0.0397 m = **40 mm**

H_2f_2 = n_3/D_{eq} = 1.33/25.173 = 0.053 m = **53 mm**

$H_1N_1 = H_2N_2 = H_2f_2 - f_1H_1$ = 53 – 40 = **13 mm**

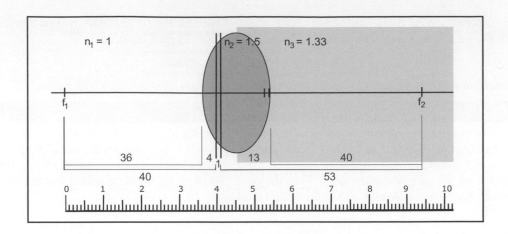

Our image size and placement formulas will change slightly: p and q are to be measured *from the nodal points,* and the formula relating p and q becomes

$$\frac{f_1 H_1}{q} = 1 - \frac{H_2 f_2}{p}$$

Look at the drawing to see that
p = image distance to V_1 + distance from V_1 to H_1 + distance from H_1 to N_1
  = 50 + 4 + 13 = **67 mm**
$f_1 H_1$ = 40
$H_2 f_2$ = 53

$$\frac{f_1 H_1}{q} = 1 - \frac{H_2 f_2}{p};$$

$$\frac{40}{q} = 1 - \frac{53}{67} = 1 - 0.79 = 0.21;$$

$q = 40/0.21 =$ **190 mm**
$\mathbf{M} = -q/p = -190/67 =$ **–2.8**
$\mathbf{I} = (M)(O) = (-2.8)(11) =$ **–31 m**
q is measured to N_2. Again look at the drawing to see that the distance between V_2 and image is
190 + 13 – 13 = 190 mm; the **image is located 190 mm inside the water, is real and inverted, and is 31 mm long**.

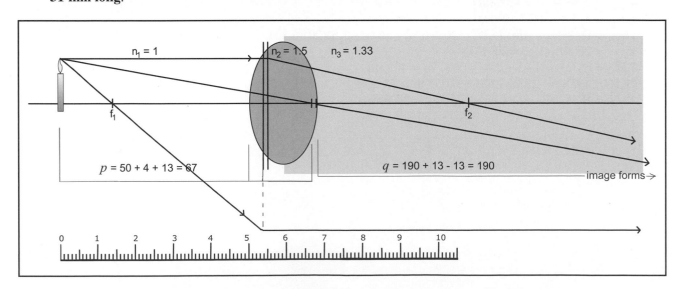

11. A thick lens made of flint glass, $n_2 = 1.70$, separates air, $n_1 = 1$, from plastic, $n_3 = 1.50$. The lens has a maximum thickness of 20 mm, the surface facing air has a radius of curvature of 17.5 mm, and the surface facing plastic is plano. A 20-mm object is placed 50 mm from the front vertex of the lens. Where does the image form and what is its size?

DIAGRAM OF THE HUMAN EYE

Below is a schematic diagram of the human eye. Made up of several different refracting surfaces and indices, the eye can be considered a complex system of lenses with $n_1 = 1$, $n_2 = 1.37$, $n_3 = 1.33$, $n_4 = 1.42$, and $n_5 = 1.33$. Or, the eye can be considered as one optical lens consisting of the cornea and crystalline lens. In either case it is possible to construct one set of principal planes and nodal points that can be used to mathematically model what happens to the rays of light that enter the eye.

The measurements in the drawing below are based on Helmholtz's schematic eye. This diagram is for the emmetropic eye with no accommodation. The drawing is not to scale. It was redrawn from Pedrotti FL, Pedrotti LS: *Introduction to Optics,* ed 2, Englewood Cliffs, NJ, 1992, Prentice-Hall.

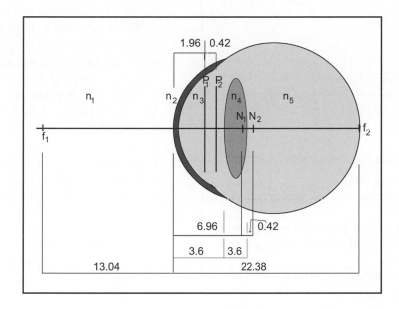

The questions with an asterisk (*) in front of the question number are advanced questions. They are not likely to be on the ABO exam but might be on the ABOM exam or the COT exam.

The questions are not presented in the order of the subjects in the section. Some of these questions may require you to think about what you have read in the section, and some may depend on material covered in previous sections.

1. In the standard drawing of a thin plus lens the primary focal point is
   a. on the same side as the center of curvature.
   b. on the right side of the lens.
   c. at the point where the axis meets the lens.
   d. on the left side of the lens.

2. You are looking at yourself in a plane (flat) reflecting surface that is 2.0 feet away. Your image in the mirror is
   a. 7.6 feet from you.
   b. 4.0 feet from you.
   c. 3.5 feet from you.
   d. 2.0 feet from you.

3. The angle of reflection is measured
   a. between the surface and the normal to the surface.
   b. between the reflecting ray and the surface.
   c. between the reflecting ray and the normal to the surface.
   d. between the incident ray and the reflecting ray.

4. A plane (flat) reflecting surface
   a. does not change the vergence of the rays reflecting from it.
   b. adds positive vergence to the rays reflecting from it.
   c. adds negative vergence to the rays reflecting from it.
   d. demonstrates total internal reflection.

5. The law of reflection states that
   a. the angle of reflection is greater than the angle of incidence.
   b. the angle of reflection is determined by Snell's Law.
   c. the angle of reflection is equal to the angle of incidence.
   d. the angle of reflection is determined by the normal to the surface.

6. A concave reflecting surface
   a. does not change the vergence of the rays reflecting from it.
   b. adds positive vergence to the rays reflecting from it.
   c. adds negative vergence to the rays reflecting from it.
   d. always creates virtual images.

7. If an object is 6 inches in front of a plane (flat) reflecting surface, the image will form
   a. 6 inches from the object.
   b. 18 inches from the object.
   c. 12 inches behind the reflecting surface.
   d. 6 inches behind the reflecting surface.

*8. An object is placed 25 cm to the left of a thin lens that has a power of +5.00D. The image will be
   a. real, inverted, and magnified.
   b. real, erect, and magnified.
   c. virtual, inverted, and magnified.
   d. virtual, inverted, and magnified.

*9. In the standard ray tracing diagram the focal point of a concave reflecting surface is
   a. on the tangent to the surface.
   b. to the left of the surface.
   c. to the right of the surface.
   d. at the vertex of the surface.

*10. A lens has a power of −15.00D. The primary focal point in a standard ray tracing drawing will be
   a. 67 cm to the left of the lens.
   b. 67 cm to the right of the lens.
   c. 67 mm to the right of the lens.
   d. 67 mm to the left of the lens.

*11. In ray tracing formulas we define a positive direction as the direction that the ray of light travels.
   a. True
   b. False

*12. For a curved mirror ray tracing, the ray that travels through the center of curvature
   a. reflects through the focal point, or reflects as if it came from the focal point.
   b. reflects parallel to the axis.
   c. reflects back on itself.
   d. reflects the same distance below the axis as the incident ray is above the axis.

*13. If an object is placed 12 cm from a convex mirror that has a focal length of 15 cm, the image will form
   a. 60 cm to the left of the mirror.
   b. 60 cm to the right of the mirror.
   c. 6.7 cm to the left of the mirror.
   d. 6.7 cm to the right of the mirror.

*14. A ray of light that travels through the focal point of a concave mirror
    a. reflects through the focal point, or reflects as if it came from the focal point.
    b. reflects back on itself.
    c. reflects the same distance below the axis as the incident ray is above the axis.
    d. reflects parallel to the axis.

*15. In the standard ray tracing diagram the focal point of a convex reflecting surface is
    a. on the tangent to the surface.
    b. to the left of the surface.
    c. to the right of the surface.
    d. at the vertex of the surface.

*16. A concave mirror has a focal length of 10 cm. If the object is placed 20 cm to the left of the surface of the mirror, the image forms
    a. 6.7 cm to the right of the mirror.
    b. 6.7 cm to the left of the mirror.
    c. 20 cm to the right of the mirror.
    d. 20 cm to the left of the mirror.

*17. A curved mirror has a focal length of +25 cm. An object placed 6 cm to the left to the mirror will form an image that is
    a. virtual, to the right of the mirror, and magnified.
    b. virtual, to the left of the mirror, and minified.
    c. real, to the right of the mirror, and magnified.
    d. real, to the left of the mirror, and minified.

*18. A ray traveling parallel to the axis of a curved mirror
    a. reflects through the focal point, or reflects as if it came from the focal point.
    b. reflects parallel to the axis.
    c. reflects the same distance below the axis as the incident ray is above the axis.
    d. reflects back on itself.

*19. In using the formula for image size and placement for a particular curved mirror, you determine that the magnification, M, is −1.5. This means that
    a. the image is inverted and larger than the object.
    b. the image is above the axis and smaller than the object.
    c. the image is below the axis and smaller than the object.
    d. the image is above the axis and larger than the object.

*20. In the standard ray tracing a positive image size for a curved mirror means that
    a. the image forms to the right of the mirror.
    b. the image forms to the left of the mirror.
    c. the image forms below the axis.
    d. the image forms above the axis.

*21. An object placed between the center of curvature and the focal point of a converging mirror will form an image that is
    a. real, to the left of the mirror, and minified.
    b. real, to the left of the mirror, and magnified.
    c. virtual, to the right of the mirror, and minified.
    d. virtual, to the left of the mirror, and minified.

*22. A convex reflecting surface
    a. does not change the vergence of the rays reflecting from it.
    b. adds positive vergence to the rays reflecting from it.
    c. adds negative vergence to the rays reflecting from it.
    d. usually creates real images.

*23. In tracing rays to construct the image location for a curved mirror, the ray that is incident at the vertex of the mirror
    a. reflects through the focal point, or reflects as if it came from the focal point.
    b. reflects parallel to the axis.
    c. reflects the same distance below the axis as the incident ray is above the axis.
    d. reflects back on itself.

*24. In a standard ray tracing drawing a curved mirror has the center of curvature 8 cm to the right of the mirror. The power of the mirror is
    a. +8.00D.   c. −12.50D.
    b. +12.50D.   d. −25.00D.

*25. On a crown glass lens with a front surface power of +12.25, a back surface power of −2.25, and a thickness of 15 mm, the principal planes will be
    a. at about the center of the lens.
    b. closer to the −2.25 surface than to the +12.25 surface.
    c. closer to the +12.25 surface than to the −2.25 surface.
    d. at the front and back vertex points.

*26. An object is placed 25 cm to the left of a thin lens that has a power of +5.00D. The image will form
    a. 100 cm to the left of the lens.
    b. 100 cm to the right of the lens.
    c. 4.2 cm to the right of the lens.
    d. 4.2 cm to the left of the lens.

*27. A lens made from Trivex has a front surface radius of curvature of 15 cm and a back surface radius of curvature of 35 cm. The lens is 5.5 mm thick at the center point. What is the front vertex power of the lens?
    a. +5.06D
    b. +2.00D
    c. +2.03D
    d. +2.51D

*28. The ray that travels through the primary focal point for a thin converging lens
a. emerges parallel to the axis.
b. travels through the lens undeviated.
c. emerges from the lens traveling toward the secondary focal point.
d. will demonstrate total internal reflection.

*29. A lens has a focal length of 55 cm in air. When immersed in water the lens will have a focal length of
a. 36 cm.
b. 41 cm.
c. 55 cm.
d. 73 cm

*30. An object is placed 15 cm to the left of a thin –2.50 lens. The image will form
a. 3 cm to the left of the lens.
b. 11 cm to the left to the lens.
c. 24 cm to the right of the lens.
d. 24 cm to the left to the lens.

*31. On a ray tracing the image distance is 23 cm and the object distance is 42 cm. The image will be
a. magnified and will form to the right of the lens.
b. minified and will form to the right of the lens.
c. magnified and will form to the left of the lens.
d. minified and will form to the left of the lens.

*32. On a ray tracing the image distance is 23 cm and the object distance is 42 cm. The image will be
a. virtual and erect.
b. virtual and inverted.
c. real and erect.
d. real and inverted.

*33. A lens made from Trivex has a front surface radius of curvature of 15 cm and a back surface radius of curvature of 35 cm. The lens is 5.5 mm thick at the center point. What is the equivalent power of the lens?
a. +2.51D
b. +2.04D
c. +2.01D
d. +1.95D

*34. In the standard ray tracing a positive image distance for a curved mirror means that
a. the image forms to the right of the mirror.
b. the image forms above the axis.
c. the image forms below the axis.
d. the image forms to the left of the mirror.

*35. In the standard drawing of a thin minus lens the secondary focal point is
a. on the right side of the lens.
b. on the left side of the lens.
c. on the same side as the center of curvature.
d. at the point where the axis meets the lens.

*36. A lens made from Trivex has a front surface radius of curvature of 15 cm and a back surface radius of curvature of 35 cm. The lens is 5.5 mm thick at the center point. What is the back vertex power of the lens?
a. +2.01
b. +2.07D
c. +2.51
d. +2.95

*37. The focal point for a curved reflecting surface is
a. one-third the distance from the vertex to the center of curvature.
b. to the left of the center of curvature.
c. at the center of curvature.
d. one-half the distance from the vertex to the center of curvature.

*38. A curved mirror has a power of +5.00D.
a. The mirror is concave and has a focal length of 40 cm.
b. The mirror is concave and has a focal length of 20 cm.
c. The mirror is convex and has a focal length of 40 cm.
d. The mirror is convex and has a focal length of 20 cm.

*39. A plano-convex lens of +5.00 OU is mounted on a scuba mask with the plano surface cemented to the mask. If the lens were diagrammed to show where the image of a fish swimming in front of the scuba diver would form, the nodal points would be
a. displaced toward the water side of the mask.
b. displaced toward the air side of the mask.
c. at the vertex points of the lens.
d. at the eye and the outside surface of the mask.

*40. The rearview mirror on the passenger side of many cars has a warning printed on it: objects are closer than they appear in the mirror. This mirror makes the images of the other cars look smaller, and it has a larger field of view than the mirror on the driver's side.
a. This is a convex converging mirror.
b. This is a convex diverging mirror.
c. This is a concave converging mirror.
d. This is a concave diverging mirror.

Appendix 1
BASIC GLOSSARY

A MEASUREMENT   The distance from lens edge to lens edge, measured horizontally.

ABBÉ NUMBER   A measurement of the ability of a material to disperse white light into its component colors; also called nu value, or v. It is also the inverse of relative dispersion, δ.

ABERRATIONS   Properties of the lens material or lens design that result in distorted or blurred images.

ABSORPTION   The conversion of one form of energy into a different form of energy. Generally, light is absorbed as heat, although it may result in a chemical or electrical reaction.

AMBLYOPIA   A condition in which the eye does not have good correctable vision but has no physical anomaly.

AMETROPIA   A condition in which the eye has a refractive error.

ANGLE OF INCIDENCE   The angle between a ray of light incident on a surface and the normal (or perpendicular line) to the surface at the point of incidence.

ANGLE OF REFRACTION   The angle between a ray of light after refraction into a material and the normal (or perpendicular line) to the surface.

ANGLE OF REFLECTION   The angle between a ray of light after reflection from a surface and the normal (or perpendicular line) to the surface.

ANGULAR MAGNIFICATION   The ratio of the angle subtended by the image to the angle subtended by the object when projected on the retina.

ANISOMETROPIA   An unequal refractive condition between a person's two eyes. The person is considered ANISOMETROPIC.

APPARENT DEPTH   The distance an imbedded object appears to be from the surface of the material, when viewed from another material. The approximation given is closest to accurate when the line from the observer (in one material) to the object (in another material) is perpendicular to the surface of the second material. As an example, the distance that a fish in an aquarium appears to be from the side of the aquarium is the distance that the image of the fish is from the side of the aquarium if the person observing the fish is at the same level as the fish.

ASTHENOPIA   A general feeling of discomfort in or around the eyes, or a general discomfort as a result of conditions in or around the eyes.

ASTIGMATIC INTERVAL   The distance between the two focal lengths of a toric or astigmatic lens or system.

ASTIGMATISM   Literally, "not a point focus." Usually refers to two line foci for a single lens.
Regular astigmatism: The focal lines are at right angles to each other.
Irregular astigmatism: The focal lines are not at right angles to each other. Irregular astigmatism is usually the result of injury or disease.
With the rule astigmatism: The shorter of the two focal lengths is vertical, and the correcting lens has the axis of the minus cylinder within 30° of the 0-180 meridian. When the vertical meridian of the cornea or crystalline lens is steeper than the horizontal meridian, with the rule astigmatism is the result.
Against the rule astigmatism: The shorter of the two focal lengths is horizontal, and the correcting lens has the axis of the minus cylinder within 30° of the 090 meridian. When the horizontal meridian of the cornea or crystalline lens is steeper than the vertical meridian, against the rule astigmatism is the result.
Oblique astigmatism: The two focal lines are between the 31° and 59° meridian, and between the 121° and 149° meridian.

AXIS   (of a lens). The ray that passes through the centers of curvature of both surfaces.

The *axis of a curved mirror* is any ray that travels through the center of curvature of the mirror. A curved mirror has an infinite number of potential axes.

The *axis of a cylinder* is the meridian of plano power or no power.

The *axis of a prescription* is the meridian on the lens where there is no cylinder power; it is the direction of the sphere power alone.

B MEASUREMENT   The distance from lens edge to lens edge, measured vertically.

BACK FOCAL LENGTH   The distance from the back surface vertex of a lens to the secondary focal point.

BACK VERTEX POWER   The inverse of the back focal length in meters; it is a measurement of the ability of the lens to converge or diverge light rays. This is the power that the wearer sees and is what is measured in the focimeter or lensmeter.

BASE CURVE   The curve on a lens that is used to calculate the other curves on the lens. Three different curves on a lens could be called the base curve:
- The curve on the lens that is molded, or the curve on the first surface that is ground and polished. For sphero-cylindrical lenses ground in minus cylinder form, this is usually the spherical front surface curve.
- The curve on the surface of the lens that contains the multifocal segment.
- The flattest curve on the toric surface of a spherocylindrical lens. Also called the toric base curve.

BOXING SYSTEM   A system for standardizing lens and frame measurements. All measurements are in millimeters. The first step in this system is to draw a box around the lens(es) and determine the geometric center of the lens.

BRIDGE   The glasses frame part that connects the right and left lenses.

CARDINAL POINTS   The primary and secondary focal points, the principal points (where the principal planes intersect with the optical axis), and the nodal points. On a single thin lens the principal points and the nodal points coincide at the optical center of the lens.

CHROMATIC ABERRATION   Occurs because light waves of different frequencies are slowed to different extents by a material. Only in a vacuum do all frequencies of the electromagnetic spectrum travel at the same speed. This property of lens materials causes images of different colors to form on different planes, resulting in slight blurring of images containing more than one frequency of light.

CIRCLE OF LEAST CONFUSION   The plane where an astigmatic or toric lens shows the least distortion. Its distance from the lens is the inverse of the spherical equivalent of the toric lens.

COMA   A lens aberration that occurs when wide beams of light travel obliquely through a lens. It results in an elongated, blurred image. In the eye the iris generally limits the aberration.

CONCAVE   1. A hollow surface. 2. A lens surface with negative power. 3. A lens with negative power. 4. A diverging refracting element. 5. A converging reflecting surface.

CONSTRUCTIVE INTERFERENCE   Occurs when two waves are in phase with each other and therefore compound each other.

CONVERGENCE   A measurement of the relative direction of travel of two light rays that are traveling toward each other. The amount of convergence of two rays at a particular plane indicates the distance the rays would have to travel from that plane in order to cross paths. Also called POSITIVE VERGENCE.

CONVEX   1. A bulging surface. 2. A lens surface with positive power. 3. A lens with positive power. 4. A converging refracting element. 5. A diverging reflecting surface.

CORRECTED CURVE   In lens design the base curve is chosen to minimize the peripheral aberrations that occur in common eyeglass lens.

CROSS CURVE   The steepest curve on a toric surface.

CURVATURE OF FIELD, also called CURVATURE OF IMAGE   A lens aberration that occurs because the focal plane of a lens is curved, not flat. Most corrected curve lens designs strive to reduce or eliminate this aberration.

CYLINDER   A surface or lens with no curvature or power in the meridian called the axis and with either positive or negative curvature or power in the meridian 90° from the axis.

D MEASUREMENT   The horizontal measurement of a lens at its midpoint. It is part of the DATUM SYSTEM of frame and lens measurement.

DATUM LINE   The same as D MEASUREMENT.

DBL   The distance between lenses.

DESTRUCTIVE INTERFERENCE   Occurs when two waves are out of phase with each other and therefore cancel each other.

DEVIATION   A change of direction.

DIFFRACTION   The bending of a wave of light when it passes through a very narrow slit or past the edge of an opaque object.

DIFFUSION   The scattering of light rays by an irregular surface or a non-homogeneous material.

DIOPTER   A measurement of vergence, or a measurement of the ability of a lens, prism, or mirror to change the direction of travel of incident light rays.

DIPLOPIA   Double vision.

DISPERSION   The breaking of light into its component colors. A material's ability to disperse light is related to the different speeds of various wavelengths of visible light in the material. For some materials, such as crown glass, dispersion is minimal. Other materials, such as flint glass, have a larger dispersive ability. See ABBÉ NUMBER.

DISPLACED   Moved or shifted to another position. For a ray of light, displaced means that it emerges in a different position from where it entered, although it may continue to travel in the original direction.

DISTORTION   A lens aberration resulting from the increasing amounts of prism present as gaze is directed away from the optical center of a lens. This aberration is the only one of the major aberrations that does not result in a blurring of the image.
>   *Barrel distortion* is seen in minus power lenses. Base-out prism amount increases as the line of gaze travels away from the center of the lens, causing straight lines to appear to be concave toward the center of the lens.
>   *Pincushion distortion* is seen in plus power lenses. Base-in prism amount increases as the line of gaze travels away from the center of the lens, causing straight lines to appear to be convex toward the center of the lens.

DIVERGENCE   A measurement of the relative direction of travel of two light rays that are traveling away from each other. The amount of divergence of two rays at a given plane indicates the distance the rays have traveled from their source, or since they crossed paths. Also called NEGATIVE VERGENCE.

EFFECTIVE DIAMETER (ED)   Twice the longest radius of a lens, measured from the geometric center of the lens to the farthest point on the lens edge.

EMMETROPIA   A condition of the eye in which parallel incident rays of light come to a point focus on the retina when the eye is not accommodating. Does not require corrective lenses for distance vision.

EQUIVALENT POWER   (of a thick lens). The power of a single infinitely thin lens needed to provide the same convergence or divergence supplied by the thick lens. This concept is used to find the locations of the principal planes.

EYEWIRE   The glasses frame part that holds a lens.

FOCAL POINT   See PRIMARY FOCAL POINT or SECONDARY FOCAL POINT.

FOCIMETER   An instrument used to measure the back focal length of a lens. This is the generic term, replacing lensmeter. LENSOMETER and VERTOMETER are trade names.

FREQUENCY   The number of occurrences in a unit of time. For light, it is the number of waves of light that pass a particular point in one second. Measured in hertz (Hz).

FRONT FOCAL LENGTH   The distance from the front surface vertex to the primary focal point.

FRONT VERTEX POWER   The inverse of the front focal length in meters. Used to measure Add power for multifocal lenses, and used in contact lens design.

GEOMETRIC CENTER   (of a lens). The midpoint of the horizontal and vertical measurements of the lens. This point is determined by means of the boxing system.

ILLUMINATION   The intensity of visible light incident on the surface of an object.

INCIDENCE   See ANGLE OF INCIDENCE.

INCIDENT SIDE   The side from which the light is traveling; used in discussion of the change in direction or speed of a wave of light or a photon as it travels from one material to another.

INDEX OF REFRACTION   Usually represented by n or μ; the ratio of the speed of light in a vacuum to the speed of yellow light (588 nm) in a material.

INTERFERENCE   Occurs when two waves with the same frequency either cancel or compound each other. See CONSTRUCTIVE INTERFERENCE and DESTRUCTIVE INTERFERENCE.

INTERVAL OF STURM   (for a *toric lens* or for an *astigmatic eye*). The distance between the two focal planes.

KERATOMETER   An instrument used to measure the curvature of the front surface of the cornea of the eye.

LENSMETER   An instrument used to determine glasses lens power. See FOCIMETER.

LENSOMETER   The American Optical trade name for a focimeter, the instrument used to determine lens power.

LONGITUDINAL WAVE MOTION   Occurs when the individual particles in the supporting material travel parallel to the direction of the propagation of the wave.

LUMINOSITY   The ability of an object to emit photons or waves of light.

MAGNIFICATION   The relationship between the image and the object.
   Linear magnification: the ratio of the size of the image to the size of the object. This is used in designing optical instruments but is not a useful ratio for spectacles. An image that is larger than the object but also appears to be at a distance behind the object may not appear to be bigger when viewed by the eye.
   Angular magnification: the ratio of the size of the image that is projected on the retina when one is looking at the object through a magnifying lens or a spectacle lens to the size of the object projected on the retina if the magnifying or spectacle lens is not present.

MAGNIFICATION, SPECTACLE   The change in image size on the retina for a corrected ametropic eye over the size of the image for an emmetropic eye. The spectacle magnification is the result of the combination of base curve, thickness, vertex distance, and material of the spectacle lens. In the form in which spectacle magnification is usually expressed, 1 means no magnification change from that seen by the emmetropic eye at the same eye-to-object distance, greater than 1 means that the image is magnified on the retina, and between 0 and 1 means that the image is smaller than that seen by the emmetropic eye.

MARGINAL ASTIGMATISM   Also called OBLIQUE ASTIGMATISM or RADIAL ASTIGMATISM. A lens aberration that occurs because waves with a horizontal orientation have a different focal length from waves with a vertical orientation when they enter a spherical lens obliquely (not perpendicular to the surface of the lens). This aberration causes the lens to induce unwanted cylinder power when the wearer looks through the lens at an angle. See the section on Martin's formula for tilt, p. 161. Corrected curve design lenses attempt to reduce or eliminate this aberration.

MERIDIAN   Any straight line on the surface of the lens, going through the optical center of the lens.

n   See INDEX OF REFRACTION.

NEGATIVE VERGENCE   See DIVERGENCE.

OBLIQUE ASTIGMATISM   See MARGINAL ASTIGMATISM.

OD   The right eye. OD is an abbreviation for the Latin words *oculus dexter.*

OPACITY   A measurement of the ability of a material to absorb or reflect visible light.

OPTICAL CENTER (OC)   In a thin lens, the point on the optical axis where any ray of light incident on the lens passes through the lens undeviated (but possibly displaced). It may be in the lens or on a surface of the lens, or it may be outside of the lens altogether. In common usage on the thin lens the OC is the thickest part of a plus lens or the thinnest part of a minus lens. Or, the lens OC is the point on a lens surface where there is no prism power.

OPTICAL INFINITY   20 feet or more, or 6 meters or more. Rays or waves of light that *originate* 20 feet or 6 meters or more from the observer are considered to be traveling parallel to each other when they reach the observer.

OS   The left eye. OS is an abbreviation for the Latin words *oculus sinister.*

OU   Both eyes. OU is an abbreviation for the Latin words *oculus uterque.*

PARALLEL RAYS   Rays of light that will never meet when extended in either direction. In optics, rays of light that are coming from an object 6 or more meters away are considered to be traveling parallel. For the purpose of defining parallel rays, optical infinity is defined as 6 meters.

PARAXIAL RAYS   Rays that are traveling close to the axis of a lens or mirror.

PATTERN DIFFERENCE   The difference between the A measurement and the B measurement on a lens. The closer a lens is to square or circular, the smaller the P measurement is.

PENCIL   A group of rays diverging from or converging on a single point of 0 dimension.

PHOTON   The basic particle of the electromagnetic spectrum. Used in quantum physics to describe some of the properties of the electromagnetic spectrum.

PLANO   A surface that is flat or has no curvature, or a lens with no refractive power.

POLARIZED LIGHT   Light in which all of the light waves are oscillating in only one plane. This is LINEAR POLARIZATION or PLANE POLARIZATION. (Linear is preferred.) PARTIAL POLARIZATION occurs when the oscillations are not completely confined to one plane.

POSITIVE VERGENCE   See CONVERGENCE.

PRIMARY FOCAL POINT   For a *converging lens or mirror,* the point on the optical axis from which diverging light rays will be refracted or reflected parallel to the axis as a result of the lens or mirror. For a *diverging lens or mirror,* the point on the optical axis toward which light rays will be converging in order for them to be refracted or reflected parallel to the axis.

PRINCIPAL PLANES   Imaginary planes that can be used to describe the refraction occurring within a lens. Their positions with respect to the front and back vertices of a lens can be determined by use of the FRONT and BACK VERTEX POWER FORMULAS and the EQUIVALENT POWER FORMULA.

PRINCIPAL POINTS   The points where the principal planes cross the axis of the lens.

PUPILLARY DISTANCE (PD)   The distance in millimeters between the visual axes of the person's eyes, generally near the center of the pupil.

RAY   The path of a single photon of light.

REAL IMAGE   An image that is formed by converging rays after refraction or reflection. This image will form on a screen or film.

REFLECTION   Occurs when a ray of light falling on a surface or an interface between two materials is turned back into the incident material.

REFRACTION   Occurs when a ray of light entering a material changes direction because of the difference in optical density between the incident and refracting materials.

RECTILINEAR PROPAGATION OF LIGHT   The law that says that light traveling through a homogeneous material travels in a straight line.

SAGITTAL DEPTH, or SAG   On a curve that has two endpoints, the least distance from the plane of the endpoints to the point of the curve farthest from this plane.

SECONDARY FOCAL POINT   The point on the optical axis toward which incident parallel paraxial rays will converge, or from which incident parallel paraxial rays appear to diverge, as a result of the lens or mirror.

SPECULAR REFLECTION   Reflection from a surface that is smooth or polished.

SPHERICAL ABERRATION   The blurring of images that results from spherical lenses and mirrors having different focal lengths for rays of light that are not paraxial, or traveling near the axis. Peripheral rays come to a focus closer to the plane of the lens or mirror than paraxial rays do. This aberration is a problem only in optical systems with a large aperture. The iris of the eye, by limiting the size of the beam of light entering the eye, largely eliminates this aberration in ophthalmic applications. This aberration is a problem in instruments with wide aperture such as telescopes.

TEMPLE   The portion of the frame that attaches to the frame front at the sides and goes back toward the ear. The temple may curve around behind the ear, or it may continue straight back.

TORIC   A lens or surface that has different powers or curvatures in different meridians.

TORIC BASE CURVE   The flatter of the two curves on a toric surface.

TRANSPARENCY   The attribute of a material that allows transmission of light to occur through the material without scattering the light.

TRANSVERSE WAVE MOTION   Occurs when the individual particles in the supporting material travel perpendicular to the direction of the propagation of the wave.

VERGENCE   A measurement of the relative direction of travel of two light rays. Vergence is the inverse of the distance the rays would have to travel in order to cross paths. See CONVERGENCE and DIVERGENCE.

VERTEX   The point where the axis of the lens or mirror intersects with the surface (either front or back) of the lens or mirror.

VERTOMETER   Bausch & Lomb trade name for a focimeter, the instrument used to determine lens power.

VIRTUAL IMAGE   An image that appears to be in a particular position but is not, because the rays that form the image *appear* to be diverging from that position. This image will not form on a screen or film.

WAVELENGTH   The distance from a point on a wave to the corresponding point on the next wave.

Appendix 2
ANSI STANDARDS Z80.1–1999
(PROPOSED 2005 REVISIONS ARE GRAYED)

— PRESCRIPTION OPHTHALMIC LENS TOLERANCE RECOMMENDATIONS —

1. Tolerance for lens power (ANSI Z80.1–2005 section 5.1.1.1and 5.1.1.2):
   a. Definition: DISTANCE REFRACTIVE POWER: Measures the power on the meridian of highest absolute power. **Example:** –6.00 –4.00 ×090: the –10.00 power on the 180 meridian is the highest meridian power.
   b. Method of measurement: Focimeter, back or ocular surface of lens toward the lens stop. Power in the meridian of highest power must meet the following tolerance, based on the strongest power on the lens. In the example above, the power on the 180 meridian must fall within ±0.20D (2% of 10.00D).
   c. Tolerance: Individual single vision and traditional multifocal lenses:

Meridian of Highest Power	Tolerance on Meridian of Highest Power
0.00 up to 6.50D	±0.13D
Above 6.50D	±2%

Tolerance: Progressive lenses:

Meridian of Highest Power	Tolerance on Meridian of Highest Power
0.00 up to 8.00D	±0.16 D
Above 8.00D	±2%

Note: If the power has been compensated for wearing vertex distance, the compensated power will be used to determine tolerances and the acceptable powers and the documentation will indicate the compensated powers.
Note: The test that was used in the 1995 standards for ensuring that the sphere power and cylinder amount erred in the same direction has been replaced by the use of the highest meridian power for the meridional power tolerance instead of using the sphere power of the written prescription.

2. Tolerance for cylinder power (ANSI Z80.1–2005 section 5.1.1.1 and 5.1.1.2):
   a. Definition: CYLINDER POWER: "The difference (plus or minus) between powers measured in the two principal meridians of a spherocylinder lens" (ANSI Z80.1–1999 section 3.19.1). A lens with only spherical power is considered to have a cylinder of 0.00D.
   b. Method of measurement: Focimeter, back surface of lens toward the lens stop. The difference between the two principal powers must meet the following tolerances, based on the amount of the cylinder power. **Example:** for –6.00 –4.00 ×090, the difference between the 090 and 180 axis powers must be within ±0.15D.
   c. Individual single vision and traditional multifocal designs:

Amount of Cylinder	Tolerance on Nominal Value of the Cylinder
0.00 up to 2.00D	±0.13D
Above 2.00D up to 4.50D	±0.15D
Above 4.50D	±4%

Progressive lenses:

Amount of Cylinder	Tolerance on Nominal Value of the Cylinder
0.00 up to 2.00D	±0.16D
Above 2.00D up to 3.50D	±0.18D
Above 3.50D	±5%

3. Tolerance for cylinder axis (ANSI Z80.1–2005 section 5.1.2):
   a. Definition: CYLINDER AXIS: "The principal meridian which contains only the spherical power component of a spherocylinder lens" (ANSI Z80.1–1999 section 3.3.1).
   b. Method of measurement: Focimeter, back surface of lens toward the lens stop. **Example:** for –6.00 –4.00 ×090, the axis must be within 2 degrees of the 90th meridian.
   c. Tolerances:

Nominal Value of the Cylinder Power	Tolerance of the Axis
Up to 0.25D	±14 degrees
Above 0.25D up to 0.50D	±7 degrees
Above 0.50D up to 0.75D	±5 degrees
Above 0.75D up to 1.50D	±3 degrees
Above 1.50D	±2 degrees

4. Tolerance for addition power for multifocal and progressive addition lenses (ANSI Z80.1–2005 section 5.1.3):
   a. Definition: ADDITION: "The difference in vertex power, normally referred to the surface containing the add, between the reading, or intermediate portion of a multifocal lens and its distance portion" (ANSI Z80.1–1999 section 3.2).
   b. Method of measurement: Focimeter, *surface of lens that contains the segment* toward the lens stop. Read either the sphere or cylinder power that gives target lines the closest to vertical for the distance, then the same lines for the near or intermediate portion. The difference between these two readings is the near addition. The distance reading should be taken as far above the DRP as the near reading is below the DRP, and outset the same amount as the near inset.

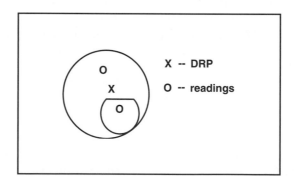

   c. Tolerances:

Nominal Value of Addition Power	Tolerance on the Addition Power
Up to 4.00D	±0.12D
Above 4.00D	±0.18D

Note: If the addition power is compensated for wearing position or multifocal style, the tolerance applies to the compensated value, and this compensated value must be documented. **Example:** If the addition for a progressive lens is ordered 0.25 strong because of the progressive design, this compensation must be documented, and the tolerance applies to the new add power.

5. Tolerance for prismatic power on a single lens (ANSI Z80.1–2005 section 5.1.4):
   a. Definitions:
   - PRISM REFERENCE POINT (PRP): "That point on a lens as specified by the manufacturer at which the prism value of the finished lens is to be measured" (ANSI Z80.1–1999 section 3.21.4).
   - FITTING POINT: "That point on a lens specified by the manufacturer which is used as a reference point for positioning the lens in front of a patient's eye" (ANSI Z80.1–1999 section 3.21.2).
   - DISTANCE REFERENCE POINT (DRP): "That point on a lens as specified by the manufacturer at which the distance sphere power, cylinder power and axis shall be measured" (ANSI Z80.1–1999 section 3.21.1).
   b. Method of measurement: For progressive addition lenses the PRP is the point specified by the manufacturer at which the prism is verified, usually the dot below the fitting cross. For all other single vision and multifocal lenses, the PRP is the DRP. This point should be centered in the focimeter and the amount of prism present noted.

   i. VERTICAL IMBALANCE: The difference between the prism reference point height for the lenses must be no more than 1 mm. If it is more than 1 mm, the induced prism resulting from different heights must be no more than $1/3^\Delta$.

   METHOD: Determine which of the two lenses has the greater absolute power on the 90th meridian. If powers are similar, determine which lens has the highest prescribed prism. Place this lens in the focimeter with the prism reference point centered and raise the lens table to the bottom of the glasses. Without changing the position of the lens table, move to the other lens and read the amount of vertical prism at that height. If there is more than $1/3^\Delta$, or, for prescribed prism, if the prism amount is more than $1/3^\Delta$ off, dot at this height, move this lens until the prism reference point is centered, and redot. If the dots are more than 1 mm apart, the glasses do not meet specifications.
   See p. 104 in the text for a diagram of this method.

   ii. HORIZONTAL IMBALANCE: The difference between the prism reference points must be within 2.5 mm of specification. If it is more than 2.5 mm from specification, there may be up to $2/3^\Delta$ of unprescribed horizontal prism.

   METHOD: Dot prism reference points. If measurement is more than 2.5 mm from the specified amount, dot $1/3^\Delta$ of prism in each eye. (If measurement is too large, decenter lenses in for dotting. If measurement is too small, decenter lenses out for dotting.) Remeasure new dots. If new measurement is what was specified, or errs in the opposite direction from the original measurement, the mounted pair is acceptable.
   See p. 104 in the text for a diagram of this method.

Vertical Power	Vertical
0.00 to 3.37D	0.33^Δ in weaker lens
Above 3.37D	1 mm difference in heights
PROGRESSIVE ADDITION LENSES	
Horizontal Power	**Horizontal**
0.00 to 3.37D	0.67^Δ total on 180 meridian
Above 3.37D	1.0 mm difference from specified PD
NON–PROGRESSIVE ADDITION LENSES	
Horizontal Power	**Horizontal**
0.00 to 2.75D	0.67^Δ total on 180 meridian
Above 2.75D	2.5 mm difference from specified PD

   c. Tolerances for mounted lenses:

Note: Prism thinning is considered to be prescribed prism. For progressive addition lenses with power greater than 3.375D, the *combined* vertical variation between the requested PRP may not exceed 1 mm.

6. Tolerance for BASE CURVE (ANSI Z80.1-2005 section 5.1.5):
   a. Definition: "The standard or reference curve in a lens or series of lenses, for example the manufacturer's marked or nominal tool surface power of the finished surface of a semi-finished spherical lens or the marked minimum tool surface power of the finished surface of a semi-finished toric lens" (ANSI Z80.1–1999 section 3.7.1).
   b. Method of measurement: For spherical surfaces, any method that is accurate to ±0.25D. Non-aspheric and progressive design lenses might require calculations based on back surface curves, lens thickness, back vertex power, index of refraction (and the wavelength used to calculate the index of refraction).
   c. Tolerances: ±0.75D.

7. Tolerance for CENTER THICKNESS (ANSI Z80.1–2005 section 6.1.3):
   a. Definition: "The thickness of a lens at the prism reference point" (ANSI Z80.1–1999 section 3.2.6). This tolerance is in effect when the thickness is specified by the prescriber or agreed to by the prescriber. This tolerance is *NOT* an acceptable deviation from the safe thickness specified by the lens manufacturer for exemption of plastic lenses from impact resistance testing.
   b. Method of measurement: The thickness should be measured normal to the convex surface at the PRP.
   c. Tolerances: ±0.3 mm

8. Tolerance for SEGMENT POSITION (ANSI Z80.1-2005 section 6.2.3 and 6.2.4):
   a. Definition of segment: "A specified area of a multifocal lens having a different refractive power from the distance portion" (ANSI Z80.1–1999 section 3.2.3).
   b. Method of measurement: Based on the boxing system of measurement.
   c. Tolerances:
      i. Vertical placement:
         • The segment top for a non-progressive addition lens, or the fitting cross of a progressive addition lens, must be within ±1 mm of specification.
         • The difference between the two segment heights in a mounted pair may not exceed 1 mm unless specified otherwise.
      ii. Horizontal placement:
         • For a mounted pair, the centers of the tops of the segments must be within ±2.5 mm of the near interpupillary distance specification. There is no 0.67^Δ exemption for the placement of the multifocal segment in low-power non-progressive addition lenses.
         • The segments will appear symmetric unless requested otherwise.
         • For progressive addition lenses, the fitting cross and the distance interpupillary distance will be used, and each individual lens will vary by no more than 1 mm from the monocular specification.
      iii. Tilt:
         • The top of traditional multifocal segments and the reference lines of progressive addition lenses will have no more than 2 degrees of tilt from the 180 meridian.

9. Requirements for claiming UV protection (ANSI Z80.1–2005 section 7.2):
   a. Definitions: UV_B is between 290 and 315 nm. UV_A is between 315 and 380 nm (ANSI Z80.1–1999 section 3.16.23).
   b. Method of measurement: Mathematical. Practical method not specified.
   c. Specifications: "Manufacturers of lenses who claim specific ultraviolet attenuating properties shall state the average percent transmittance between 290 and 315 nm (UV_B) and between 315 and 380 nm (UV_A)" (ANSI Z80.1–1999 section 7.2).

10. Warpage and waves (ANSI Z80.1–2005 section 6.2.2):
   a. Definitions: A wave would cause a straight line to appear curved when viewed through the lens. Warpage is a lens defect resulting from improper processing or mounting.
   b. Method of measurement: Looking at a grid of straight lines through the lens held at either arm's length or with the inspector's eye at 12 inches (for weak power lenses) or at the focal length of the lens will aid the inspector in noticing areas that should be checked in the focimeter. Warpage can be checked with a lens clock or sagitta gauge.
   c. Tolerances:
      • Noticeable focimeter target distortion or blur is not acceptable within 15 mm radius of the DRP in any direction.

- If the segment is more than 30 mm, there should be no distortion or blur within 15 mm of the center of the top of the segment. For segments smaller than 30 mm there may be no distortion or blur over the whole area of the segment.
- Warpage of the base curve that is the result of finished processing will not exceed 1D.
- Distortion or blur is acceptable outside the optical area of both lenticular lenses and progressive power lenses.
- These requirements are waived within 6 mm of the edge of the lens.

11. IMPACT RESISTANCE (ANSI Z80.1–2005 section 6.1.1):
   a. Definition: "All lenses must conform to the impact resistance requirements. ... Laminated, plastic and raised-ledge multifocal lenses may be certified by the manufacturer as conforming to the initial design testing or statistically significant sampling. ... All monolithic (not laminated) glass lenses shall be treated to be resistant to impact" (ANSI Z80.1–1999 section 6.1.1.1).
   b. Method of measurement: A 5/8-inch (15.9-mm) diameter steel ball weighing not less than 0.56 oz (16 grams) is dropped from no less than 50 inches (127 cm). The lens should be centered, but multifocal lenses may be decentered so that the impact of the ball will not be on the segment. Lenses should not be clamped. The lens may be covered by or placed in a polyethylene bag, no heavier than 0.076 mm or thicker than 0.003 inch. This protection should be in contact with the lens surface during the test.
   c. Exemptions: The following are exempted from the drop-ball technique of testing (ANSI Z80.1–1999 section 6.1.1.2):
      - Prism segment multifocal lenses
      - Slab-off prisms
      - Lenticular cataract lenses
      - Iseikonics
      - Depressed segment one-piece multifocal lenses
      - Biconcave, myodisc, and minus lenticular lenses
      - Custom laminates and cemented assemblies

Annex D Optical and Mechanical Tolerances Summary (Informative)						
		Measure	**Power Range**	**Tolerance**	**Section**	**Comments**
General optical tolerances, individual lenses (edged or uncut)	Distance refractive power	Highest meridian for SV and MFs	≥0.00D, ≤±6.50D >±6.50D	±0.13D ±2%	5.1.1.1	2% of meridian power
		Highest meridian for progressives	≥0.00D, ≤±8.00D >±8.00D	±0.16D ±2%	5.1.1.2	2% of meridian power
		Cylinder power for SV and MFs	≥0.00D, ≤2.00D >2.00D, ≤4.50D >4.50D	±0.13D ±0.15D ±4%	5.1.1.1	2% of cylinder power
		Cylinder power for progressives	≥0.00D, ≤2.00D >2.00D, ≤3.50D >3.50D	±0.16D ±0.18D ±5%	5.1.1.2	2% of cylinder power
		Cylinder axis	>0.00D, ≤0.25D >0.25D, ≤0.50D >0.50D, ≤0.75D >0.75D, ≤1.50D >1.50D	±14° ±7° ±5° ±3° ±2°	5.1.2	
	Add	Add power	≤+4.00D >+4.00D	±0.12D ±0.18D	5.1.3	
	△	Prism		0.33△ at PRP	5.1.4	
		PRP location		≤1.0 mm from specified PRD		
		Base curve		±0.75D	5.1.5	When specified

Continued.

Annex D   Optical and Mechanical Tolerances Summary (Informative)—Cont'd.

		Measure	Power Range	Tolerance	Section	Comments
Mounted SV and multifocal	Δ imbalance	Vertical prism	≥0.00D, ≤±3.37D >±3.37D	0.33Δ ≤1 mm difference in height of PRPs	5.2.1.1	
		Horizontal prism	≥0.00D, ≤±2.75D >±3.37D	0.67Δ PRPs ≤±2.5 mm from specified distance interpupillary distance	5.2.1.1	
	Segment	Segment tilt		±2°	6.2.4	Measured from 180°
		Vertical location		±1.0 mm	6.2.3.1	Each lens
		Vertical difference		1.0 mm		Between lenses
		Horizontal location		±2.5 mm	6.2.3.1	From specified near interpupillary distance
Mounted PAL	Δ imbalance	Vertical prism (PAL imbalance)	≥0.00D, ≤±3.37D >±3.37D	0.33Δ ≤1 mm difference in height of PRPs	5.2.1.1	Between lenses
		Horizontal prism (PAL imbalance)	≥0.00D, ≤±3.37D >±3.37D	0.67Δ PRPs ≤±2.5 mm from specified monocular interpupillary distance	5.2.1.1	
	Fitting point	Vertical location		1.0 mm	6.2.3.2	Each lens
		Vertical difference		1.0 mm		Between lenses
		Horizontal location		±1.0 mm	6.2.3.2	From specified near interpupillary distance
		Horizontal axis tilt		±2 degrees	6.2.4	Using the permanent horizontal reference markings
Misc		Center thickness		±0.3 mm	6.1.3	When specified
		Segment size		±0.5 mm	6.1.4	
		Warpage		1.00D	6.2.2	Cylinder induced on front

From ANSI Z80.1–2005 Annex D, p 41 (draft document).

Appendix 3
OPTICAL SYMBOLS AND FORMULAS

The following symbols are used in the formulas in this appendix. Any other symbols used in a formula are defined in the formula. Page references are to the beginning of the discussion of the formula.

SYMBOLS

$\angle a$ = apical angle.

d = distance in mm or m.

D = diopters.

$\angle d$ = angle of deviation.

f = focal length in meters.

$\angle i$ = angle of incidence.

I = intensity of light.

λ = wavelength of a light wave in nm.

M = magnification in decimal form.

n = refractive index.

p = object distance.

P = prism diopters.

q = image distance.

$\angle r$ = angle of refraction or angle of reflection.

r = radius of curvature in meters.

t = thickness in meters.

FORMULAS

Abbé Value, p. 36

$$v = \frac{n_{yellow} - 1}{n_{blue} - n_{red}}$$

v = *nu* value or constringence

Above

See SEGMENT DROP or BELOW.

Anti-Reflective Coatings, p. 174

$(n_{coating})^2 = n_{lens}$ This is an attribute of ideal coating material; it is not practical.

coating thickness $= \dfrac{m}{\lambda}$ λ is the wavelength of a particular wave; m = 1,3,5,7...; m = 1 is ideal.

Angular Magnification, p. 169

Nominal magnification = 1/4 D

Conventional magnification, or maximum angular magnification = 1/4 D + 1

Actual angular magnification will be between 1/4 D and 1/4 D + 1, depending on the position of the eye and the position of the object with respect to the focal length of the magnifying lens.

Apparent Depth, p. 33

$$\text{apparent depth} = (n_1)\frac{\text{actual depth}}{n_2}$$

n_1 is the index of the material of the observer.
n_2 is the index of the material containing the object.

Apparent Thickness, p. 34

$$\text{apparent thickness} = \frac{\text{actual thickness}}{n \text{ of the material}}$$

Back Vertex Power, p. 84

$$D_{back} = D_2 + \frac{D_1}{1 - \left(\frac{t}{n}\right)D_1} \quad \text{(exact formula; t is thickness in meters)}$$

$$D_{back} \approx D_1 + D_2 + \left(\frac{t}{n}\right)(D_1)^2 \quad \text{(approximation; t is thickness in meters)}$$

See also EQUIVALENT POWER, FRONT VERTEX POWER.

Base Curve or Vogel's Rule, p. 146

Plus lens: front base curve = spherical equivalent + 6.00
Minus lens: front base curve = 1/2 spherical equivalent + 6.00

Below

See SEGMENT DROP.

Brewster's Angle, p. 179

$$\tan \angle i = \frac{n_i}{n_r}$$

Cardinal Points

See EQUIVALENT POWER, FRONT and BACK VERTEX POWER, NODAL POINTS, PRINCIPAL PLANE.

Center Thickness

See THICKNESS FORMULA.

Circle of Least Confusion

See SPHERICAL EQUIVALENT.

Compensated Power, p. 81

$$D_{new} = \left(\frac{D_{Rx}}{1 - dD_{Rx}}\right) \quad \text{(where d is the change in meters in vertex distance; it is negative if lens is moved away from the eye, positive if lens is moved toward the eye)}$$

Approximate change in power: $dD^2/1000$ (for the approximation formula, d is the change in millimeters in vertex distance)
See also EFFECTIVE POWER.

Critical Angle, p. 31

$$\text{critical angle} = \sin^{-1}\left(\frac{n_r}{n_i}\right)$$

See also SNELL's LAW.

Crossed Cylinders

See THOMPSON'S FORMULA.

Decentration, p. 138

Binocular decentration: where wearer's PD is binocular and per-lens decentration is symmetric:

per lens decentration = 1/2 (DBC – PD$_{binocular}$)

Monocular decentration: where wearer's PD is monocular:

per lens decentration = 1/2 DBC – PD$_{monocular}$

Diffraction, p. 19

$$\lambda = \frac{dy}{l}$$

d = distance between slits in diffraction grating, meters

y = distance between first two areas of constructive interference

l = distance from diffraction grating to screen, meters

Deviating Angle, Prism

See PRISM.

Diopters of Prism

See PRISM.

Dispersive Power

Inverse of ABBÉ NUMBER.

Displacement

See LATERAL DISPLACEMENT.

Drop

See SEGMENT DROP.

Edge Thickness

See THICKNESS FORMULA.

Effective Power, p. 79

$$D_{effective} = \left(\frac{D_{Rx}}{1 + dD_{Rx}}\right)$$

(where d is the change in vertex distance; it is negative if lens is moved away from the eye, positive if lens is moved toward the eye)

Approximate change in power: $dD^2/1000$

See also COMPENSATED POWER.

Equivalent Power, p. 196

$$D_{eq} = D_1 + D_2 - \left(\frac{t}{n}\right)D_1 D_2 \quad \text{(t is thickness in meters)}$$

See also BACK and FRONT VERTEX POWER.

Focal Length Formula, p. 45

$$D = \frac{n_i}{f} \qquad f = \frac{n_i}{D} \qquad f = \frac{40(n_i)}{D} \quad \text{for f in inches}$$

When the lens is in air, $n_i = 1$.

Fresnel's Equation for Reflection, p. 172

$$I_r = \frac{(n - 1)^2}{(n + 1)^2}$$

I_r = amount of light reflected from one surface, in decimal form.

Front Vertex Power, p. 85

$$D_{front} = D_1 + \frac{D_2}{1 - \left(\frac{t}{n}\right)D_2} \quad \text{(exact formula; t is thickness in meters)}$$

$D_{front} \approx D_1 + D_2 + \left(\dfrac{t}{n}\right)(D_2)^2$ (approximation; t is thickness in meters)

See also EQUIVALENT POWER, OPTICAL CENTER, BACK VERTEX POWER.

Illumination, p. 23

$E = \dfrac{I}{d^2}$

E = illumination on object in lux (or foot candles)
I = light emitted or reflected from source
d = distance of object from source in meters (or feet)

Image Placement, Lens or Spherical Mirror, p. 187

$\dfrac{1}{f} = \dfrac{1}{q} + \dfrac{1}{p}$

where:

p = object distance

q = image distance

See also LINEAR MAGNIFICATION. See p. 204 for the more general form used for thick lenses.

Index of Refraction, p. 27

$n = \dfrac{\text{speed of light in vacuum}}{\text{speed of light in material}}$

Also called mu, μ.

Inset

See SEGMENT INSET.

Lambert's Equation for Lens Transmission, p. 177

$I_2 = I_1 T_q$

where:

I_2 = transmission through an absorptive glass lens

I_1 = percent of light entering the absorptive glass lens

T = transmission per 2 mm of lens material

q = (thickness of lens in mm)/2

Lateral Displacement, p. 35

displacement = thickness $\left(\dfrac{\sin\angle d}{\cos\angle r}\right)$, where thickness and displacement have the same units

Lensmaker's Equation, p. 51

$D = +/-\dfrac{n-1}{r_1} + /-\dfrac{n-1}{r_2}$ (+ for convex surfaces, – for concave surfaces)

General case, in which lens is surrounded by air.
See also SURFACE POWER FORMULA.

Linear Magnification, p. 188

$M = -\dfrac{q}{p} = \dfrac{I}{O}$ (lenses and mirror linear magnification)

where:

p = object distance

q = image distance

I = image height

O = object height

See also IMAGE PLACEMENT, SPECTACLE MAGNIFICATION.

Magnification, Angular

See ANGULAR MAGNIFICATION.

Magnification, Linear

See LINEAR MAGNIFICATION.

Magnification, Spectacle

See SPECTACLE MAGNIFICATION.

Malus' Law, p. 180

$I_2 = I_1 \cos^2 \theta$ (θ is the difference in orientation of two polarizing filters to each other)

Martin's Formula for Pantoscopic Tilt, p. 161

$$D_{sph} = D\left(1 + \frac{\sin^2\alpha}{2n}\right)$$

    where:

    D_{sph} = induced sphere

    α = degrees of tilt

    D = sphere power on the 180 meridian

$D_{cyl} = D_{sph} \tan^2\alpha$

    where D_{cyl} = induced cylinder on the 180 meridian

    To eliminate unwanted induced power and cylinder, lower OC 1 mm for every 2° pantoscopic tilt.

Minimum Blank Size, p. 144

minimum blank size = ED + total decentration + 2 (for binocular measurements)

                     = ED + 2 × (one-lens decentration) + 2 (for monocular measurements)

Used when MRP is centered in the lens blank. Does not take position of longest radius into account.

Mirrors

See IMAGE PLACEMENT and LINEAR MAGNIFICATION.

n

See INDEX OF REFRACTION.

Nodal Points, p. 202

$HN = H_2 f_2 - f_1 H_1$

HN is the distance from the principal point to the corresponding nodal point (see text).

See also PRINCIPAL PLANE, EQUIVALENT POWER, and FRONT and BACK VERTEX POWER.

Nominal Power Formula, p. 50

$D_n = D_1 + D_2$ (D_1 and D_2 are front and back surface powers)

Oblique Meridian, p. 75

$D_T = D_{sph} + D_{cyl}(\sin \alpha)^2$ (α = difference between axis of Rx and oblique meridian wanted)

Obliquely Crossed Cylinders

See THOMPSON'S FORMULA.

Pantoscopic Tilt

See MARTIN'S FORMULA.

Polarizing Filters

See MALUS' LAW and BREWSTER'S EQUATION.

Prentice's Law, p. 99

$P = \dfrac{dD}{10}$ (where d is decentration in mm)

$P = cD$ (where c is centration in cm)

Principal Plane, p. 195

$V_1H_1 = f - f_1$
$V_2H_2 = f_2 - f$

   where:
   f is derived from D_{eq}; f_1 is derived from D_F, f_2 is derived from D_B
   V_1H_1 = distance, front vertex to first principal plane
   V_2H_2 = distance, back vertex to second principal plane

Prism, pp. 94, 96

$\angle d = \angle a(n - 1)$

   where:
   $\angle d$ is angle of deviation
   $\angle a$ is apical angle

$$P = \frac{\text{displacement of image in centimenters}}{\text{distance from prism in meters}}$$

$P = 100 \tan \angle d = 100 \tan [\angle a(n - 1)]$

See also PRENTICE'S LAW, PRISM THICKNESS, RESULTANT PRISM, RESOLVING PRISM.

Prism Thickness, p. 153

$$t = \frac{dP}{100(n - 1)}$$

$$P = \frac{t(100[n - 1])}{d}$$

   where:
   t = base to apex difference, in mm
   d = lens diameter, mm.

(Note: For a 50 mm blank, if n = 1.50, there is 1 mm thickness per 1^Δ prism.)
See also PRISM.

Recomputed Power

See EFFECTIVE POWER and COMPENSATED POWER.

Reflection, Law of, p. 25

angle of incidence = angle of reflection
See also FRESNEL'S EQUATION FOR REFLECTION.

Reflection from a Lens Surface

See FRESNEL'S EQUATION FOR REFLECTION.

Refraction, Law of

See SNELL'S LAW.

Refractive Power Formula, p. 148

$$\frac{D_{(marked)}}{D_{(refractive)}} = \frac{0.530}{n - 1}$$

or

$$D_{(refractive)} = \frac{n - 1}{0.530} D_{(marked)}$$

or

$$D_{(marked)} = \frac{0.530}{n - 1} D_{(refractive)}$$

Resolving Prism, p. 125

$V = (P)(\sin a)$
$H = (P)(\cos a)$

where:
a = angle of orientation of prism)
V = vertical component of prism
H = horizontal component of prism
Ignore sign of H and V.

See also RESULTANT PRISM.

Resultant Prism, p. 122

$P^2 = V^2 + H^2$
$\tan a = \dfrac{V}{H}$

See also RESOLVING PRISM.

Sagittal Depth, or Sag, p. 149

$\text{sag} = r - \sqrt{\left(r^2 - \left[\dfrac{d}{2}\right]\right)}$ (where d is eye size, minimum blank size, or diameter of the lens, and all measurements are in the same unit)

Approximation formula:

$\text{sag} \approx \dfrac{(d/2)^2 D}{2000(n-1)}$ (where d is eye size, minimum blank size, or diameter of the lens, in millimeters)

See also THICKNESS FORMULA.

Segment Drop or Below, p. 141

drop = segment height – 1/2 B

Negative drop means the segment height is below the 1/2 B line, typical for traditional bifocal segments. Positive drop means the segment height is above the 1/2 B line; this usually occurs in progressive addition lenses and is also called ABOVE or SEGMENT RAISE.

Segment Inset, p. 142

Binocular measurements:
    Segment inset = 1/2 ($PD_{distance} - PD_{near}$)
    Total inset   = 1/2 ($DBC - PD_{near}$)
or
                     = decentration + segment inset

Monocular measurements:
    Segment inset = $PD_{distance} - PD_{near}$
    Total inset   = 1/2 $DBC - PD_{near}$
or
                     = decentration + segment inset

Snell's Law, p. 29

$n_i(\sin \angle i) = n_r(\sin \angle r)$
$\angle i = \angle r + \angle d$
See also CRITICAL ANGLE.

Spectacle Magnification, p. 164

$SM = \dfrac{1}{1 - \left(\dfrac{t}{n}\right)D_1} \times \dfrac{1}{1 - hD}$ (where h = vertex distance + 0.003, in meters)

Change in magnification, approximations (All measurements in millimeters. Gives approximate change in percent magnification, based on single changes. See text for explanations. Δ means "change in."):

$$\Delta\%SM = \frac{\Delta D_1 t}{15}$$

$$\Delta\%SM = \frac{D_1 \Delta t}{15}$$

$$\Delta\%SM = \frac{\Delta h D}{10}$$

Spherical Equivalent, p. 68

$$D_{sph.eq.} = D_{sphere} + \frac{D_{cyl}}{2}$$

Surface Power Formula, p. 48

$$D = \frac{n_r - n_i}{r}$$ (r is + if center of curvature is to the right of the surface; r is – if center of curvature is to the left of the surface.)

See also LENSMAKER'S EQUATION.

Thickness Formula, p. 153

No prism present at MRP, spherical lens:
    Plus lens: center thickness = edge thickness + sag_{lens}
    Minus lens: edge thickness = center thickness + sag_{lens}
With prism present at MRP, spherical lens:
    Plus lens: center thickness = edge thickness + sag_{lens} + 1/2 prism base thickness
    Minus lens: edge thickness = center thickness + sag_{lens} + 1/2 prism base thickness
See also SAGITTAL, PRISM THICKNESS.

Thick Lens Formula

See BACK and FRONT VERTEX POWER, EQUIVALENT POWER, NODAL POINTS, and PRINCIPAL PLANES.

Thin Lens

See IMAGE PLACEMENT and MAGNIFICATION.

Thompson's Formula for Obliquely Crossed Cylinders, p. 170

$$C^2 = C_1^2 + C_2^2 + 2C_1 C_2 \cos 2\gamma$$

$$S = S1 + S2 + \frac{C_1 + C_2 - C}{2}$$

$$\tan 2\theta = \frac{C_2 \sin 2\gamma}{C_1 + C_2 \cos 2\gamma}$$

Convert both prescriptions to plus cylinder.
Label the Rx with the lower axis $s_1 c_1 axis_1$ and the Rx with the higher axis $s_2 c_2 axis_2$.
γ is $axis_2 - axis_1$.
θ is added to $axis_1$.
See pp. 170 to 172 for more explanation.

Tilt

See MARTIN'S FORMULA.

Transmission

See LAMBERT'S EQUATION FOR TRANSMISSION.

True Power

See REFRACTIVE POWER.

Vergence, p. 22

Vergence is the inverse of distance. The distance is represented by a small letter, the vergence by a large letter. Thus D = 1/d, V = 1/v, etc.

Vogel's Rule, p. 146

Plus lens: front base curve = spherical equivalent + 6.00
Minus lens: front base curve = 1/2 spherical equivalent + 6.00

See SPHERICAL EQUIVALENT.

Wave Formula, p. 18

$v = f\lambda$

v = velocity of light in the medium, in meters/second.
f = frequency of the wave in Hz (waves/second).
λ = wavelength of the wave in the medium, in meters/wave.

Appendix 4
TRIGONOMETRIC TABLES

angle (sin)	sine (cos)	cosine (tan)	tangent	angle (sin)	sine (cos)	cosine (tan)	tangent
0	0.00000	1.00000	0.00000				
1	0.01745	0.99985	0.01746	46	0.71934	0.69466	1.03553
2	0.03490	0.99939	0.03492	47	0.73135	0.68200	1.07237
3	0.05234	0.99863	0.05241	48	0.74315	0.66913	1.11061
4	0.06976	0.99756	0.06993	49	0.75471	0.65606	1.15037
5	0.08716	0.99619	0.08749	50	0.76604	0.64279	1.19175
6	0.10453	0.99452	0.10510	51	0.77715	0.62932	1.23490
7	0.12187	0.99255	0.12278	52	0.78801	0.61566	1.27994
8	0.13917	0.99027	0.14054	53	0.79864	0.60181	1.32705
9	0.15643	0.98769	0.15838	54	0.80902	0.58778	1.37638
10	0.17365	0.98481	0.17633	55	0.81915	0.57358	1.42815
11	0.19081	0.98163	0.19438	56	0.82904	0.55919	1.48256
12	0.20791	0.97815	0.21256	57	0.83867	0.54464	1.53987
13	0.22495	0.97437	0.23087	58	0.84805	0.52992	1.60034
14	0.24192	0.97030	0.24933	59	0.85717	0.51504	1.66428
15	0.25882	0.96593	0.26795	60	0.86603	0.50000	1.73205
16	0.27564	0.96126	0.28675	61	0.87462	0.48481	1.80405
17	0.29237	0.95630	0.30573	62	0.88295	0.46947	1.88073
18	0.30902	0.95106	0.32492	63	0.89101	0.45399	1.96261
19	0.32557	0.94552	0.34433	64	0.89879	0.43837	2.05031
20	0.34202	0.93969	0.36397	65	0.90631	0.42262	2.14451
21	0.35837	0.93358	0.38386	66	0.91355	0.40674	2.24604
22	0.37461	0.92718	0.40403	67	0.92051	0.39073	2.35586
23	0.39073	0.92050	0.42448	68	0.92718	0.37461	2.47509
24	0.40674	0.91355	0.44523	69	0.93358	0.35837	2.60509
25	0.42262	0.90631	0.46631	70	0.93969	0.34202	2.747481
26	0.43837	0.89879	0.48773	71	0.94552	0.32557	2.90422
27	0.45399	0.89101	0.50953	72	0.95106	0.30902	3.07769
28	0.46947	0.88295	0.53171	73	0.95630	0.29237	3.27086
29	0.48481	0.87462	0.55431	74	0.96126	0.27564	3.48742
30	0.50000	0.86603	0.57735	75	0.96593	0.25882	3.73206
31	0.51504	0.85717	0.60086	76	0.97030	0.24192	4.01079
32	0.52992	0.84805	0.62487	77	0.97437	0.22495	4.33149
33	0.54464	0.83867	0.64941	78	0.97815	0.20791	4.70464
34	0.55919	0.82904	0.67451	79	0.98163	0.19081	5.14457
35	0.57358	0.81915	0.70021	80	0.98481	0.17365	5.67130
36	0.58779	0.80902	0.72654	81	0.98769	0.15643	6.31378
37	0.60182	0.79864	0.75355	82	0.99027	0.13917	7.11540
38	0.61566	0.78801	0.78129	83	0.99255	0.12187	8.14439
39	0.62932	0.77715	0.80978	84	0.99452	0.10453	9.51442
40	0.64279	0.76604	0.83910	85	0.99619	0.08716	11.43014
41	0.65606	0.75471	0.86929	86	0.99756	0.06976	14.30080
42	0.66913	0.74314	0.90040	87	0.99863	0.05234	19.08137
43	0.68200	0.73135	0.93252	88	0.99939	0.03490	28.63679
44	0.69466	0.71934	0.96569	89	0.99985	0.01745	57.29215
45	0.70711	0.70711	1.00000	90	1.00000	0.00000	not defined

angle (sin)	sine (cos)	cosine (tan)	tangent	angle (sin)	sine (sin)	cosine (cos)	tangent (tan)
91	0.99985	−0.01745	−57.28996	136	0.69466	−0.71934	−0.96569
92	0.99939	−0.03490	−28.63625	137	0.68200	−0.73135	−0.93252
93	0.99863	−0.05234	−19.08114	138	0.66913	−0.74314	−0.90040
94	0.99756	−0.06976	−14.30067	139	0.65606	−0.75471	−0.86929
95	0.99619	−0.08716	−11.43005	140	0.64279	−0.76604	−0.83910
96	0.99452	−0.10453	−9.51436	141	0.62932	−0.77715	−0.80978
97	0.99255	−0.12187	−8.14435	142	0.61566	−0.78801	−0.78129
98	0.99027	−0.13917	−7.11537	143	0.60182	−0.79864	−0.75355
99	0.98769	−0.15643	−6.31375	144	0.58779	−0.80902	−0.72654
100	0.98481	−0.17365	−5.67128	145	0.57358	−0.81915	−0.70021
101	0.98163	−0.19081	−5.14455	146	0.55919	−0.82904	−0.67451
102	0.97815	−0.20791	−4.70463	147	0.54464	−0.83867	−0.64941
103	0.97437	−0.22495	−4.33148	148	0.52992	−0.84805	−0.62487
104	0.97030	−0.24192	−4.01078	149	0.51504	−0.85717	−0.60086
105	0.96593	−0.25882	−3.73205	150	0.50000	−0.86603	−0.57735
106	0.96126	−0.27564	−3.48741	151	0.48481	−0.87462	−0.55431
107	0.95630	−0.29237	−3.27085	152	0.46947	−0.88295	−0.53171
108	0.95106	−0.30902	−3.07768	153	0.45399	−0.89101	−0.50953
109	0.94552	−0.32557	−2.90421	154	0.43837	−0.89879	−0.48773
110	0.93969	−0.34202	−2.74748	155	0.42262	−0.90631	−0.46631
111	0.93358	−0.35837	−2.60509	156	0.40674	−0.91355	−0.44523
112	0.92718	−0.37461	−2.47509	157	0.39073	−0.92050	−0.42447
113	0.92050	−0.39073	−2.35585	158	0.37461	−0.92718	−0.40403
114	0.91355	−0.40674	−2.24604	159	0.35837	−0.93358	−0.38386
115	0.90631	−0.42262	−2.14451	160	0.34202	−0.93969	−0.36397
116	0.89879	−0.43837	−2.05030	161	0.32557	−0.94552	−0.34433
117	0.89101	−0.45399	−1.96261	162	0.30902	−0.95106	−0.32492
118	0.88295	−0.46947	−1.88073	163	0.29237	−0.95630	−0.30573
119	0.87462	−0.48481	−1.80405	164	0.27564	−0.96126	−0.28675
120	0.86603	−0.50000	−1.73205	165	0.25882	−0.96593	−0.26795
121	0.85717	−0.51504	−1.66428	166	0.24192	−0.97030	−0.24933
122	0.84805	−0.52992	−1.60033	167	0.22495	−0.97437	−0.23087
123	0.83867	−0.54464	−1.53986	168	0.20791	−0.97815	−0.21256
124	0.82904	−0.55919	−1.48256	169	0.19081	−0.98163	−0.19438
125	0.81915	−0.57358	−1.42815	170	0.17365	−0.98481	−0.17633
126	0.80902	−0.58779	−1.37638	171	0.15643	−0.98769	−0.15838
127	0.79864	−0.60182	−1.32704	172	0.13917	−0.99027	−0.14054
128	0.78801	−0.61566	−1.27994	173	0.12187	−0.99255	−0.12278
129	0.77715	−0.62932	−1.23490	174	0.10453	−0.99452	−0.10510
130	0.76604	−0.64279	−1.19175	175	0.08716	−0.99619	−0.08749
131	0.75471	−0.65606	−1.15037	176	0.06976	−0.99756	−0.06993
132	0.74314	−0.66913	−1.11061	177	0.05234	−0.99863	−0.05241
133	0.73135	−0.68200	−1.07237	178	0.03490	−0.99939	−0.03492
134	0.71934	−0.69466	−1.03553	179	0.01745	−0.99985	−0.01746
135	0.70711	−0.70711	−1.00000	180	0.00000	−1.00000	0.00000

Optical Formulas Tutorial

Appendix 5
OBLIQUE MERIDIAN TABLE

Degrees Difference from the Axis of the Rx	Percent of Cylinder in Effect		Increment in Second Column
	%	Decimal	
0	0	0.00	1
5	1	0.01	2
10	3	0.03	4
15	7	0.07	5
20	12	0.12	6
25	18	0.18	7
30	25	0.25	8
35	33	0.33	8
40	41	0.41	9
45	50	0.50	9
50	59	0.59	8
55	67	0.67	8
60	75	0.75	7
65	82	0.82	6
70	88	0.88	5
75	93	0.93	4
80	97	0.97	2
85	99	0.99	1
90	100	1.00	

How to Use the Table

1. Determine the difference between the meridian requested and the axis of the Rx. Subtract the smaller from the larger.
2. Find the line in the first column that is closest to the difference.
3. Determine the percent of cylinder in effect for that difference.
4. Multiply the percent in decimal form times the cylinder amount of the Rx.
5. Add the sphere power of the Rx.

EXAMPLES:

A5-1. The Rx is +1.00 –2.50 ×125. What is the approximate power on the 180 meridian?
   The difference between the meridian requested and the axis of the Rx is 180 – 125 = 55.
   55 is an entry in the first column of the table.
   The percent that goes with 55 is 67%, or 0.67.
   (0.67)(–2.50) = –1.675
   –1.675 + (+1.00) = –0.675 = –0.68. **The power on the 180 meridian is –0.68**.
A5-2. For the Rx –5.25 –1.50 ×013, what is the power on the 90 meridian?
   The difference between the meridian requested and the axis of the Rx is 90 – 13 = 77.
   77 is between 75 and 80 and is closer to 75. Use the row of the table that has 75 in the first column.
   The percent that goes with 75 is 93%, or 0.93.
   (0.93)(–1.50) = –1.395
   –1.395 + (–5.25) = –6.645 = –6.65. **The power on the 90 meridian is a little more minus than –6.65.**
If desired, do the same for the 80° line: The percent that goes with 80 is 97%, giving a power of –6.71, so the approximate answer is between –6.65 and –6.71. **The answer found by using the formula is –6.67.**

How to Create the Table

You might want to create the table when taking a test in which you are not allowed a calculator, such as the ABO or some state licensing examinations. Here's how to do it:

The last column is the increment of the percent column from one line to the next.

Memorize the following number: **124567889** (*Note that this is just ascending numbers with 3 missing and 8 repeated.*)

Start by creating the first column: Starting with 0, increment the first column by 5 degrees.

Create the increment column: it is the number that you memorized in step 1, and then the number in reverse.

Create the percent column: Start with 0 for the first entry. Add the increment column to get the second entry. Example:

First entry is 0. The increment column entry is 1, so add:

0 + 1 = 1 for the second row. The third column entry is 2, so add:

1 + 2 = 3 for the third row. The third column entry is 4, so add:

3 + 4 = 7 for the fourth row. . . .

Now convert your percentages in column two to decimals by moving the decimal point two places to the left.

Appendix 6
REFERENCES

American National Standards Institute: *ANSI standards, Z80.1-1999.* (Available from: American National Standards Institute, Attn.: Customer Service, 11 W. 42nd St., New York, NY10036.)

American Optical four-book set of programmed instruction. *Basic Optical Concepts; Normal and Abnormal Vision; The Human Eye; Lenses, Prisms and Mirrors,* Southbridge, Mass, 1986, American Optical.

Brooks CW: *Essentials of Ophthalmic Lens Finishing,* ed 2, Boston, 2003, Butterworth-Heinemann.

Brooks CW: *Understanding Lens Surfacing,* Boston, 1992, Butterworth-Heinemann.

Brooks CW, Borish IM: *System for Ophthalmic Dispensing,* ed 2, Boston, 1995, Butterworth-Heinemann.

Bruneni J: Ask the labs, *EyeCare Business,* April 1998, p 40.

Coletta VP: *College Physics,* St Louis, 1995, Mosby.

Crummett WP, Western AB: *University Physics: Models and Applications,* Dubuque, Iowa, 1994, WC Brown.

Epting JB, Morgret FC Jr: *Ophthalmic Mechanics and Dispensing,* Radnor, Pa, 1964, Chilton.

Ervin F, ed: *The Masters Review,* Landover, Md, 1994, National Academy of Opticianry.

Fannin T, Grosvenor T: *Clinical Optics,* ed 2, Boston, 1996, Butterworth-Heinemann.

Farrell TK: *The Glossary of Optical Terminology,* New York, 1986, Professional Press.

FRAMES Data, Inc: *Lenses Product Guide,* XXXI (33), Winter 2004, Jobson. www.FRAMESdata.com.

Freeman MH: *Optics,* ed 10, London, 1990, Butterworths.

Jalie M: *The Principles of Ophthalmic Lenses,* London, 1980, Association of Dispensing Opticians.

Janney GD, Tunnacliffe AH: *Worked Problems in Ophthalmic Lenses,* London, 1979, Eastern.

Jenkins FA, White HE: *Fundamentals of Optics,* New York, 1957, McGraw-Hill.

Keeney AH, Hagman RE, Fratello CJ: *Dictionary of Ophthalmic Optics,* Landover, Md, 1995, National Academy of Opticianry.

Loshin DS: *The Geometrical Optics Workbook,* Boston, 1991, Butterworth-Heinemann.

Meyer-Arendt JR: *Introduction to Classical and Modern Optics,* ed 4, Englewood Cliffs, NJ, 1995, Prentice-Hall.

National Academy of Opticianry: *Career Progression Program,* Landover, Md, National Academy of Opticianry.

Pedrotti L, Pedrotti F: *Introduction to Optics,* Englewood Cliffs, NJ, 1993, Prentice-Hall.

PPG Industries, Pittsburgh, Pa. http://corporate.ppg.com/PPG/opticalprod/en/monomers/products/Properties.htm.

Rubin ML: *Optics for Clinicians,* ed 2, Gainesville, Fla., 1977, Triad.

Saude T: *Ocular Anatomy and Physiology,* Boston, 1993, Blackwell.

Stein HA, Slatt BA, and Stein RM: *Fitting Guide for Rigid and Soft Contact Lenses,* St Louis, 1990, Mosby.

Appendix 7
ANSWERS TO EXERCISES AND REVIEW QUESTIONS

Section I

Exercises

1. +2.00
2. –2.00
3. +4.50
4. +1.50
5. –6.50
6. –2.50
7. +1.50
8. +4.87
9. –14.50
10. +8.00
11. 0
12. 0
13. +1.50
14. +4.50
15. –2.50
16. –6.50
17. +13.50
18. –11.37
19. –5.50
20. +5.50
21. +1.00
22. +1.00
23. +4.50
24. –4.50
25. +9.00
26. –9.00
27. –45.00
28. –26.39
29. +45.00
30. +8.4375
31. +1.00
32. +1.00
33. +2.00
34. –2.00
35. +2.25
36. –2.25
37. –1.25
38. –0.40
39. +2.22
40. +5.40
41. +5.0189… .
42. +10
43. +5.1009… .
44. +6.2807… .
45. –5.0505… .
46. 132.57
47. 0.46
48. 1.56
49. 6
50. 4
51. 9
52. 186,282
53. 186,280
54. 186,300
55. 186,000
56. 5,000 mm
57. 200 cm
58. 500 mm
59. 0.2 cm
60. 0.00245 m
61. 45 mm
62. 0.045 m
63. 0.0805 m

(In 64 to 71, some answers depend on whether you use 39.37 or 40 for the conversion from feet to meters.)

64. 6.10 in or 6.2 in
65. 0.51 ft or 0.52 ft
66. 1.83 or 1.80 m
67. 6.10 m or 6.00 m
68. 4.7 in
69. 41 cm
70. 0.76 m or 0.75 m
71. 3.3 ft
72. 0.58779
73. 0.01745
74. 0.01746
75. 0
76. –0.80902
77. –28.63625
78. 36 degrees
79. 54 degrees
80. 20 degrees
81. –20 from calculator, 160 from tables
82. 99 degrees
83. 30 degrees. The tables also give 150 degrees.
84. 0.5000
85. 3.00×10^6 m/sec
86. 1.86×10^5 miles/sec
87. 7.45×10^{14} waves/sec
88. 3.80×10^{-7} m

89. 0.000,000,001 m
90. 540,000,000,000,000 Hz
91. 299,792,000 m
92. 49.6×10^8 or 4.96×10^9
93. 41.6×10^8 or 4.16×10^9
94. $70 \times 10^{-8} = 7.0 \times 10^{-7}$
95. 4.55×10^{14}

Section II

Exercises

1. 5.10×10^{14}
2. 3.71×10^{-7} or 371 nm
3. 4.43×10^{-7} or 443 nm
4. 3.60×10^{-7} or 360 nm; UV-A
5. 550 nm; yellow or yellow-green
6. 0.1666....
7. Y = 1/y
8. 0.2 meter, or 20 cm, or 200 mm
9. a. 63 lux
   b. 40 lux
10. a. 3,333,333 lux
    b. 1,875,000 lux
11. $\angle r = 15°$
12. $\angle i = 15°$
13. $\angle d = -18°$; ray is leaving the denser material or going from slow to fast.
14. $\angle r = 29°$
15. n = 1.58; 1.90×10^8
16. n = 1.71; 1.75×10^8
17. 122,000 mps or 1.96×10^8
18. 1.66; 112,000 miles/sec
19. 131,000 miles/sec; 2.11×10^8 m/sec
20. 61°
21. 18°
22. 28°
23. 17°
24. 1.61
25. 36°
26. a. 23°
    b. 39°
    c. 59°
    d. total internal reflection
    e. total internal reflection
27. 33°
28. 1.89 in
29. 10.6 in
30. 2.82 mm
31. 3.05 mm
32. 5.63 in
33. Abbé number = 29; n = 1.72

Review Questions

1. b
2. c
3. a
4. d
5. a
6. b
7. c
8. c
9. c
10. d
11. b
12. b
13. d
14. b
15. c
16. a
17. c
18. a
19. d
20. a
21. d
22. b
23. c
24. d
25. a
26. c
27. b
28. d
29. c
30. d
31. a
32. b
33. b
34. d
35. a
36. b
37. b
38. a
39. c
40. d
41. c
42. d
43. a
44. b
45. a
46. a
47. b
48. b
49. b
50. a
51. b
52. d

53. d
54. a
55. c
56. d
57. c
58. d
59. a
60. c

Section III

Exercises

1. +20.00D
2. +10 in (actual 9.8 in)
3. −0.2 m, −20 cm, −200 mm, −7.87 in, or −8 in
4. +2.50D
5. +10.00D
6. +5.00D (actual +4.92D)
7. +9.96D
8. −1.61D
9. 0.156 m or 15.6 cm or 156 mm
10. a. −20.92D
    b. −28.00D
    c. −19.37D and −25.93D
11. −60.88D
12. a. longer: 7.76 mm
    b. −60.57D
13. +3.25; flat; plano-convex
14. +6.00; flat; bi-convex, equi-convex
15. −4.75; flat; bi-concave
16. −4.75; bent; meniscus, true meniscus, periscopic
17. +7.25; bent; meniscus
18. +9.75; flat; bi-convex
19. +4.75
20. +7.62D
21. −5.25D
22. +5.00D
23. −6.00D
24. −5.62D
25. −1.87 (periscopic)
26. +3.50D in n = 1.60; +2.87 in CR-39

27-32. Any notation as long as the pairs are correct

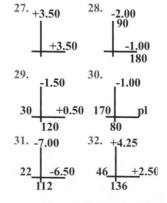

33. −0.50 −0.50 ×135
    −1.00 +0.50 ×045
34. +3.00 −4.50 ×080
    −1.50 +4.50 ×170
35. −0.50 −1.00 ×090
    −1.50 +1.00 ×180
36. +3.50 −1.00 ×110
    +2.50 +1.00 ×020
37. +2.12 −2.00 ×175
    +0.12 +2.00 ×085
38. +12.00DS
39. −0.50 × 045 ◯ −1.00 ×135
40. +3.00 × 170 ◯ −1.50 ×080
41. −0.50 × 180 ◯ −1.50 ×090
42. +3.50 × 020 ◯ +2.50 ×110
43. +0.12 × 175 ◯ +2.12 ×085
44. +12.00 DS
45. a. +1.00 −1.50 ×120
    b. +4.00 −3.00 ×045
    c. −0.87 −1.50 ×160
46. a. −1.00 +3.00 ×150
    b. −1.75 +0.75 ×050
    c. −3.37 +1.75 ×155
47. a. −1.00 × 180 ◯ +1.00 ×090
    b. +2.50 × 040 ◯ −1.12 ×130
    c. +1.00 × 006 ◯ −0.50 ×096
48. a. +2.00 −3.00 ×110
    b. +3.25 −2.25 ×170
    c. +10.50 −1.00 ×103
49. +4.00 −3.00 ×180 or +1.00 +3.00 ×090
50. −4.00 −2.00 ×180 or −6.00 +2.00 ×090
51. +1.00 −3.50 ×090 or −2.50 +3.50 ×80
52. +1.50 −0.50 ×135 or +1.00 + 0.50 ×045
54. +8.50 −1.00 ×015
55. ±3.50 +1.50 ×135 (call the prescriber)
56. −0.37 −1.50 ×008
57. correct
58. +3.75D or +3.75 DS
59. pl +0.62 ×010
60. correct
61. −3.00 ±0.75 ×015 (call the prescriber)
62. correct
63. correct
64. −7.50D or −7.50 DS
65. +0.62 −0.62 ×010
66. −3.12 +3.12 ×067
67. −1.12D or −1.12 DS
68. +0.50 −0.50 ×030
69. correct
70. −1.25D
71. −1.00D
72. +0.50D

73. –0.62D
74. +2.00D
75. +0.25D
76. +2.50D
77. –1.62D
78. –1.37D
79. –2.50D
80. MA
81. M
82. CMA
83. SHA
84. H
85. CHA
86. emmetropia
87. SMA
88. CMA
89. SMA
90. MA
91. SMA
92. CHA
93. MA
94. CHA
95. CMA
96. CHA
97. SHA
98. WR
99. O
100. WR
101. AR
102. WR
103. O
104. WR
105. WR
106. O
107. AR
108. –0.50D
109. –6.00D
110. +2.25D
111. +1.00 DC (power is –1.50D)
112. +4.71D
113. –9.48D
114. OD –5.26D
     OS –6.95D
115. OD +5.15 +2.16 ×090
     OS +6.22 +2.74 ×145
116. OD –4.75D
     OS –6.00 (rounded; –6.12 not available)
117. OD +4.87 +1.87 ×090
     OS +5.75 +2.25 ×145
118. +10.31 either method; rounds to +10.25 or
     +10.37
119. a. –6.38 –1.91 ×090
        –8.05 –0.24 ×090

b. –6.62 –2.12 ×090
   –8.50 –0.25 ×090
c. –6.00 –1.75 ×090
   –7.75 DS (if available)
d. –6.75 –2.25 ×090
   –8.75 –0.25 ×090
120. nominal pl
     back +0.06D
     front +0.06D
121. nominal +5.00D
     back +5.41D
     front +5.10D
122. nominal +10.00D
     back +10.95D
     front +10.03D

Review Questions

1. b
2. c
3. b
4. a
5. d
6. d
7. d
8. d
9. b
10. c
11. d
12. c
13. c
14. c
15. b
16. b
17. a
18. d
19. a
20. c
21. c
22. b
23. b
24. d
25. c
26. a
27. c
28. a
29. a
30. b
31. d
32. d
33. d
34. d
35. a
36. a

37. b
38. d
39. a
40. b
41. c
42. c
43. b
44. b
45. a
46. b
47. b
48. a
49. c
50. d
51. b
52. a
53. a
54. a
55. d
56. c
57. a
58. d
59. d
60. a
61. d
62. c
63. a
64. d
65. b
66. c
67. b

Section IV

Exercises

1. $\angle d = 11.9°$
2. $\angle a = 36.1°$
3. n = 1.60
4. 1^Δ base to the right
5. 8 cm (movement is down)
6. 1.5 m, base up
7. 2.0°
8. 4.0°
9. n = 1.60
10. 0.8^Δ BU
11. 0
12. 1.4^Δ BO
13. 2.8^Δ BU
14. OD 0.7^Δ BI
    OS 0.4^Δ BO
    total prism 0.3^Δ BI OD; yes
15. total 0.1^Δ BI; yes
16. total 2.8^Δ BI; yes
17. 1.3^Δ BU OD or BD OS

18. 0.6^Δ BI; yes
    1.5^Δ BI; no
19. OD 1.5^Δ BU
    OS 1.5^Δ BD
20. OD 2^Δ BI
    OS 2^Δ BI
21. OD 1.5^Δ BO
    OS 1.5^Δ BO
22. OD 2.5^Δ BU
    OS 2.5^Δ BD
23. 1.3^Δ BD OU
24. 0
25. round 22:
    OD 2.5^Δ BD
    OS 3.3^Δ BD
    round 28:
    OD 3.2^Δ BD
    OS 4.2^Δ BD
26. 1.3^Δ BU OD or BD OS
27. 0.1^Δ BU OS
28. 1.7^Δ BD OD
29. total 2.6^Δ BD OD
    order 2.6^Δ slab-off OD or 2.6^Δ reverse slab-off OS (or the closest available to 2.6^Δ)
30. total 3.2^Δ BU OD
    order 3.2^Δ slab-off OS or 3.2^Δ reverse slab-off OD (or the closest available to 3.2^Δ)
31. total 2.8^Δ BD OS
    order 2.8^Δ slab-off OS or 2.8^Δ reverse slab-off OD (or the closest available to 2.8^Δ)
32. 26. regular slab-off OS, reverse slab-off OD (but may not be needed)
    27. none
    28. regular slab-off OD, reverse slab-off OS
33. imbalance 1.25^Δ; need about 6 mm difference; some possibilities:
    a. OD ST 40 OS ST 25/28
    b. OD ST 25/28 OS round 22
34. imbalance 2.6^Δ; need about 12 mm; possibilities:
    a. OD round 22 OS ST 40
    b. OD Ultex OS ST 25/28
35. 1.4^Δ BU OS imbalance.
36. Franklins: 2.6^Δ imbalance; round 22 2.0^Δ imbalance
37. a. 1.2^Δ BD OD; (slab-off OD if needed)
    b. 2.1^Δ BD OD; slab-off OD
    c. 0.6^Δ BD OD; no slab-off needed
    ST 40/Franklin style has the least imbalance at reading level.
38. a. 3.0^Δ BU OD; slab-off OS
    b. 2.1^Δ BU OD; slab-off OS
    c. 3.6^Δ BU OD; slab-off OS
    round 22 has the least imbalance at reading level.
39. 3.2^Δ BU & I @ 45 or 3.2^Δ @ 45; Q1

40. 2.2^Δ BU & I @ 117 or 2.2^Δ @ 117; Q2
41. 5^Δ BD & I @ 127 or 5^Δ @ 307; Q4
42. 3.6^Δ BD & I @ 34 or 3.6^Δ @ 214; Q3

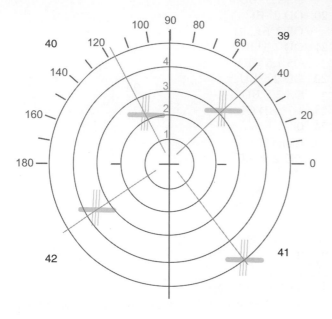

43. 2.2^Δ BD & 0.6^Δ BO
44. 3^Δ BD & 3^Δ BI
45. 2.3^Δ BU & O @ 50 becomes 1.8^Δ BU & 1.5^Δ BO

Review Questions

1. c
2. a
3. a
4. a
5. d
6. a
7. a
8. c
9. c
10. d
11. c
12. b
13. b
14. a
15. a
16. a
17. d
18. d
19. a
20. d
21. d
22. c
23. a
24. b
25. b
26. c
27. c
28. b
29. c
30. c
31. c
32. d
33. d
34. b
35. a
36. b
37. a
38. d
39. c
40. d
41. b
42. d
43. d
44. b
45. c
46. b
47. b
48. a
49. d
50. b
51. a
52. b
53. a
54. d
55. d
56. c
57. d
58. a

Section V

Exercises

In Answers 1 to 3, because of the difficulties of measuring from the page, if your ruler matches the one in the diagrams, your measurement should be within 1 mm of mine.

1. a. A = 62 mm
      B = 31 mm
      DBL = 15 mm
      FCD = 77 mm
      ED = 62 mm
      frame difference = 31
   b. D = 62 mm
      DBL = 15 mm
   c. seg height = 13 mm
      drop = –2.5 mm
   d. 6 mm in OU
   e. 4.5/7.5 in
   f. seg inset 2.5 mm OU
      total inset 8.5 mm OU

g. seg inset 3/2
total inset 7.5/9.5

2. a. A = 43 mm
B =32 mm
DBL = 14 mm
FCD = 57 mm
ED = 46 mm
frame difference = 11

b. D = 41.5 mm
DBL = 17.5 mm

c. seg height = 11.5 mm
drop = –4.5 mm

d. 1 mm OU in

e. 4.5/1.5 in

f. seg inset 1.5 mm OU
total inset 1.5 mm OU

g. seg inset 1.5/2.5
total inset 4/3.5

3. a. A = 46 mm
B = 27 mm
DBL = 17 mm
FCD = 63 mm
ED = 47 mm
frame difference = 20

b. D = 46 mm
DBL = 17 mm

c. seg height = 16.5/13 mm
3/–0.5 (OD above 31)

d. 26/28 mm
5.5/3.5 in

4. 67 mm

5. 56 mm

6. 65/65

7. +4.00; +4.25

8. +8.25 or +6.25; +7.75

9. +3.00; +2.25

10. +4.25//–6.25 $\bigcirc$ –7.75

11. +6.00 $\bigcirc$ +6.50 //–6.00

12. +10.25//–3.75 $\bigcirc$ –5.25

13. +2.00//–10.50D $\bigcirc$ –11.75

14. –3.59D

15. +10.10D

16. –6.62D

17. –4.00D

18. a. +1.56

b. +1.56//–10.06 $\bigcirc$ –12.06

c. +1.25//–8.12 $\bigcirc$ –9.62 (In some laboratories this will be rounded up to –9.75.)

The power of a lens with the surfaces found in c, if made from a material with index of refraction of 1.530, would be –6.87 –1.50 ×090.

19. 4.0 mm

20. a. BC +8.25D:
b. true curves +7.75 and –5.25
c. sag_{front} = 6.5 mm
sag_{back} = 4.2 mm
d. ct = 4.3 mm

21. edge 3.8 mm, center 5.1 mm

22. edge 4.7 mm, center 6.3 mm

Review Questions

1. c
2. b
3. a
4. d
5. c
6. b
7. a
8. a
9. b
10. b
11. d
12. b
13. d
14. a
15. d
16. a
17. a
18. a
19. c
20. c
21. c
22. d
23. c
24. c
25. d
26. a
27. c
28. d
29. c
30. b
31. a
32. d
33. b
34. b
35. b
36. d
37. c
38. c
39. a; selection b is the result of the approximation formula
40. b
41. b
42. a

Section VI
Exercises

1. $-6.22 - 0.82 \times 180$
2. $+10.02 + 0.08 \times 180$
3. $+4.67 + 0.62 \times 090$
4. as is: OD -14.7%

            OS -10.6%

   difference 4.1%

   a. change t: OD 0.1%

   b. change vd: OD 1.5%

                 OS -2.0%

   c. change BC: OD 0.1%

                 OS -0.1%

Using those changes:

   OD -13.4%

   OS -12.2%

   Difference 1.2%

In Exercise 4, just moving the bevel of the OS 2 mm toward the back of the lens, which will move the lens forward in the frame and increase the OS vd by 2 mm, will drop the magnification difference significantly. This may be the most practical solution for this pair of glasses.

5. OD 0.5%

   OS 1.4%

   Difference 0.9%

6. Conventional magnification of $1.5\times$
7. $-10.50 + 2.12 \times 134$ (rounded) or $-8.37 - 2.12 \times 044$
8. $+10.12 + 1.75 \times 144$ or $+11.87 - 1.75 \times 054$
9. front reflects 4.0%

   back reflects 3.8%

   transmission 92.2%

   total transmission 92.4%

10. front reflects 5.1%

   back reflects 4.9%

   transmission 90.0%

   total transmission 90.2%

11. front reflects 6.2%

   back reflects 5.8%

   transmission 88.0%

   total transmission 88.4%

12. 74.8%
13. center 83.6%

   edge 62.9%

14. a. 0.778

   b. 0.403

   c. 31.3%

   d. 0.751

   e. 58.4%

15. $33°$
16. 21%

Review Questions

1. d
2. d
3. c
4. c
5. a
6. d
7. a
8. b
9. c
10. b
11. d
12. d
13. c
14. c
15. d
16. b
17. c
18. b
19. a
20. a
21. d
22. d
23. b
24. b
25. a
26. a
27. c
28. b
29. a
30. a
31. c
32. b
33. a
34. a
35. c

Section VII
Exercises

1. a. $p = 100$

     $q = 67$

     $M = -0.67$

     $I = -13$

   b. $p = 80$

     $q = 80$

     $M = -1$

     $I = -20$

   c. $p = 60$

     $q = 120$

     $M = -2$

     $I = -40$

   d. $p = 40$

     $q = $ infinity

M = n.a.

I = n.a.

e. $p = 20$

$q = -40$

M = 2

I = 40

2. a. $p = 80$

$q = -27$

M = 0.34

I = 7

b. $p = 40$

$q = -20$

M = 0.5

I = 10

c. $p = 20-$

$q = -13$

M = 0.65–

I = 13

3. $1/f = 0 = 1/p + 1/q$

$1/p = - 1/q$

$p = -q$

$M = -q/p = (-q)/(-q) = 1$

4. The image forms to the left of the mirror, it is inverted, real, and magnified.

5. a. $p = 100$

$q = 67$

M = –0.67

I = –13

b. $p = 40$

q = infinity

M = n.a.

I = n.a.

c. $p = 20$

$q = -40$

M = 2

I = 40

6. a. $p = 80$

$q = -27$

M = 0.34

I = 7

b. $p = 60$

$q = -24$

M = 0.4

I = 8

c. $p = 20$

$q = -13$

M = 0.65

I = 13

7. $D_1 = +35D$

$D_2 = +1D$

n = 1.50

t = 0.035 m

$r_1 = +0.014$ m

$r_2 = -0.5$ m

$D_F = +36.02$

$f_1 = 28$ mm

$D_B = +191.91D$

$f_2 = 5$ mm

$D_{eq} = 35.18D$

$f_{eq} = 28$ mm

8. $r_1 = +0.02$ m

$r_2 = +0.05$ m

n = 1.50

t = 0.05 m

$D_1 = +25D$

$D_2 = -10D$

$D_F = +17.50$

$f_1 = 57$ mm

$D_B = +140D$

$f_2 = 7$ mm

$D_{eq} = 23.33D$

$f_{eq} = 43$ mm

9. a. $p = 60$

$q = 53$

M = –0.88

I = –13

b. $p = 28$

q = infinity

M = n.a.

I = n.a.

c. $p = 15$

$q = -32$

M = 2.2

I = 32

10. a. $p = 60$

$q = -25$

M = 0.42

I = 6

b. $p = 30$

$q = -18$

M = 0.59

I = 9

11.

$n_1 = 1.00$

$n_2 = 1.70$

$n_3 = 1.50$

t = 20 mm = 0.02 m

$r_1 = 0.0175$ m

r_2 = infinity

$D_1 = +40D$

$D_2 = pl$

$D_B = +75.56$

$f_2V_2 = 20$ mm

$D_F = +40D$

$f_1V_1 = 25$ mm

$D_{eq} = +40D$

$f_1H_1 = 25$ mm

$H_2f_2 = 38$ mm

HN = 13 mm
p = 50 + 13 = 63 mm
q = 63 mm
IV$_2$ = 63 + 13 – 18 = 58 mm
M = –1.0

O = 20 mm
I = –20 mm
The 20-mm-high image is real and inverted and forms 58 mm inside the 1.50 plastic.
See diagram below.

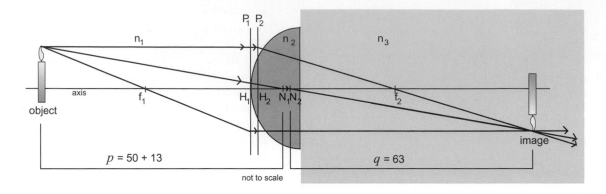

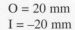

Review Questions

1. d
2. b
3. c
4. a
5. c
6. b
7. d
8. a
9. b
10. c
11. a
12. c
13. d
14. d
15. c
16. d
17. a
18. a
19. a
20. d
21. b
22. c
23. c
24. d
25. c
26. b
27. c
28. a
29. d
30. b
31. a
32. d
33. b
34. d
35. b
36. b
37. d
38. b
39. a
40. b

INDEX

Center of curvature, 186, 192
Center thickness, 150, 151, 152-153
    for prism, 154-155
Centimeters, 8
Centrad, 95
CHA (compound hyperopic astigmatism), 71
Chromatic aberrations, 36
Circle of least confusion, 66-69
CMA (compound myopic astigmatism), 71
Coatings, anti-reflective, 174-175, 221
Colmascope, 181
Color perception, 25
Compensated power, 81-84, 222
Compound hyperopic astigmatism (CHA), 71
Compound lens, 53
    circle of least confusion for, 67-68
    optical cross of, 55
Compound myopic astigmatism (CMA), 71
Compounding situations, with prism, 103
Concave lens, 44-45
Concave mirror, 185-186
Concave surface, 47
Constringence, 37
Constructive interference, 17, 20, 174-175
Conventional magnification, 169
Convergent lines, 21
Converging rays, 21, 43
Conversions, 8-10
Convex lens, 43-44
Convex mirror, 186
Convex surface, 47
Cord, 150
Cord diameter, 150
Corrected curve design lenses, 146
Cosine (cos), 9-12
Critical angle, 31-33, 222
Cross cylinder form, for taking Rx from optical cross, 60-62
Cross cylinder transposition, 63
Curvature
    center of, 186, 192
    of field, 146
Cylinder(s)
    amount of, 54
    axis of, 53
    and lenses, 52-53
    obliquely crossed, Thompson's formula for, 170-172
    optical cross of, 54
Cylinder notation, 65
Cylindrical amount, 54
Cylindrical surface, 53

D

Datum (D) measurement, 138
Datum system, 138
DBL (distance between lenses), 137
Decentration, 138-140, 223
    total, 141-143
Decimeters, 8

Depth
    apparent, 33-34, 222
    in boxing system, 137
Destructive interference, 18, 20, 174-175
Deviating angle, 94-95
    prism diopter and, 96-97
Deviation, angle of, 26
Diffraction, 19-20, 223
Diffuse reflection, 24
Diopter(s), 45, 46-47
    prism, 95-96
Diplopia, 102, 111
Dispersion, 17, 36-37
    defined, 93
    of light by prism, 93
Dispersive value, 37
Displacement
    lateral, 35-36, 224
    by prism, 93-94
Distance between lenses (DBL), 137
Divergence, of wave, 17
Divergent lines, 21
Diverging rays, 21-22, 43
Division
    on scientific calculator, 6
    in scientific notation, 14
    of signed numbers, 3-4
Double vision, 102, 111

E

Edge thickness, 151, 152-153
    for prism, 154-155
Effective diameter (ED), 140
Effective power, 77-81, 223
Electromagnetic spectrum, 15
    wavelength and frequency in, 16
Emmetropic eye, 69
English-metric conversions, 9
Equivalent power, 85, 196, 223
Equivalent power formula, 196
Exact numbers, 7
Executive-style bifocal, 114
Exercising prism, 93
Exponents, 12-14
Eye, diagram of, 205
Eye size, 137

F

Face form, 161, 163
Farsightedness, 69
FCD (frame center distance), 138
Filter(s), polarizing, 179-181
Finishing. See Surfacing and finishing.
Flat lens, 47
Flat transposition, 62-63
Focal length, 43
    formula for, 45-46, 223
    of mirror, 186